Essentials in Ophthalmology

Medical Retina

Frank G. Holz Richard Spaide
Editors

Essentials in Ophthalmology

G. K. Krieglstein R. N. Weinreb
Series Editors

Glaucoma

Cataract and Refractive Surgery

Uveitis and Immunological Disorders

Vitreo-retinal Surgery

Medical Retina

Oculoplastics and Orbit

Pediatric Ophthalmology,
Neuro-Ophthalmology, Genetics

Cornea and External Eye Disease

Editors Frank G. Holz
Richard Spaide

Medical Retina

Focus on Retinal Imaging

Springer

Series Editors

Günter K. Krieglstein, MD
Professor and Chairman
Department of Ophthalmology
University of Cologne
Joseph-Stelzmann-Straße 9
50931 Köln
Germany

Robert N. Weinreb, MD
Professor and Director
Hamilton Glaucoma Center
Department of Ophthalmology
University of California at San Diego
9500 Gilman Drive
La Jolla, CA 92093-0946
USA

Volume Editors

Frank G. Holz, MD
Professor and Chairman
Department of Ophthalmology
University of Bonn
Ernst-Abbe-Straße 2
53127 Bonn
Germany

Richard Spaide, MD
Private Practice
Vitreous, Retina, and Macula
Consultants of New York
460 Park Avenue
New York, NY 10022
USA

ISSN: 1612-3212 e-ISSN: 1612-3212

ISBN: 978-3-540-85539-2 e-ISBN: 978-3-540-85540-8

DOI: 10.1007/978-3-540-85540-8

Springer Heidelberg Dordrecht London New York

Library of Congress Control Number: 2009934507

Cover design: wmx-Design, Heidelberg

Printed on acid-free paper

9 8 7 6 5 4 3 2 1

(www.springer.com)

Foreword

The Essentials in Ophthalmology series represents an unique updating publication on the progress in all subspecialties of ophthalmology.

In a quarterly rhythm, eight issues are published covering clinically relevant achievements in the whole field of ophthalmology. This timely transfer of advancements for the best possible care of our eye patients has proven to be effective. The initial working hypothesis of providing new knowledge immediately following publication in the peer-reviewed journal and not waiting for the textbook appears to be highly workable.

We are now in the third cycle of the Essentials in Ophthalmology series, having been encouraged by readership acceptance of the first two series, each of eight volumes. This is a success that was made possible predominantly by the numerous opinion-leading authors and the outstanding section editors, as well as with the constructive support of the publisher. There are many good reasons to continue and still improve the dissemination of this didactic and clinically relevant information.

G. K. Krieglstein
R. N. Weinreb
Series Editors

Preface

Ocular imaging started with drawings and paintings that were used to show representative examples of diseases affecting the fundus. These were typically reproduced as lithographic plates in early texts. Although expensive to produce and not necessarily correct, they were often pleasing to the eye. With the advent of fundus photography, specific images of patients could be recorded, stored, and indexed at low cost. Photography provided a way to record topographic representations of the fundus. This opened many possibilities: specific patients could easily be recorded and catalogued, interval changes could be documented, and later retrieval of images could foster scientific research. Fluorescein angiography was first performed by a medical student, Harold Novotny, and an intern, David Alvis. They were initially trying to determine the levels of oxygenation in the retina, but they immediately realized that this new technique could document the circulation in the eye. The paper describing their technique and findings was rejected by a leading peer-reviewed ophthalmology journal. Even so, the use of fluorescein angiography rapidly expanded not only because of its ability to evaluate the circulation of the eye, but also because consequences of breakdowns of the blood–ocular barrier could be visualized. Fluorescein angiography provided information not only about anatomy, but also about the physiology of the eye. Early investigators integrated anatomic, physiologic, and histopathologic information together to form the foundations of field, medical retina. With further technological innovations, scanning laser ophthalmoscopy and optical coherence tomography were introduced in ophthalmology to obtain high-resolution two-dimensional and cross-sectional images of the fundus. An even more complete understanding of pathologic processes arose with the integration of information from other forms of ocular imaging with that of optical coherence tomography. New developments are underway that allow for visualization of biochemical processes in the retina. Molecular imaging has the potential to gauge the amount of oxygen in the retina, measure levels of compounds such as macular pigment, and identify disease-specific molecules to allow for earlier diagnosis and individualized therapy.

In retrospect, many, if not most, of the major advances in medical retina were made because of advances in ophthalmic imaging technology. All these advances required integration of more than one source of information. So it is fitting that this edition in the Medical Retina series is devoted to ocular imaging. This volume reviews some of the established forms of imaging and concentrates on the new – in isolation and also as integrated into a larger process aimed at giving information to clinicians and researchers alike. The chapters of this book have been written by international leaders at the forefronts of their fields. The result is a state-of-the-art overview of retinal imaging that should be interesting and useful for everyone interested in the retina. It has been our pleasure to have the opportunity to work with the authors and the publisher to produce this book.

Bonn, Germany **Frank G. Holz**
New York, NY, USA **Richard Spaide**

Contents

Chapter 13
Spectral Domain Optical Coherence Tomography for Macular Holes
Jerzy Nawrocki and Zofia Michalewska

Chapter 14
Combined Spectral-Domain Optical Coherence Tomography/Scanning Laser Ophthalmoscopy Imaging of Vitreous and the Vitreo-Retinal Interface
Jerry Sebag and Michelle Y. Wang

Chapter 15
Choroidal Imaging with Optical Coherence Tomography
Richard Spaide

Contributors

Tos T. J. M. Berendschot
Department of Ophthalmology, University of Maastricht, Maastricht NL-6202 AZ, The Netherlands, t.berendschot@ohk.unimaas.nl

Francesca M. Cordeiro
UCL Institute of Ophthalmology, 11-43 Bath Street, London, EC1V 9EL, UK
Western Eye Hospital, 153-173 Marylebone Road, London, NW1 5QH, UK
m.cordeiro@ucl.ac.uk

François C. Delori
Schepens Eye Research Institute, Harvard Medical School, 20 Staniford Street, Boston, MA 02114, USA, francoisdelori@schepens.harvard.edu

Wolfgang Drexler
School of Optometry and Vision Sciences, Cardiff University, Maindy Road, Cathays, Cardiff CF24 4LU, UK
drexlerw@cardiff.ac.uk

Teodoro Evans
Apdo 144–1225 Plaza Mayor, San Jose, Costa Rica

Howard F. Fine
Department of Ophthalmology, Robert Wood Johnson University Medical Center, New Brunswick, NJ 08901, USA
hffine@gmail.com

Fred W. Fitzke
UCL Institute of Ophthalmology, 11-43 Bath Street, London EC1V 9EL, UK
f.fitzke@ucl.ac.uk

Monika Fleckenstein
Department of Ophthalmology, Ernst-Abbe-Str. 2 University of Bonn, 53127 Bonn, Germany

Thomas Friberg
UPMC Eye Institute, University of Pittsburgh Medical Center, 203 Lothrop Street, Suite # No. 824, Pittsburgh, PA 15213, USA
fribeg@pitt.edu

Sarah Harmon
Ocular Oncology Service, Suite 1440, Wills Eye Institute, 840 Walnut Street, Philadelphia, PA 19107, USA

Hans-Martin Helb
Department of Ophthalmology, Ernst-Abbe-Str. 2 University of Bonn, 53127 Bonn, Germany

Christoph K. Hitzenberger
Center for Biomedical Engineering and Physics, Medical University of Vienna, Vienna, Austria

Frank G. Holz
Department of Ophthalmology, Ernst-Abbe-Str. 2 University of Bonn, 53127 Bonn, Germany
frank.holz@ukb.uni-bonn.de

Carel B. Hoyng
Department of Ophthalmology, Radboud University Nijmegen Medical Centre, Philips van Leydenlaan 15, 6525 EX Nijmegen, The Netherlands

Peter Charbel Issa
Department of Ophthalmology, Ernst-Abbe-Str. 2 University of Bonn, 53127 Bonn, Germany
Nuffield Laboratory of Ophthalmology, Oxford University, Oxford, UK
peter.issa@ukb.uni-bonn.de

Claudia N. Keilhauer
Department of Ophthalmology, University Hospital, Josef-Schneider-Str. 11, 97080 Würzburg, Germany, c. strachwitz@augenklinik.uni-wuerzburg.de

Jeroen B. Klevering
Department of Ophthalmology, Radboud University Nijmegen Medical Centre, Philips van Leydenlaan 15, 6525 EX Nijmegen, The Netherlands

Leanne Labriola
Retina Service (LTL, TF),
UPMC Eye Center, University of Pittsburgh Medical Center, 203 Lothrop Street, Suite 824, Pittsburgh, PA, USA

Sara Lally
Ocular Oncology Service, Suite 1440, Wills Eye Institute, 840 Walnut Street, Philadelphia, PA 19107, USA

Rainer Leitgeb
Center for Biomedical Engineering and Physics, Medical University of Vienna, Vienna, Austria

Francesca Menchini
Department of Ophthalmology, University of Udine, Piazza della Misericordia, 15 c/o Pad. Petracco, 33100 Udine, Italy
francescamenchini@gmail.com

Carsten H. Meyer
Augenklinik, Universität Bonn, Ernst-Abbe-Straβe 2, 53127 Bonn, Germany

Zofia Michalewska
Ophthalmic Clinic "Jasne Blonia", ul. Rojna 90. Lodz, 91–162, Poland
zosia_n@yahoo.com

Jerzy Nawrocki
Ophthalmic Clinic "Jasne Blonia", ul. Rojna 90. Lodz, 91–162, Poland
jerzy_n@poczta.onet.pl

Mariacristina Parravano
Ophthalmology, Fondazione G.B. Bietti per lo studio e la ricerca in Oftalmolologia-IRCCS, Via Livenza n 3, 00198 Rome, Italy
criparra@tin.it

Jonathan L. Prenner
Department of Ophthalmology, Robert Wood Johnson University Medical Center, New Brunswick, NJ 08901, USA

Aparna Ramasubramanian
Ocular Oncology Service, Suite 1440, Wills Eye Institute, 840 Walnut Street, Philadelphia, PA 19107, USA

Daniel Roth
Department of Ophthalmology, Robert Wood Johnson University Medical Center, New Brunswick, NJ 08901, USA

Sandeep Saxena
Department of Ophthalmology, King George´s Medical University, Chowk, Lucknow, India 226003
sandeepsaxena2020@yahoo.com

Steffen Schmitz-Valckenberg
Department of Ophthalmology, University of Bonn, Ernst-Abbe-Str. 2, 53127 Bonn, Germany
steffen.schmitz-valckenberg@ukb.uni-bonn.de

Hendrik P.N. Scholl
Department of Ophthalmology, Ernst-Abbe-Str. 2 University of Bonn, 53127 Bonn, Germany

Dietrich Schweitzer
Department of Ophthalmology, Friedrich-Schiller-University of Jena, Bachstr. 18, 07743 Jena, Germany
dietrich.schweitzer@med.uni-jena.de

Jerry Sebag
University of Southern California and VMR Institute, 7677 Center Avenue, Suite 400, Huntington Beach, CA 92647, USA
jsebag@vmrinstitute.com

Carol L. Shields
Ocular Oncology Service, Suite 1440, Wills Eye Institute, 840 Walnut Street, Philadelphia, PA 19107, USA
carol.shields@shieldsoncology.com

Richard Spaide
The Vitreous-Retina-Macula Consultants of New York, 460 Park Avenue, 5th Floor, New York, NY 10022, USA
rickspaide@yahoo.com

Thomas Theelen
Department of Ophthalmology, Radboud University Nijmegen Medical Centre, Philips van Leydenlaan 15, 6525 EX Nijmegen, The Netherlands,
t.theelen@ohk.umcn.nl

Gianni Virgili
Department of Ophthalmology, University of Florence, Piazza San Marco 4, Florence 50121, Italy
gianni.virgili@unifi.it

Michelle Y. Wang
University of Southern California and VMR Institute, 7677 Center Avenue, Suite 400, Huntington Beach, CA 92647, USA

Sebastian Wolf
Department of Ophthalmology, Inselspital, University of Bern, Freiburgstr., 3010 Bern, Switzerland
sebastian.wolf@insel.ch

Lihteh Wu
Apdo 144–1225 Plaza Mayor, San Jose, Costa Rica,
lw65@cornell.edu

Chapter 1

Common Pitfalls in the Use of Optical Coherence Tomography for Macular Diseases[1]

1

Lihteh Wu and Teodoro Evans

Core Messages

- Optical coherence tomography (OCT) is a valuable and indispensable tool in the current management of macular diseases.
- As in other imaging modalities, artifacts occur with both time-domain and spectral/Fourier-domain OCT imaging.
- Recognition of these artifacts will improve the management of macular diseases and prevent treatment decisions based on erroneous data.
- Stratus® OCT retinal thickness measurements are more to error in eyes with subretinal pathology when compared with eyes with intraretinal pathology.
- In time-domain OCT, the topographic maps are derived from the individual radial scans; thus, maps should never be interpreted for artifacts without examining the individual scans.
- Despite the inherent advantages of spectral/Fourier-domain OCT over the time-domain Stratus® OCT, the Stratus® OCT remains quite useful for the day-to-day clinical practice.

1.1 Introduction

Optical coherence tomography (OCT) is a noninvasive medical diagnostic imaging modality that utilizes light to image tissue using low coherence interferometry [1]. It measures the echo time delay and intensity of light that is reflected back from different structures in a tissue. In the OCT machine, a beam of light from a superluminescent diode is divided through a beam splitter into sample and reference beams. Light from the sample beam is directed toward the tissue of interest and depending on the composition of the internal tissular structures, the sample beam will be reflected with different echo time delays. Light from the reference beam is reflected from a reference mirror located at a known distance. Both the reflected reference and sample beams are combined by a modified Michelson interferometer and detected by the OCT [1, 2]. Detection of these beams is based on time-domain or spectral-domain protocols.

The most widely used OCT machine, Stratus® OCT (Carl Zeiss–Meditec, Dublin, California, USA), is based on time-domain detection. In time-domain OCT, the position of the reference mirror is adjusted, creating different time delays for the echoes of the reference beam. Axial scans (A scan) are obtained by directing the sample beam at different tissue depths and recording the reflected light echoes. The Stratus® OCT can make from 128 to 768 A scans in a single scan pass. Each A scan has 1,024 data points and is 2 mm long. By scanning the sample beam of light in a transverse direction, a cross-sectional OCT (B scan) image is obtained. Once the information is obtained, a tomogram is constructed using a false color scale that represents the amount of light backscattering from microstructures at different depths of the imaged tissue. In the false color scale, bright colors such as red to white represent high reflectivity and dark colors such as blue to black represent minimal or no reflectivity. The ganglion cell layer, the inner and outer nuclear layers have a low reflectivity, and therefore appear blue–black in the false color scale. Conversely, the retinal pigment epithelium (RPE)/choriocapillaris and the nerve fiber layer exhibit a high reflectivity [2, 3]. The hyperreflective band

[1]The authors have no financial or propietary interest in any of the products or techniques mentioned in this chapter.

at the level of the RPE/choriocapillaris is actually composed of two highly reflective lines separated from each other by one thin layer of low to moderate reflectivity. The inner highly reflective line most likely corresponds to the junction of the photoreceptor's outer and inner segments. The outer highly reflective line possible corresponds to the RPE/choriocapillaris [4–6].

In Spectral or Fourier domain OCT, all echoes of light composing the interference spectrum of echo time delays are measured simultaneously by a spectrometer and a high-speed charge coupled device. The interference spectrum is made up of oscillations whose frequencies are proportional to the echo time delay. By calculating the Fourier transform, the machine calculates the axial scan measurements without adjusting the reference mirror. The Fourier transform is a mathematical procedure that extracts the frequency spectrum of a signal. This results in an improvement over time-domain OCT in sensitivity and image acquisition speed [7–9].

Despite the introduction of spectral-domain OCT into clinical practice over the past 2 years, many retina practices throughout the world continue to rely on the Stratus® OCT. Since its approval by the FDA on January 2002, more than 6000 Stratus® OCT systems have been installed worldwide. It is estimated that 37,000 daily scans are performed in the United States. Today, OCT has become a valuable and indispensable adjunct to clinical practice. For instance, OCT has been shown to have a higher sensitivity than stereoscopic biomicroscopy for the detection of diabetic macular edema [10]. In addition, a more reliable diagnosis in the early stages of macular holes can be made with the help of an OCT [11]. OCT has also introduced new clinical concepts such as stage "0" macular hole [12].

Summary for the Clinicians

- OCT is a noninvasive, noncontact transpupillary imaging modality that uses light waves to obtain high-resolution cross-sectional images of the retina creating an in vivo optical biopsy of the macula.
- Currently, there are two types of OCT machines commercially available: the time-domain Stratus® OCT and multiple spectral/Fourier-domain OCT.
- Spectral/Fourier-domain OCT acquires images much faster than time-domain OCT, improving the resolution of the images obtained and decreasing the number of artifacts.

1.2 Limitations of Time-Domain OCT

In spite of its enormous utility and ease of use, the Stratus® OCT machine can deliver inaccurate results if the clinician is not aware of the basic software functions and algorithms. Artifacts are commonly encountered in OCT imaging [13, 14]. Common errors in the daily use of the Stratus can be classified into two major groups: acquisition errors and interpretation errors.

1.2.1 Acquisition Errors in the Stratus® OCT

The image obtained should be of sufficient quality (a signal strength of five or more) to minimize artifacts and avoid misdiagnosis. The quality of the image is dependent on the speed of image acquisition and the presence or absence of media opacities. One of the major pitfalls of the Stratus® OCT is that the image acquisition is dependent on the patient's fixation. The highest resolution scan of 6 mm of retina takes a little under 2 s to perform. Even in eyes with good fixation, it is difficult to remain motionless for this amount of time. The eye movements increase dramatically in eyes with poor fixation due to poor visual acuity. This can affect the precision of measurements and OCT images at the subsequent follow-up scans. If the fellow eye maintains fixation, the use of the external fixation LED can be helpful.

Obtaining a good image in an eye with optical aberrations such as high myopia, hypermetropia, or astigmatism is a challenge. If the image appears degraded, one must make sure that the best focus is in place by dialing the focusing knob. At times, asking the patient to wear their contact lenses may improve the image. Staphylomatous changes in highly myopic eyes make perpendicularity of the examining beam to the macula very difficult or nearly impossible to achieve (Fig. 1.1). The optical aberrations induced by these eyes prevent good images even in eyes with clear media.

In the older OCT machines, a pupillary dilation of at least 5 mm in diameter was necessary to achieve a good image. With the Stratus® OCT, the pupil needs to be at least 3 mm in size, otherwise vignetting may occur. Vignetting refers to the partial blockage of the OCT imaging beam by the iris. This results in an image with a loss of signal over a specific portion of the OCT image.

Media opacities can affect the strength of the signal resulting in an inaccurate interpretation. Any pathological condition that affects corneal transparency, including drying of the pre-corneal tear film, will adversely affect image quality. Therefore, we find it important to keep the cornea lubricated with artificial tears and asking the patient to

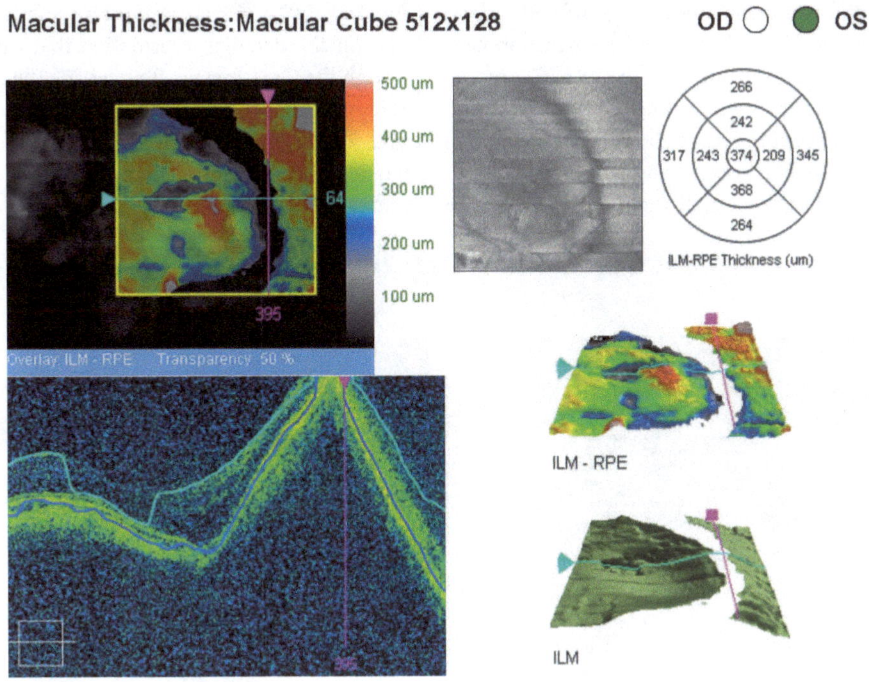

Fig. 1.1 A highly myopic eye with clear media illustrating a mirror artifact in a spectral-domain OCT scan. When the signal reaches the end of the screen (*vertical purple line*), it appears to bounce and create a mirror image. The maps are inaccurate as they have no data points in parts of the map (seen as a *white crescent*)

blink between scans. Since the examining beam of light is emitted in the near infrared, mild to moderate nuclear sclerosis does not affect much the OCT images. However, cortical and posterior subcapsular opacities do affect the quality of the images obtained (Fig. 1.2). Vitreous opacities also degrade the OCT images. OCT images with low signals are characterized by a washed out and dim appearance. If the strength of the signal is low enough, even highly reflective structures such as the RPE/choriocapillaris and the nerve fiber layer may become much less reflective and induce errors during retinal thickness analysis.

In 2005, Ray et al. [13] reported that poor scan acquisition was probably responsible for an artifact in approximately 11% of the topographic maps examined at a tertiary referral center. These artifacts included *"out of register" artifacts (a scan that was shifted superiorly such that the inner retina was truncated), "cut edge" artifacts (a scan that occurred when the edge was truncated inappropiately), and "off center" artifacts (when the foveal center was misidentified)* [13]. It must be noted that the operators of the OCT in this study were experienced technicians, but they did not benefit from the latest OCT software. In fact, prior to version 4.0, the analysis of confidence function was not available, so the operator is not warned by the machine that a problem exists with the current scan [13, 15]. As Hee [15] pointed out, the fact that the fast macular thickness map protocol was chosen rather than the macular thickness map protocol also increases the incidence of acquisition artifacts. In the fast macular thickness protocol, all six radial scans are performed simultaneously. Thus, if only one of the six scans has an artifact, the resulting map will also have an artifact. In contrast, in the macular thickness map protocol, each of the six radial scans are performed individually. Thus, if the operator realizes that one of the scans is faulty, the scan can be repeated. The advantage of the fast macular thickness map is that it is quicker to obtain and in patients who have a hard time fixating and who tire easily, it might be the best option to obtain an adequate scan.

1.2.2 Interpretation Errors with the Stratus® OCT

The analyzing software for retinal scans includes an automated correction for movement and an algorithm for retinal thickness measurements, both of which can produce errors during the analysis of the scans. The purpose of the movement correction is to straighten the RPE layer in case of fluctuations related with eye movement during the scan. This software can mask certain alterations of the

RPE related to different pathologies. In age-related macular degeneration (AMD), the movement correction can hide the presence of drusen and alter the retinal contour or can flatten retinal pigment epithelium detachments (PED). Similarly, in central serous chorioretinopathy, the movement correction can also flatten the presence of the typical rounded PED or even hide them if they are small (Fig. 1.3). In these patients, the usefulness of the OCT relies on the detailed information that can be obtained through the OCT images. To override the morphological alterations in the RPE of the movement correction software, we recommend one to evaluate the unprocessed images found under the "scan profile" analysis or the "scan selection" section.

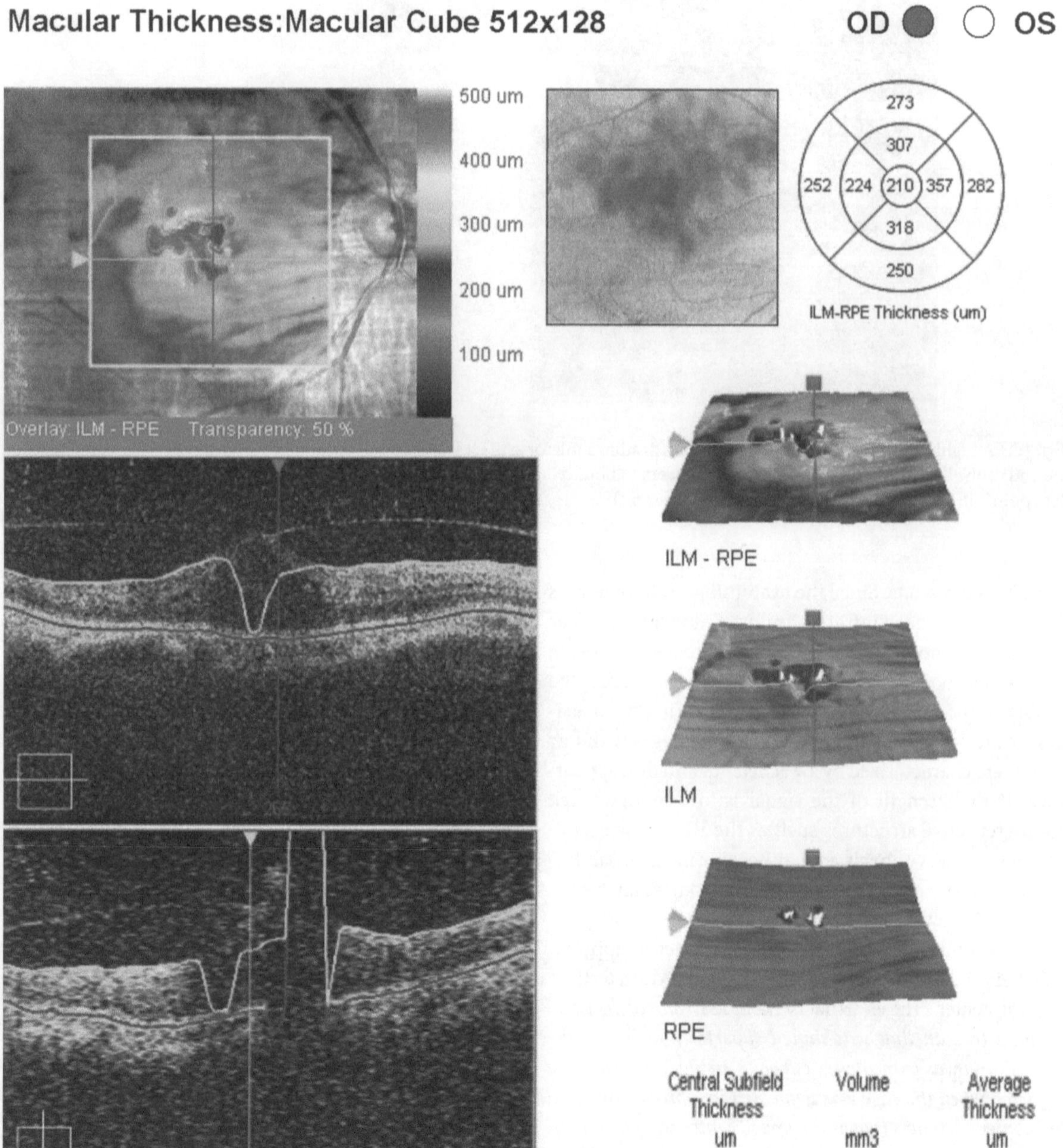

	Central Subfield Thickness um	Volume mm3	Average Thickness um
ILM - RPE	210	9.5	264

Fig. 1.2 An eye with a moderate posterior subcapsular cataract and vitreomacular traction syndrome. Notice how the media opacities distort the positioning of the boundary lines used in the measurement of the retinal thickness in this Cirrus® spectral-domain OCT scan

One of the most useful and powerful properties of the OCT is its ability to measure retinal thickness in a reproducible fashion. With the advent of retinal pharmacotherapy, central macular thickness has become an important endpoint of treatment. Measurements of the retinal thickness algorithm are based on the automated capability of the OCT of identifying the internal limiting membrane (inner retinal boundary) and the hyperreflective band of the RPE-choriocapillaris (outer retinal boundary). Once these two boundaries are mapped, the

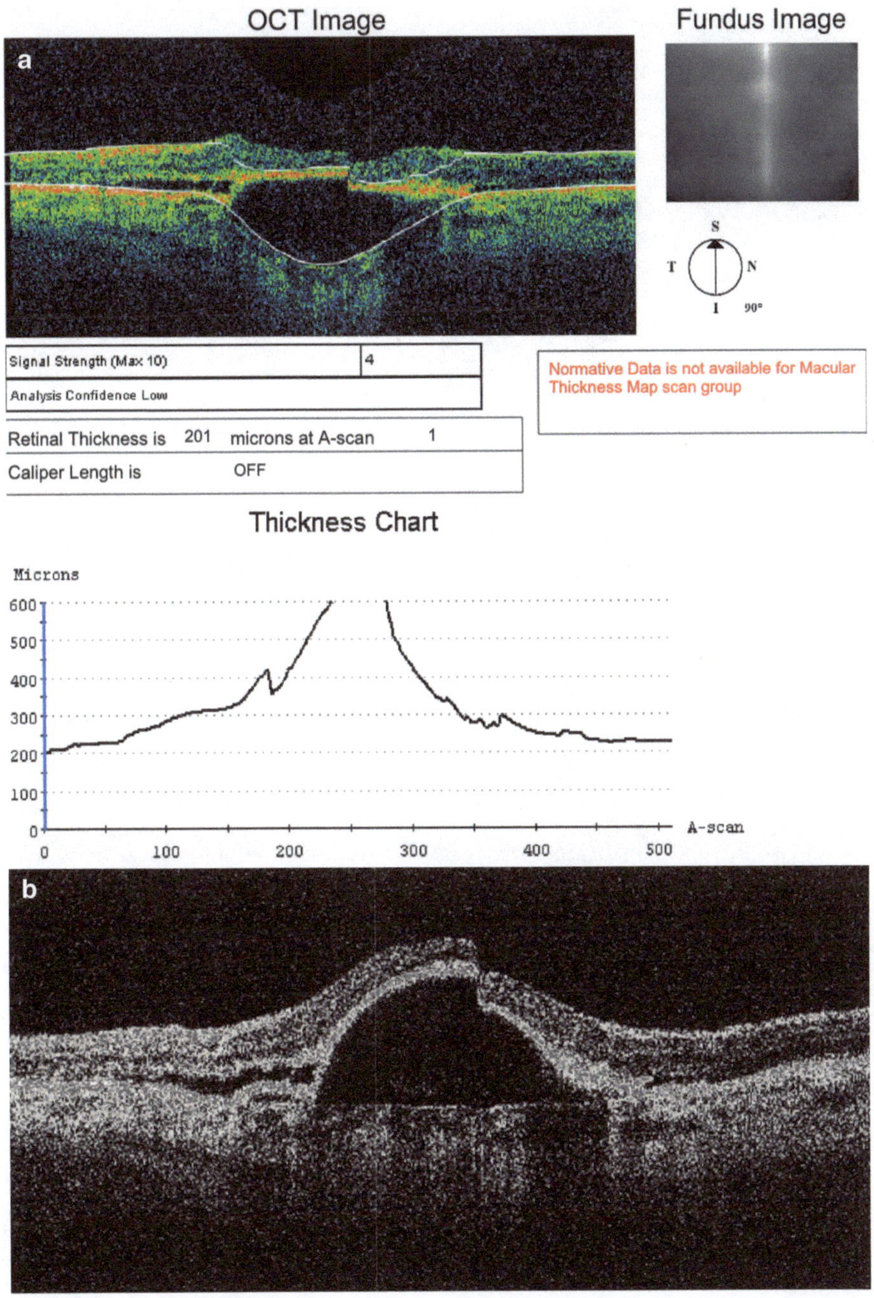

Fig. 1.3 A 45-year-old man with a pigment epithelial detachment (PED) secondary to central serous chorioretinopathy. (**a**) Stratus® OCT retinal thickness report demonstrating flattening of the PED. Notice the incorrect placement of both inner and outer retinal boundary lines. (**b**) Stratus® OCT scan profile report displaying the correct anatomic picture of the PED. (**c**) A 74-year-old female with PED secondary to exudative age-related macular degeneration. Cirrus® Spectral-domain OCT correctly places the inner and outer boundaries for retinal thickness measurement and does not flatten the PED

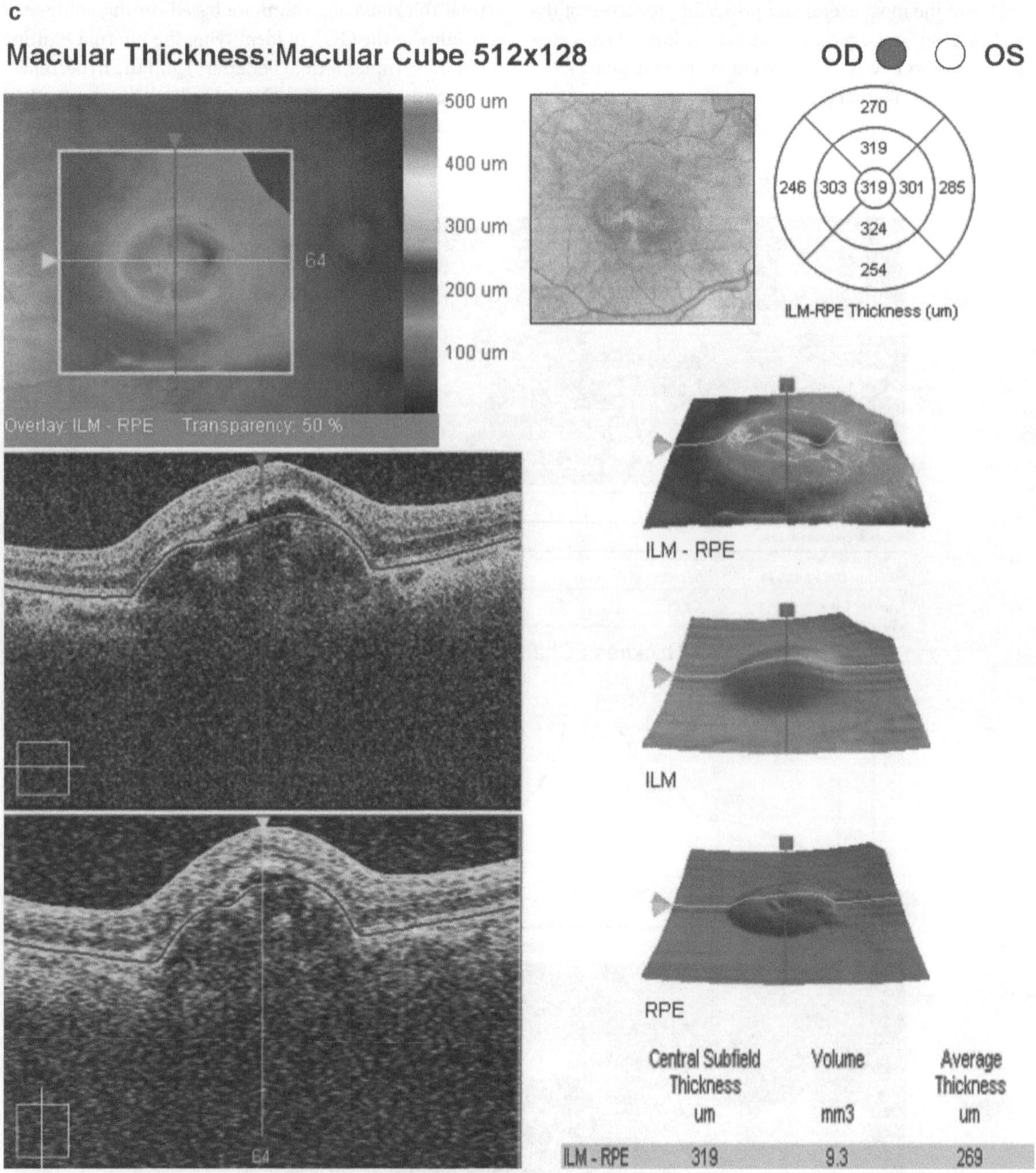

Fig. 1.3 (continued)

software measures the distance between the two boundaries and assigns this value as the retinal thickness. Errors related with this algorithm are remarkably common, but are generally detected by the software [13, 14]. The Stratus® OCT software incorrectly identifies the outer retinal boundary, as it draws this boundary at the inner highly reflective line that corresponds to the junction of the outer and inner segments of the photoreceptors rather than the outer highly reflective line [4, 5]. Thus, the Stratus® underestimates the true retinal thickness and may fail to detect retinal thickness changes between the photoreceptor outer segment and the RPE. The presence of vitreoretinal traction may cause a failure in the localization of the internal limiting membrane with misplacement of the inner boundary on the zone of vitreous traction (Fig. 1.4). The presence of a dense retinal

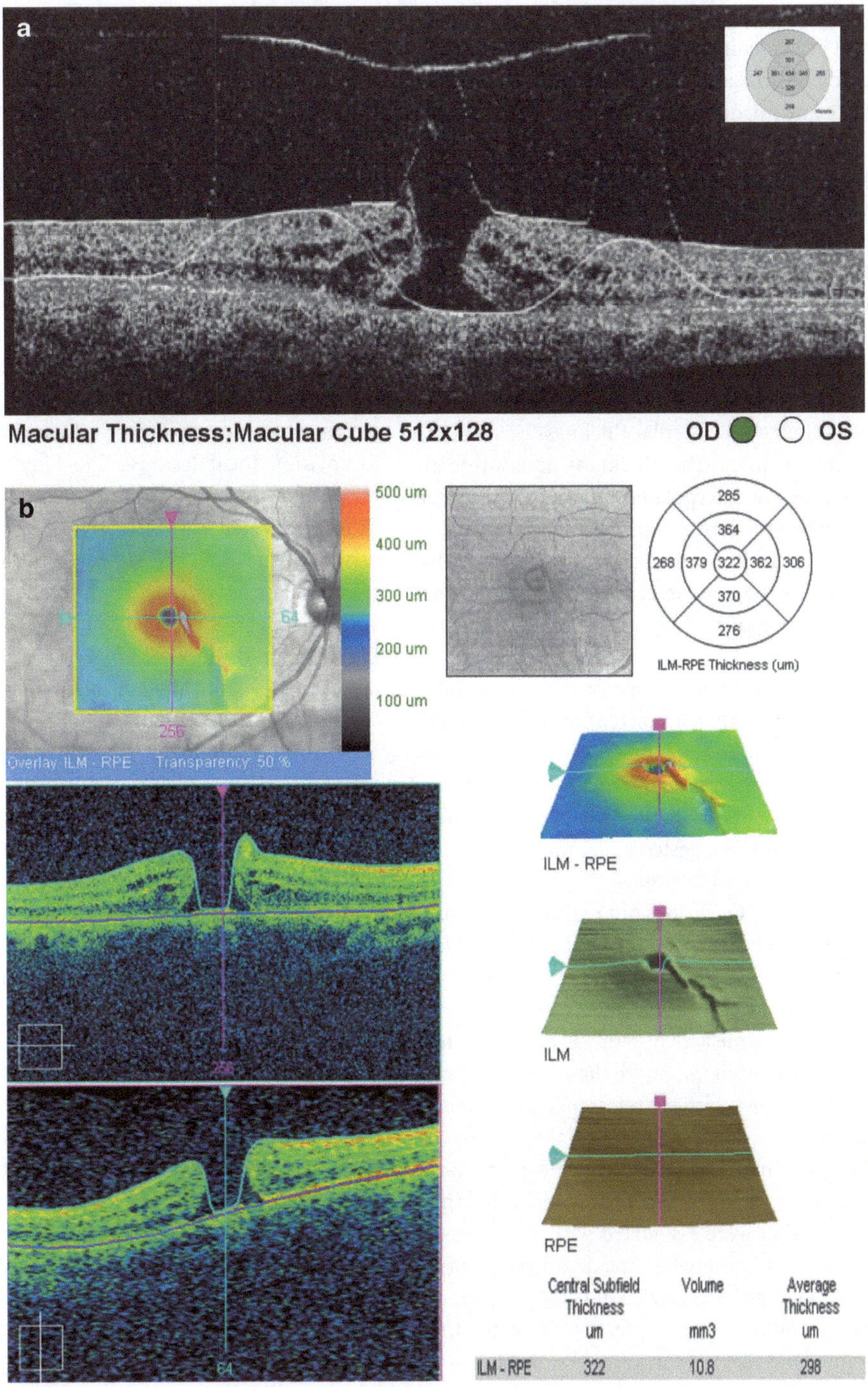

Fig. 1.4 A 62-year-old male with a full thickness macular hole on his right eye. (**a**) Stratus® OCT scan with a signal strength of 9 but an "analysis confidence low" warning on the scan message box. Stratus® OCT retinal thickness tabular report displays a foveal thickness of 454 μm (inset). Notice the segmentation algorithm lines for retinal thickness demonstrating marked errors with measurements between the internal limiting membrane and the posterior hyaloid. (**b**) Cirrus® Spectral-domain OCT of another patient with a macular hole where the retinal thickness measurement is correct. Notice that the segmentation algorithm correctly placed the inner and outer retinal boundaries

hemorrhage can obscure the RPE-choriocapillaris band producing an incorrect interpretation of the outer boundary measurement. Images with poor signal strength are also prone to cause misdirection of the automated boundary layers of the algorithm. Conditions that are characterized by the presence of subretinal fluid, such as choroidal neovascularization, are related to more severe errors than those with retinal cysts or retinal vascular diseases [14].

The Stratus® OCT can also create a topographic and volumetric map of a 6 mm diameter circle based on thickness data from six radial line scans that are evenly spaced around the circle. The two most common macular thickness protocols are the fast macular thickness map and the macular thickness map. The thickness measurements between the lines are interpolated. Therefore, if a focal lesion lies between the lines, it may not be detected in a given OCT scan resulting in sampling errors [13, 16]. Therefore, it would be a grave error for the clinician to just look at the topographic map and ignore the individual scans.

The current Stratus® software is not capable of differentiating between subretinal fluid volume and retinal volume. In eyes with subretinal fluid, the fluid is often combined with the neurosensory retina during retinal thickness measurements. This is the reason why Sadda and colleagues [6] have suggested using the term "retinal height" rather than retinal thickness.

Finally, the Stratus® OCT does not register the scans to an anatomic region on the retina. The video image that is captured as one scans the retina is not captured at the same time of the retina scan. Thus when repeating a scan, one is not sure if the same area of retina is being scanned.

Ray et al. [13] reported that more than 40% of Stratus® OCT macular scans in a tertiary referral center had artifacts. Furthermore, in more than 60% of these scans, the macular thickness map was incorrectly measured using the fast macular thickness protocol. They identified three types of artifacts that were associated with an erroneous macular thickness measurement: misidentification of the inner or outer boundaries (Figs. 1.3 and 1.4), a degraded image (Fig. 1.2) and off-center artifacts [13]. At the time, Hee [15] pointed out that the software version 4.0 had not been released and suggested that the new software version 4.0 would reduce the number of artifacts encountered in Stratus® OCT imaging. However, despite the use of software version 4.0, Sadda et al. [14] retrospectively reported errors in the detection of retinal boundaries in 92% of cases of 200 patients who underwent Stratus® OCT imaging. Moderate errors were present in 19.5% of cases and severe errors in 13.5% [14].

1.3 Advantages and Limitations of Spectral-Domain OCT

There are several spectral-domain OCTs that are currently commercially available. They are all different but in general the image acquisition is much faster and the resulting images are of a higher resolution. Since the reference mirror does not need to be adjusted during the scanning, spectral-domain OCT can produce at least 25,000 axial scans per second, which is about 50 times faster than the Stratus® OCT. This increased speed in image acquisition minimizes motion artifacts. Three-dimensional OCT data of the macula is acquired using a dense raster scan pattern, which reduces the chances of missing focal lesions. The larger number of scans allows for a greater resolution of the ensuing images. Furthermore, each OCT scan is precisely registered to the fundus image [8, 9, 17]. However, the automated segmentation algorithms are all different. For instance, the Cirrus® spectral-domain OCT (Carl Zeiss-Meditec, Dublin, California, USA) places the outer retinal boundary at the level of the RPE rather than at the junction of the outer and inner segments of the photoreceptors. The Spectralis® Heidelberg Retinal Angiography + OCT (Heidelberg Engineering, Heidelberg, Germany) appears to use the outer RPE as its outer retinal boundary [18]. Thus, retinal thickness measurements in eyes with and without posterior segment pathology are consistently higher in spectral-domain OCT than in the Stratus®; however, the retinal thickness measurement differences between the Spectralis®, Cirrus®, and Stratus® vary depending on the specific pathological process that is being imaged [15, 18]. Conversion factors between the Stratus® and the different spectral-domain OCT machines is not possible at this time, because there is poor agreement between the different OCT machines [19, 20]. Therefore, the clinician should not translate retinal thickness measurements between machines or switch from one OCT machine to another in a given patient.

Even though spectral-domain OCT systems represent a great leap forward, there are certain limitations that physicians should be aware of. Spectral-domain OCT cannot distinguish between positive and negative echo delays, which results in mirror artifacts (Fig. 1.1). Resolution limitations of the spectrometers used in spectral-domain OCT make them susceptible to measurement errors if the distance of the instrument to the eye is changed. In these cases, the retina will display different intensities. Media opacities still degrade the image obtained and can cause erroneous positioning of the inner and outer boundaries during retinal thickness measurements (Fig. 1.2).

Summary for the Clinician

- As in other imaging modalities, artifacts are fairly common with OCT.
- Artifacts can be divided into acquisition and interpretation artifacts.
- A good image is an important determinant in avoiding artifacts; however, good signal strength does not assure a reliable OCT analysis and the clinician should look for any disparity in the report, as the Stratus® software version 4.0 and above can identify the presence of artifacts.
- Retinal thickness measurements depend on automated segmentation algorithms that place a line along the inner retinal boundary and another line along the outer retinal boundary. In cases where the normal anatomy is altered, the expertise of the examiner plays a major role in the correct positioning of the line scan.
- Interpretation of OCT topographic maps should always include examination of the cross-sectional OCT scans.
- The retinal thickness measurement differences between the Spectralis®, Cirrus®, and Stratus® vary depending on the specific pathological process that is being imaged.

1.4 Conclusion

Although errors are common in the image analysis of the Stratus® OCT, the current software version 4.0 can detect and warn of their presence. The examiner must search for any incongruent information. In many pathologies, the information of the OCT images is very useful; however, images of entities with alterations of the RPE morphology are best evaluated without any analysis protocol. Spectral-domain OCT has overcome many of the weaknesses encountered with the Stratus® OCT such as fixation dependence, small scanned area, and thickness measurements, but Stratus® OCT can still be a valuable tool in the daily clinical practice if the examiner is aware of its normal functioning and pitfalls. Finally, one must not forget that despite all the advantages of the spectral-domain OCT, it can also give erroneous information. As with any other medical imaging modality, the OCT results have to be correlated with the clinical condition of the patient.

References

1. Huang D, Swanson EA, Lin CP et al (1991) Optical coherence tomography. Science 254:1178–1181
2. Hee MR, Izatt JA, Swanson EA et al (1995) Optical coherence tomography of the human retina. Arch Ophthalmol 113:325–332
3. Puliafito CA, Hee MR, Lin CP et al (1995) Imaging of macular diseases with optical coherence tomography. Ophthalmology 102:217–229
4. Costa RA, Calucci D, Skaf M et al (2004) Optical coherence tomography 3: automatic delineation of the outer neural retinal boundary and its influence on retinal thickness measurements. Invest Ophthalmol Vis Sci 45:2399–2406
5. Pons ME, Garcia-Valenzuela E (2005) Redefining the limit of the outer retina in optical coherence tomography scans. Ophthalmology 112:1079–1085
6. Sadda SR, Joeres S, Wu Z et al (2007) Error correction and quantitative subanalysis of optical coherence tomography data using computer-assisted grading. Invest Ophthalmol Vis Sci 48:839–848
7. Kaluzny JJ, Szkulmowska A, Bajraszewski T et al (2007) Retinal imaging by spectral optical coherence tomography. Eur J Ophthalmol 17:238–245
8. Wojtkowski M, Bajraszewski T, Gorczynska I et al (2004) Ophthalmic imaging by spectral optical coherence tomography. Am J Ophthalmol 138:412–419
9. Wojtkowski M, Srinivasan V, Fujimoto JG et al (2005) Three-dimensional retinal imaging with high-speed ultrahigh-resolution optical coherence tomography. Ophthalmology 112:1734–1746
10. Browning DJ, McOwen MD, Bowen RM Jr, O'Marah TL (2004) Comparison of the clinical diagnosis of diabetic macular edema with diagnosis by optical coherence tomography. Ophthalmology 111:712–715
11. Azzolini C, Patelli F, Brancato R (2001) Correlation between optical coherence tomography data and biomicroscopic interpretation of idiopathic macular hole. Am J Ophthalmol 132:348–355
12. Chan A, Duker JS, Schuman JS, Fujimoto JG (2004) Stage 0 macular holes: observations by optical coherence tomography. Ophthalmology 111:2027–2032
13. Ray R, Stinnett SS, Jaffe GJ (2005) Evaluation of image artifact produced by optical coherence tomography of retinal pathology. Am J Ophthalmol 139:18–29
14. Sadda SR, Wu Z, Walsh AC et al (2006) Errors in retinal thickness measurements obtained by optical coherence tomography. Ophthalmology 113:285–293
15. Hee MR (2005) Artifacts in optical coherence tomography topographic maps. Am J Ophthalmol 139:154–155

16. Hee MR, Puliafito CA, Duker JS et al (1998) Topography of diabetic macular edema with optical coherence tomography. Ophthalmology 105:360–370
17. Srinivasan VJ, Wojtkowski M, Witkin AJ et al (2006) High-definition and 3-dimensional imaging of macular pathologies with high-speed ultrahigh-resolution optical coherence tomography. Ophthalmology 113(2054): e2051–2014
18. Han IC, Jaffe GJ (2009) Comparison of spectral- and time-domain optical coherence tomography for retinal thickness measurements in healthy and diseased eyes. Am J Ophthalmol 147:847–858, 858 e841
19. Forooghian F, Cukras C, Meyerle CB et al (2008) Evaluation of time domain and spectral domain optical coherence tomography in the measurement of diabetic macular edema. Invest Ophthalmol Vis Sci 49:4290–4296
20. Leung CK, Cheung CY, Weinreb RN et al (2008) Comparison of macular thickness measurements between time domain and spectral domain optical coherence tomography. Invest Ophthalmol Vis Sci 49:4893–4897

Chapter 2

Simultaneous SD-OCT and Confocal SLO-Imaging

2

Peter Charbel Issa, Monika Fleckenstein, Hans-Martin Helb,
Hendrik P. N. Scholl, Steffen Schmitz-Valckenberg, and Frank G. Holz

Core Messages

- Pathological findings visible on high-resolution optical coherence tomography (OCT) can be correlated with findings on confocal scanning laser ophthalmoscopy (cSLO) imaging, including fluorescein- and ICG- angiography, fundus autofluorescence (FAF) – or reflectance images, in exact topographic correspondance. Simultaneous acquisition is time-efficient and facilitates correlation of findings in the different imaging modalities.
- Eye tracking allows for stabilizing SD-OCT scans on areas of interest and averaging of multiple scans to improve image contrast.
- Exact alignement of serial examinations at the same retinal location enables to accurately track the disease course or treatment effects.

2.1 Background

Both optical coherence tomography (OCT) and confocal scanning laser ophthalmoscopy (cSLO) are increasingly used in a routine clinical setting for diagnostic purposes and assessment of treatment effects. They have also become valuable research tools due to their ability to assess retinal morphology in vivo [1, 2].

Recently, spectral domain (SD)-OCT with its advantage of high-resolution image acquisition has become commercially available. In previous (time-domain) OCT generations, reference mirrors move mechanically, which limits imaging speed. In SD-OCT, the reference mirror is stationary, and the OCT signal is acquired either by using a spectrometer as detector or by varying the narrowband wavelength of the light source in time. The resulting high-speed scan acquisition minimizes motion artifacts and enables the acquisition of three-dimensional volume OCT scans consisting of a multitude of individual scans without major interpolation [3].

In retinal imaging, confocality allows one to record alterations of a given plane with improved contrast and detail compared with conventional fundus photography. Commercially available cSLOs allow recording of various image modalities such as fluorescein and indocyanine green (ICG) angiography, fundus autofluorescence (FAF), or blue- and near-infrared reflectance images [4]. Especially, the noninvasive methods such as FAF imaging have recently gained increasing attention since they allow assessing and following alterations of the pigment epithelium with great detail [2].

2.2 Principle of the Combined Imaging Technology

A new device for retinal imaging, the Spectralis HRA+OCT (Heidelberg Engineering, Heidelberg, Germany) combines the two techniques in one instrument with various subsequent advantages including exact correlation of tomographic and topographic findings [3]. It allows to simultaneously record SD-OCT scans with fluorescein and ICG angiography, digital infrared and blue reflectance ("redfree"), or FAF images. The optical and technical principles of the cSLO unit are identical to a recently introduced instrument for clinical use, HRA2 (Heidelberg Engineering) [4]. In brief, an optically pumped solid-state laser source is used to generate the blue light excitation wavelength of 488 nm for fluorescein angiography, blue reflectance, and FAF images. Diode laser sources of 790 and 820 nm wavelength are used for ICG angiography and infrared reflectance recordings, respectively. The light safety calculations consider the specific optical setup and computer control of the device, and maximum retinal irradiance lies below the limits established by the American National Standards

Institute (ANSI) and other international standards (The Laser Institute of America 1993). Emission is recorded between 500 and 700 nm with a detection efficiency of 85% for fluorescein angiography and FAF images, and above 810 nm with a detection efficiency of 66% for ICG recordings. In the blue reflectance and infrared reflectance mode, the barrier filter is removed and the reflected light is directly recorded.

For automated alignment of the SD-OCT with the cSLO images, the software uses a sophisticated algorithm to detect eye movements between different images. A set of hundreds of landmarks is extracted automatically for every image. A combinatorial algorithm is used to match the landmarks between the different images. Six transformation parameters (two-dimensional affine transformation) are computed from the positions of the matching landmarks using a least square algorithm resulting in subpixel accuracy. The automated alignment is used for both real-time compensation of eye movements and averaging of multiple images. Assuming a Gaussian noise distribution in the image signal over time, the signal-to-noise ratio is increased by a factor of square-root of the number of images averaged, e.g., averaging over nine images will increase the signal-to-noise ratio in the generated mean image by a factor of 3.

The new operation software (ART – "Automatic Real Time" – Module, Heidelberg Engineering) is able to track eye movements in real time based on the cSLO images. Depending on the eye movements, the OCT B-scan is repositioned and thus stabilized and frozen at the retinal location selected. B-scans recorded during movement of the eye are discarded. The software then computes and compensates for movements between the B-scan images caused by the varying blood pressure and position changes of the eye relative to the camera, and finally averages the live B-scans, and thus, greatly enhances the image quality leading to remarkable B-scan detail and contrast because of a marked reduction in speckle and other noise.

The optics of the instrument allow for compensation of between −24 and + 30 diopters of ametropia in steps of 0.25 diopters. An internal fixation target from an array of 3 × 3 blue lights can be chosen individually by the examiner. Alternatively, an external target for fixation with the fellow eye may be used. Most operation settings are controlled via an interactive touch panel.

With regard to the OCT, 40,000 A-scans are acquired per second with a 7 μm axial optical resolution and a 14 μm lateral optical resolution. OCT scans can be recoded simultaneously with fluorescein angiography, ICG angiography, FAF, infrared and blue reflectance images. For the A-scans, the scan depth is 1.8 mm/512 pixels providing a digital axial resolution of 3.5 μm/pixel.

B-scans cover a transversal range of 15, 20, or 30° field of view. In the high-speed mode, scan widths are 384, 512, and 768 A-scans per B-scan with a lateral digital resolution of 11 μm/pixel and a scan rate of 89, 69, and 48 B-scans/sec. The high-resolution modes encompass a scan width of 768, 1,024, and 1,536 A-scans per B-scan with a lateral digital resolution of 5 μm/pixel at a scan rate of 48, 37, and 25 B-scans/sec.

Sequences of B-scans can be acquired to image a full volume. A large variety of patterns may be used, differing, e.g., in scan density, resolution, and orientation. The number of B-scans per volume can be adjusted from 12 B-scans per 10° to 96 B-scans per 10°. This results in a distance between consecutive parallel B-scans of approximately 30–240 μm.

All OCT images are automatically enlarged in the axial direction to improve visualization of intraretinal layers. Evaluation of OCT B-scans is done using a gray-scale visualization with a white background, which allowed for better recognition of details, especially in comparison with color-scale visualization as commonly used in time-domain OCT imaging [5].

Summary for the Clinician

- New combined imaging instruments allow studying regions of interest located on cSLO images (reflectance images, autofluorescence imaging, fluorescein angiography, or ICG angiography) with quasi in vivo histology of high-resolution SD-OCT sections. Moreover, automatic re-alignment allows for an accurate monitoring of retinal pathologies.

2.3 Clinical Application

OCT scans are presented underneath a topographic image in which an arrow marks the location and direction of the scan. Therefore, all structures on the two imaging modalities may be matched by drawing an imaginary vertical line from a point of interest in the topographic image to the OCT scan, and vice versa.

Figure 2.1 shows normal findings in the absence of retinal disease. The line in the infrared reflectance cSLO-image indicates where the OCT cross-section was obtained. There is still debate on the correlation of the various retinal layers with histological sections. However, the assignment as shown in the figure is now widely accepted.

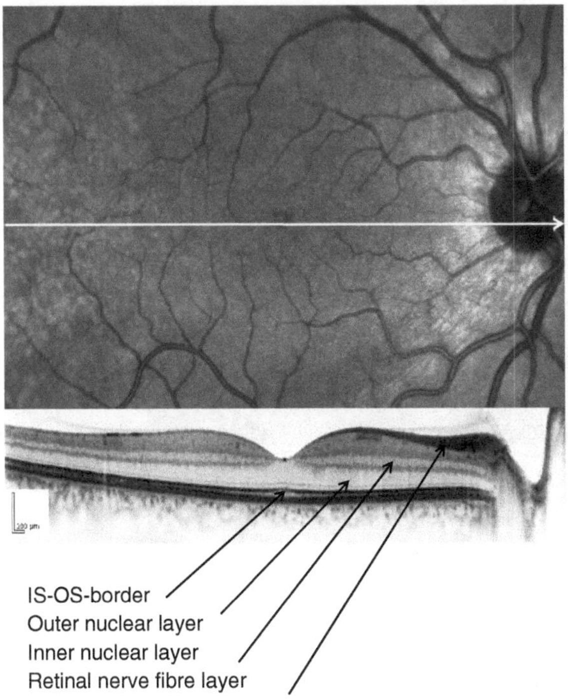

Fig. 2.1 The *white arrow* in the near-infrared confocal reflectance image shows the location where the correspondent OCT scan below is recorded. For reference, some retinal layers are assigned

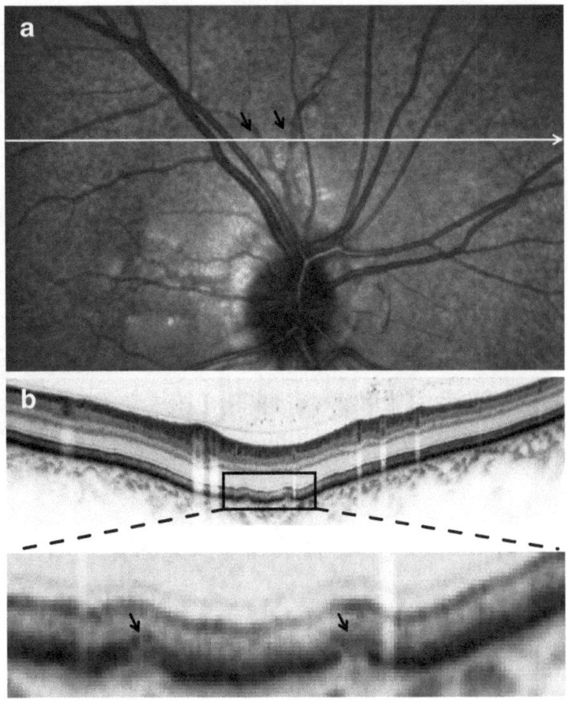

Fig. 2.2 Near-infrared reflectance image (**a**) and simultaneous OCT imaging (**b**) in a patient with peau d'orange and angioid streaks due to pseudoxanthoma elasticum. The black *arrows* point out the location of the angioid streaks

Figure 2.2 demonstrates findings on near-infrared fundus reflectance imaging in a patient with pseudoxanthoma elasticum (PXE). Near-infrared light is only marginally absorbed by the melanin in the retinal pigment epithelium (RPE). Therefore, the superior visibility of peau d'orange in this imaging mode may be explained by the location of the respective pathology below the RPE, i.e., within Bruch's membrane [6]. The simultaneously recorded SD-OCT scan crosses two angioid streaks (black arrows) and reveals a rupture in the thickened Bruch's membrane as pathological substrate. The overlying neurosensory retina appears intact.

Figure 2.3 shows the fundus of a 35-year-old myopic patient with a recent onset multiple evanescent white dot syndrome (MEWDS) in the right eye. In late-phase ICG angiography (25 min), the white dots may be better visualized than on fundus photography, fluorescein angiography, or FAF. The SD-OCT through the lesions revealed that structural alterations of the photoreceptor layer occur within the areas of white dots. This defect within the border of the inner and outer photoreceptor segments may be more widespread and persistent than expected from angiographic imaging [7, 8].

Figure 2.4 illustrates the findings on FAF and SD-OCT in a patient with severe rod-cone dystrophy due to a mutation in the MERTK gene. The MERTK protein plays a key role in the photoreceptor outer segment ingestion by the RPE during their physiological renewal [9]. In animal models with *MERTK* mutations, debris accumulates in the subretinal space due to the inability of the pigment epithelium to clear shed photoreceptor outer segments [10]. By means of SD-OCT, it was possible to detect analogous subneurosensory debris in the affected patients in vivo [11]. Moreover, simultaneous FAF imaging revealed that marked atrophy within the photoreceptor layer is associated with loss of FAF due to atrophy of the pigment epithelium.

Figure 2.5 presents serial simultaneous SD-OCT and near-infrared reflectance imaging (follow-up period 10 months) in geographic atrophy due to age-related macular degeneration (AMD). SD-OCT has recently allowed further study into the morphological changes in geographic atrophy in a quasi-histological manner [12, 13]. The exact re-location of the OCT scan in follow-up exams now enables the study of areas of geographic atrophy and their changes over time longitudinally. Within atrophic areas, the outer retina including the RPE and the outer

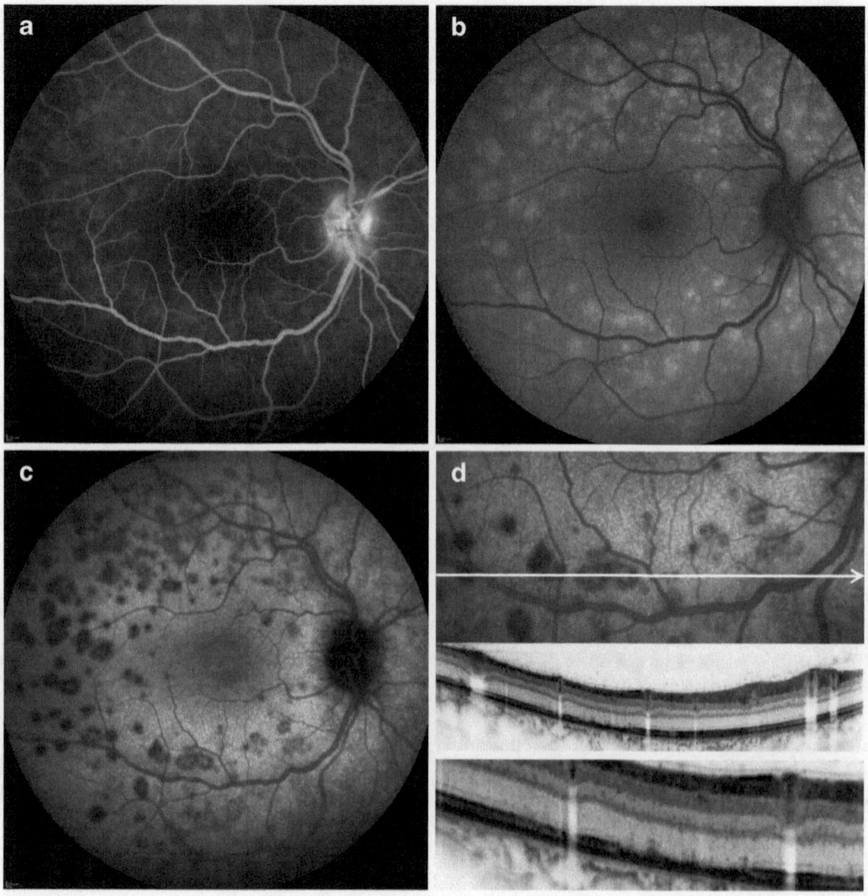

Fig. 2.3 Fluorescein angiography (**a**), FAF (**b**), late-phase (25 min) ICG angiography (**c**), and simultaneous OCT imaging (**d**) in an acute stage of MEWDS. The lesions show a superior visibility on late-phase ICG angiography. The simultaneous OCT reveals that the pathology appears to affect the outer neurosensory retina

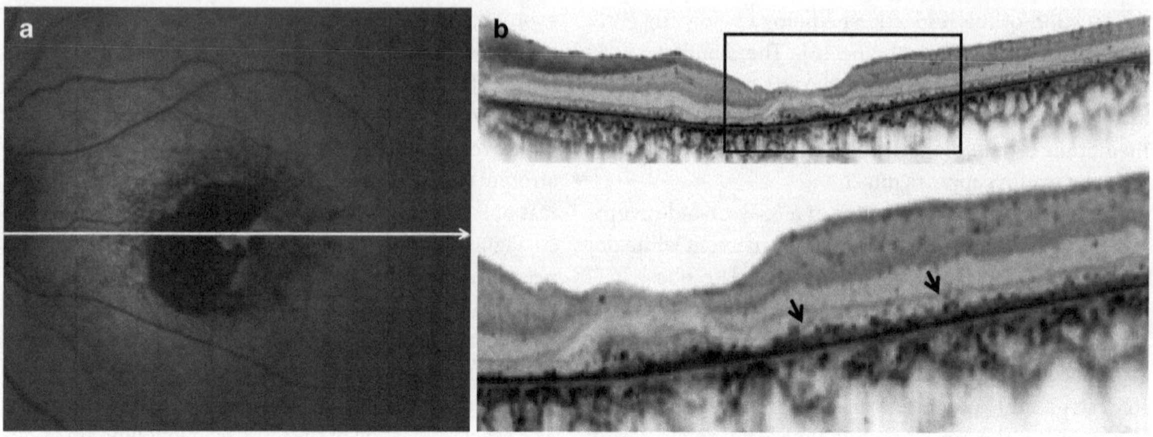

Fig. 2.4 Fundus autofluorescence (FAF) in a patient with rod-cone dystrophy due to a mutation in the MERTK gene (**a**). There was an overall reduced FAF and an area of pigment epithelial atrophy. Simultaneous SD-OCT imaging (**b**) revealed debris above the retinal pigment epithelium (black *arrows*)

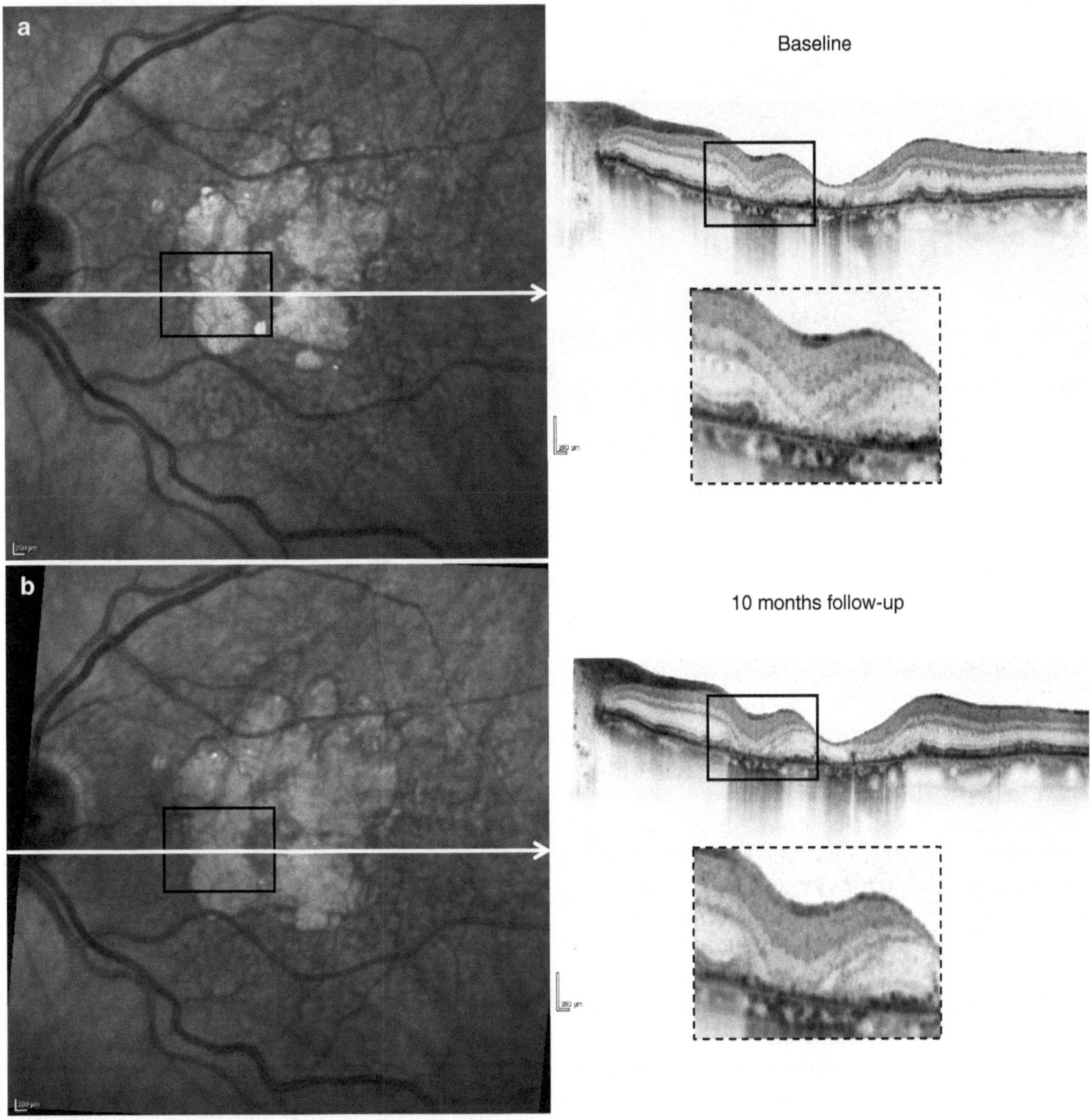

Fig. 2.5 Changes over time within a patch of geographic atrophy due to age-related macular degeneration (AMD) in a 77-year-old patient. (**a**) Infrared reflectance image and the corresponding OCT scan at baseline and (**b**) at follow-up 10 months later. Enlargement of the atrophic area occurred in conjunction with progressive atrophy within the outer retinal layers. Dashed boxes are magnifications of the boxes highlighted in the OCT scan above

nuclear layer appear atrophic on the OCT scan, resulting in close approximation of the inner retinal layers to Bruch's membrane. Compared with baseline (A), the area of outer retinal atrophy was larger at 10 months follow-up (B). The box highlights an area with enlargement of a small atrophic lesion over time.

Figure 2.6 shows a pigment epithelial detachment (PED) in a patient with neovascular AMD. It is noteworthy that the PED goes beyond the area with obvious hyperfluorescence on late-phase angiography. This is due to the masking of the angiographic leakage by macular pigment, resulting in the appearance that the foveal center would be spared.

Figure 2.7 shows the right eye of a patient with macular telangiectasia (MacTel) type 2. On ophthalmoscopy, there is often the appearance of a lamellar macular hole, which appears dark on confocal blue reflectance imaging (A). Simultaneous SD-OCT imaging reveals that the correlates on OCT imaging are foveal hyporeflective spaces within the neurosensory retina (C). In MacTel type 2, there is a

2

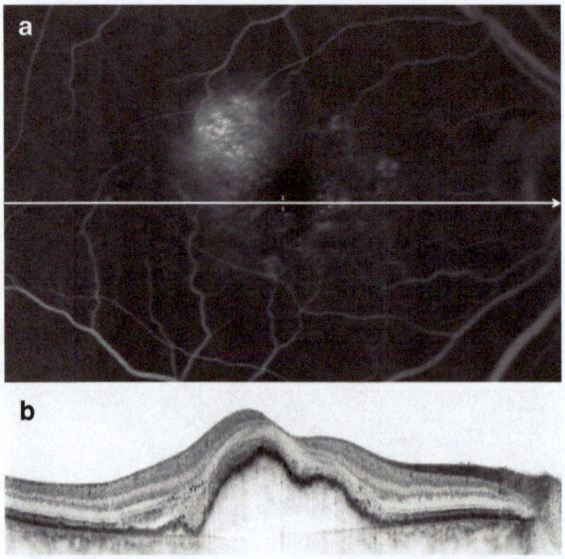

Fig. 2.6 Simultaneous fluorescein angiography and OCT examination in a patient with a pigment epithelial detachment due to AMD. Note the discrepancy between the apparent sparing of the foveal center on angiography (**a**) and the true expansion of the lesion involving the foveal center on OCT imaging (**b**)

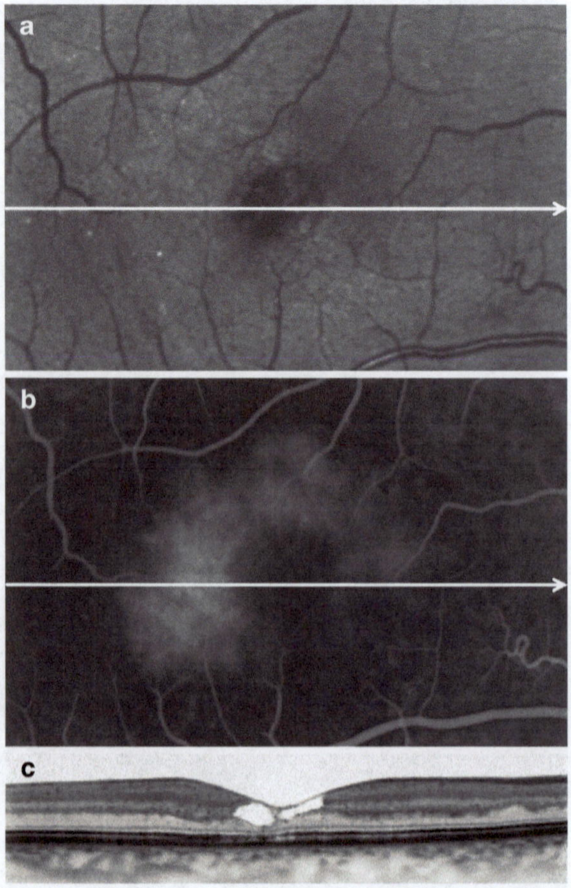

Fig. 2.7 Simultaneous confocal blue reflectance imaging (**a**) or late phase fluorescein angiography (**b**) with SD-OCT (**c**) in a patient with macular telangiectasia type 2. The small dark foveal area in (**a**) appears as a lamellar macular hole on ophthalmoscopy. The correlates on the SD-OCT scan are characteristic hyporeflective spaces within the neurosensory retina. There is no pooling of fluorescein in those cystoid spaces

characteristic late-phase leakage on fluorescein angiography within the parafoveolar area (B). The hyporeflective retinal spaces show no pooling on fluorescein angiography which is in contrast with other cystoid spaces as in exudative macular edema. These spaces have also been shown to exhibit an internal reflectivity different from exudative cystoid spaces [14]. It was concluded that hyporeflective spaces in MacTel type 2 are rather due to atrophic neurosensory alterations than having an exudative origin.

Figure 2.8 presents findings in two patients with isolated foveal hypoplasia [15]. Patient 1 was 54-year-old and presented with a visual acuity of 20/32. Patient 2 was a 9-year-old boy with bilateral unexplained low visual acuity. Visual acuity was 20/63 in the right eye and 20/50 in the left eye and a slow rotating nystagmus was present. In both patients, there was no foveolar and macular reflex. Patient 1 showed an overall light pigmentation of the peripheral fundus and a conspicuous course of the retinal vessels at the posterior pole. FAF imaging revealed a lack of macular pigment and three-dimensional OCT volume scans could not detect a foveal pit. All neurosensory retinal layers were continuous throughout the foveal center.

2.4 Conclusions

Recent improvement in OCT imaging, including increased resolution and image-contrast, a noninvasive visualization of the microstructural retinal morphology in vivo. The combination of these new OCT technologies and topographic cSLO imaging within one instrument as described here allows studying the cross-sectional structure of regions of interest on fluorescein and ICG angiography, blue or infrared reflectance, and FAF imaging. This possibility will further improve our understanding of the pathogenesis of macular pathologies and may prove to be useful for diagnosis and patient management.

There is a broad range of potential research and clinical applications for this new instrument. For example, monitoring the natural history or treatment effects in patients with AMD will be facilitated. When the patient returns for follow-up examination, it is now possible to evaluate changes on OCT imaging at precisely the same retinal location as in the previous examination due to the

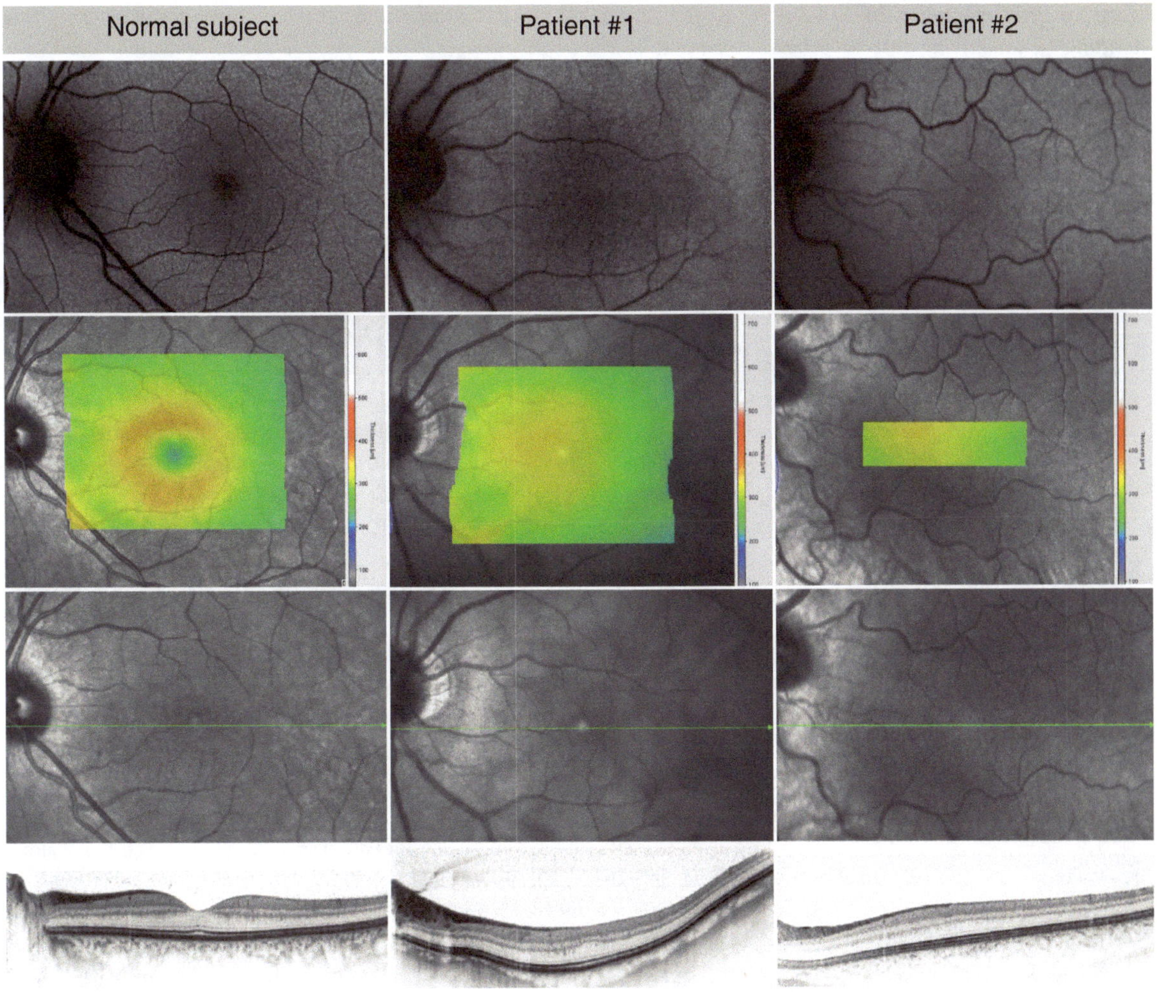

Fig. 2.8 (From Ref. [15] with permission): Left eye of a normal subject (for comparison) and two patients with foveal hypoplasia. Both patients show reduced (Patient 1) or almost absent (Patient 2) macular pigment on FAF imaging (*first row*). The color-coded retinal thickness maps reveal absence of the foveal pit in both patients. The infrared confocal reflectance image (*third row*) shows the location of the OCT-scan below (*green line*). In the patients, all retinal layers continue through the presumed foveal area on OCT scans and no foveal contour is present. Copyright © (2008) American Medical Association. All rights reserved

automated re-alignment of the OCT scans. This allows for more reliability to judge on whether or not retinal fluid accumulation has stayed the same, increased, or decreased, even if changes are only small. This information may be crucial regarding advice for re-treatment. Moreover, the combined assessment is less time-consuming and therefore more cost-effective than performing the two imaging modalities sequentially.

Besides these advantages for follow-up examinations, the automated eye-tracker allows for the averaging of multiple OCT scans at exactly the same location, resulting in a superior signal-to-noise ratio (i.e., improved image contrast) compared with nonaveraged images. It furthermore ensures that subsequent OCT scans during the acquisition of volume scans are placed at the foreseen location, independent of eye movements.

FAF imaging combined with spatially correlated OCT offers new research applications. The FAF signal mainly derives from lipofuscin granules in the RPE [16]. Excessive lipofuscin accumulation is a common pathogenetic pathway in various retinal diseases including monogenic disorders such as Stargardt's or Best's disease and complex diseases such as AMD [2, 17]. Recently, FAF imaging has been shown to be a valuable tool to analyze disease progression and it may be beneficial to monitor therapeutic interventions [18]. Correlating findings on SD-OCT with those on FAF imaging is likely to advance the understanding of underlying disease processes leading to an abnormal FAF signal. Besides FAF, other imaging modalities such as confocal blue and infrared reflectance imaging have recently been shown to reveal specific changes in different disease entities or fundus changes [19, 20]. Combined imaging with an SD-OCT will allow one to further investigate the corresponding changes on a quasi-histological level.

Summary for the Clinician

- Simultaneous recordings of SD-OCT and various cSLO-imaging modes provide a better understanding of retinal diseases. The precise correlation of topographic (cSLO) and tomographic (OCT) images, and especially the re-placement of the OCT scans at exactly the same retinal location in follow-up exams, allow a more reliable clinical evaluation of the disease evolution and treatment effects compared with the previous technologies.

References

1. Podoleanu AG, Rosen RB (2008) Combinations of techniques in imaging the retina with high resolution. Prog Retin Eye Res 27:464–499
2. Schmitz-Valckenberg S, Holz FG, Bird AC, Spaide RF (2008) Fundus autofluorescence imaging: review and perspectives. Retina 28:385–409
3. Helb HM, Charbel Issa P, Fleckenstein M et al (2009) Clinical evaluation of simultaneous confocal scanning laser ophthalmoscopy imaging combined with high-resolution spectral-domain optical coherence tomography. Acta Ophthalmologica [in press]; DOI: 10.1111/j.1755-3768.2009.01602.x
4. Jorzik JJ, Bindewald A, Dithmar S, Holz FG (2005) Digital simultaneous fluorescein and indocyanine green angiography, autofluorescence, and red-free imaging with a solid-state laser-based confocal scanning laser ophthalmoscope. Retina 25:405–416
5. Brar M, Bartsch DU, Nigam N et al (2009) Colour versus grey-scale display of images on high-resolution spectral OCT. Br J Ophthalmol 93:597–602
6. Charbel Issa P, Finger RP, Holz FG, Scholl HPN (2009) Multimodal imaging including spectral domain OCT and confocal near infrared reflectance for characterisation of outer retinal pathology in pseudoxanthoma elasticum. Invest Ophthalmol Vis Sci [in press]; DOI: 10.1167/iovs.09-3541
7. Li D, Kishi S (2009) Restored photoreceptor outer segment damage in multiple evanescent white dot syndrome. Ophthalmology 116:762–770
8. Spaide RF, Koizumi H, Freund KB (2008) Photoreceptor outer segment abnormalities as a cause of blind spot enlargement in acute zonal occult outer retinopathy-complex diseases. Am J Ophthalmol 146:111–120
9. Feng W, Yasumura D, Matthes MT, LaVail MM, Vollrath D (2002) Mertk triggers uptake of photoreceptor outer segments during phagocytosis by cultured retinal pigment epithelial cells. J Biol Chem 277:17016–17022
10. Dowling JE, Sidman RL (1962) Inherited retinal dystrophy in the rat. J Cell Biol 14:73–109
11. Charbel Issa P, Bolz HJ, Ebermann I, Domeier E, Holz FG, Scholl HP (2009) Characterization of severe rod-cone dystrophy in a consanguineous family with a splice site mutation in the MERTK gene. Br J Ophthalmol 93: 920–925
12. Fleckenstein M, Charbel Issa P, Helb HM et al (2008) High resolution spectral domain-OCT imaging in geographic atrophy associated with age-related macular degeneration. Invest Ophthalmol Vis Sci 49:4137–4144
13. Wolf-Schnurrbusch UE, Enzmann V, Brinkmann CK, Wolf S (2008) Morphologic changes in patients with geographic atrophy assessed with a novel spectral OCT-SLO combination. Invest Ophthalmol Vis Sci 49: 3095–3099
14. Barthelmes D, Sutter FK, Gillies MC (2008) Differential optical densities of intraretinal spaces. Invest Ophthalmol Vis Sci 49:3529–3534
15. Charbel Issa P, Foerl M, Helb HM, Scholl HP, Holz FG (2008) Multimodal fundus imaging in foveal hypoplasia: combined scanning laser ophthalmoscope imaging and spectral-domain optical coherence tomography. Arch Ophthalmol 126:1463–1465
16. Delori FC, Dorey CK, Staurenghi G, Arend O, Goger DG, Weiter JJ (1995) In vivo fluorescence of the ocular fundus exhibits retinal pigment epithelium lipofuscin characteristics. Invest Ophthalmol Vis Sci 36:718–729
17. Holz FG, Bellmann C, Staudt S, Schütt F, Völcker HE (2001) Fundus autofluorescence and development of geographic atrophy in age-related macular degeneration. Invest Ophthalmol Vis Sci 42:1051–1056
18. Holz FG, Bindewald-Wittich A, Fleckenstein M, Dreyhaupt J, Scholl HP, Schmitz-Valckenberg S (2007) Progression of geographic atrophy and impact of fundus autofluorescence patterns in age-related macular degeneration. Am J Ophthalmol 143:463–472
19. Charbel Issa P, Berendschot TT, Staurenghi G, Holz FG, Scholl HP (2008) Confocal blue reflectance imaging in type 2 idiopathic macular telangiectasia. Invest Ophthalmol Vis Sci 49:1172–1177
20. Weinberger AW, Lappas A, Kirschkamp T et al (2006) Fundus near infrared fluorescence correlates with fundus near infrared reflectance. Invest Ophthalmol Vis Sci 47: 3098–3108

Chapter 3

Fluorescein Angiography

3

Howard F. Fine, Jonathan L. Prenner, and Daniel Roth

Core Messages

- Fluorescein sodium is a molecule that emits photons with a wavelength of 520–530 nm (green–yellow light) following excitation with photons with a wavelength of 465–490 nm (blue light).
- Prior to fluorescein angiography, patients should be appropriately counseled on the relevant risks, which range from mild reactions such as nausea to life-threatening ones such as anaphylactic shock. Access to emergency medical supplies is crucial for angiography units.
- Knowledge of the time course of fluorescein transit in the choroid and retina as well as circulatory anatomy in normal patients is essential for the interpretation of abnormal fluorescein angiograms.
- Lesions may be hypofluorescent on angiography as a result of circulatory filling defects in arteries, capillaries, or veins; or as a result of blockage of fluorescence from overlying material such as blood, melanin, and lipid.
- Lesions may be hyperfluorescent on angiography as a result of window defect, vascular abnormality, pooling, staining, or leakage.

3.1 Principles of Fluorescein Angiography

Fluorescence is a form of luminescence, or cold-body radiation, characterized by the excitation of a material with a high energy (short wavelength) photon with subsequent release of a lower energy (longer wavelength) photon. The difference in energies is released as heat. Sodium fluorescein, $NaC_{20}H_{12}O_5$, is a hydrocarbon that is excited by wavelengths from 465 to 490 nm (blue) and emits light at a wavelength of 520–530 nm (green–yellow) [1]. It was first synthesized by Nobel laureate Johann Baeyer in 1871 [1] and introduced in ophthalmic imaging by Novotny and Alvis, two medical students, in 1961 [2]. Successful fluorescein angiography relies upon two interference filters, which allow only a narrow bandwidth of light to pass, an excitation and a barrier filter.

Sodium fluorescein is a low molecular weight molecule (367 Da) and readily diffuses through the fenestrated vessels of the choriocapillaris, but does not pass through healthy endothelial cells of nonfenestrated retinal vessels or through the retinal pigment epithelium (RPE); this property is useful diagnostically. In humans, only one-fifth of sodium fluorescein remains unbound in the bloodstream and is available for imaging; the rest remains protein-bound, primarily to albumin.

3.2 Procedures for Fluorescein Angiography

Prior to fluorescein angiography, patients should be counseled regarding the relevant risks [3]. Fluorescein may temporarily discolor the skin and urine yellow until it is eliminated, which occurs through both the kidneys and liver. Patients with renal insufficiency may therefore experience delayed elimination. Mild adverse reactions are uncommon, <5%, and include injection site reactions, nausea, and vomiting. Moderately severe reactions are infrequent, <1%, and include hives, shortness of breath, and vasovagal reactions. Life-threatening reactions are exceptionally rare, <0.001%, and include anaphylactic shock and cardiovascular collapse [4]. All units performing fluorescein angiography should have ready access to emergency medical equipment ("crash cart") in the unlikely event of life-threatening reaction. Patients with a prior history of mild or moderately severe reactions,

Table 3.1. Adverse reactions following fluorescein angiography

Mild reactions (<5%)	Injection site reaction
	Nausea
	Vomiting
Moderately severe reactions (<1%)	Urticaria
	Shortness of breath
	Vasovagal reaction
	Skin necrosis
Life-threatening reactions (<0.001%)	Anaphylactic shock
	Seizure
	Cardiovascular collapse

depending on their seriousness, may still be candidates for angiography following premedication with antihistamines such as diphenhydramine and/or corticosteroids such as prednisone. Common practice dictates the avoidance of angiography in pregnant women, especially in the first trimester [5], although evidence regarding toxicity is scant (Table 3.1).

A number of commercially available photographic systems are available, either with film or, increasingly, with digital cameras. Typical lens systems are available for 30° imaging, applicable for excellent macular detail, 60° imaging for wider field imaging, and even wide-field contact lens systems such as a 150° lens for peripheral angiography [6]. Color and/or red-free fundus photographs are obtained initially, often with stereoscopic pairs.

The typical injection procedure involves application of an upper extremity tourniquet, cannulation of an antecubital or forearm vein, tourniquet release, initiation of camera timer, and then injection of a bolus of dye, often 5 mL of 10% sodium fluorescein. Rapid injection can allow better initial images as the dye front progresses, but may increase the incidence of nausea.

Summary for the Clinician

- Patients should be informed of the relevant risks of fluorescein angiography
- Angiography units should have access to emergency medical equipment
- The typical procedure involves injection of 5 mL of 10% sodium fluorescein into an antecubital vein

3.3 Relevant Anatomy in Fluorescein Angiography

Understanding the dual circulation, choroidal and retinal, and relevant anatomic considerations are important to the interpretation of fluorescein angiography. The retinal circulation supplies the inner two-thirds of the retina, whereas the choroidal circulation supplies the outer one-third. Retinal vessels are nonfenestrated, maintaining the blood-retinal barrier via cellular tight junctions, and therefore will not leak fluorescein if healthy. Retinal vessels autoregulate such that changes in perfusion pressure have a negligible effect on blood flow. In contrast, the choroidal system does not autoregulate, has a relatively low resistance, and exhibits the highest blood flow per unit volume in the body. The choriocapillaris is fenestrated, which allows for fluorescein extravasation and diffusion through Bruch's membrane. The blood-retinal barrier of the choroid is maintained by tight junctions at the level of the RPE [7]. In addition to a myriad of other functions, the RPE is responsible for pumping fluid from the potential space below the retina. The RPE may also undergo hyperplasia and/or atrophy, affecting the amount of transmitted choroidal fluorescence. The outer plexiform layer (OPL) is the primary intraretinal interstitial space and can become edematous in a variety of pathologic conditions. The retinal vessels reside in the inner retina, from the inner nuclear layer (INL) to the internal limiting membrane (ILM). Large retinal vessels reside superficially in the nerve fiber layer (NFL), whereas fine capillaries reside deeper in the INL. Lastly, the vitreous cavity should not accumulate fluorescein unless there is a breakdown of the blood-retinal barrier.

Summary for the Clinician

- The choriocapillaris supplies the outer one-third of the retina and is fenestrated, allowing the diffusion of fluorescein to reach the outer blood-retinal barrier formed by tight junctions of RPE.
- The retinal blood vessels supply the inner two-thirds of the retina and should not leak fluorescein if healthy. The inner blood-retinal barrier is maintained by tight junctions between retinal vascular endothelial cells.

3.4 Time Course of Fluorescein Angiography

The time course inherent in normal fluorescein angiography has been described through various phases. Fluorescein travels from the internal carotid artery to the ophthalmic artery to both the posterior ciliary arteries and central retinal artery. The short posterior ciliary arteries are perfused just prior to the central retinal artery, giving rise to the choroidal phase of fluorescein angiography, typically seen at approximately 10 s following dye injection, or at 12–15 s in older patients. The initial fluorescence is termed the "choroidal flush," which is soon followed by patchy filling. If a cilioretinal artery is present (about a third of the population has one), it fills along with the choroid.

The retinal arterial phase begins 1–2 s following the choroidal phase with filling of the central retinal artery, at about 12 s following dye injection. The veins appear black, silhouetted by choroidal fluorescence. The foveal avascular zone (FAZ) appears darker than the surrounding retina because of the absence of vessels and greater thickness of RPE, which blocks choroidal fluorescence in this area. The capillary phase occurs soon after, at about 13 s following dye injection.

The transition from fluorescein filling the arterioles, then capillaries, then venules is termed as the arteriovenous phase. In the early arteriovenous phase, at about 14 s following dye injection, laminar flow is seen as fluorescein-laden blood flows slowly adjacent to the venular walls from proximal arterioles. The faster-moving blood in the center of the veins appears dark, because it arrives from more distal veins, which initially have a lower fluorescein concentration. Dye eventually fills the entire lumen during the venous stage, at roughly 16 s following dye injection.

Maximal fluorescence is observed approximately 25 s following injection, at which time the fine perifoveal capillaries can be best imaged. The recirculation phase occurs at roughly 30 s following dye injection, as blood with a concentration of fluorescein lower than that of the initial bolus returns.

The late phase of angiography occurs as the fluorescein concentration in retinal and choroidal vessels diminishes, typically 3–5 min following injection. Fluorescein that has extravasated from the choriocapillaris diffuses throughout the choroid up to the tight junctions of the RPE (Fig. 3.1) (Table 3.2).

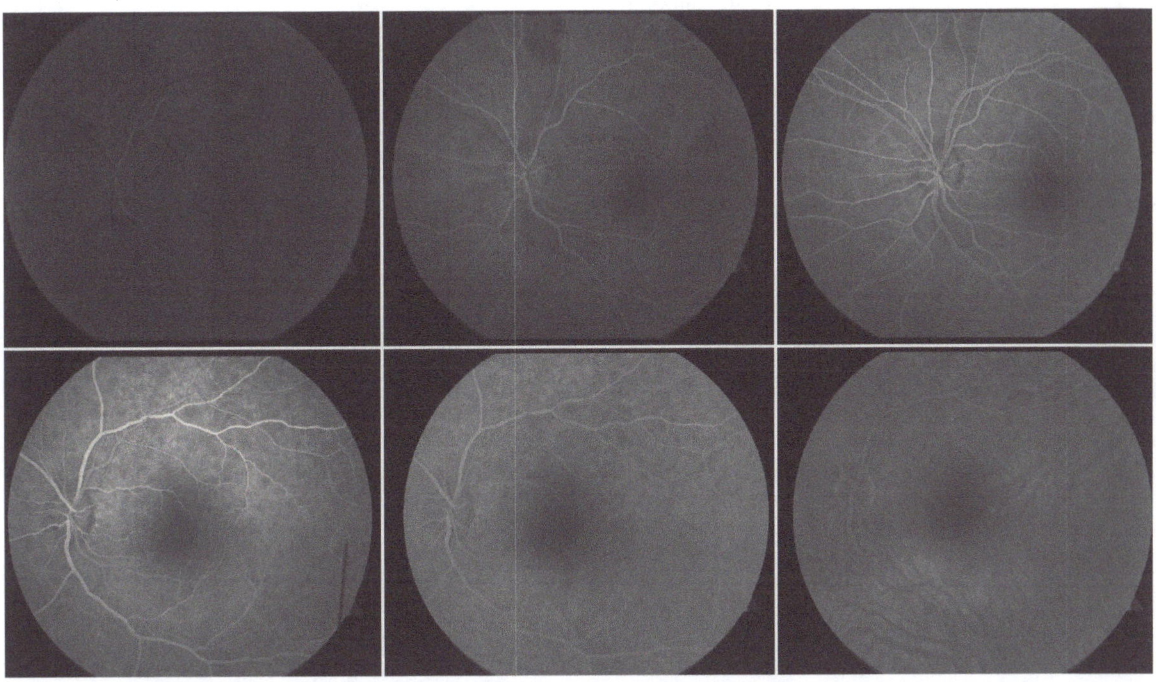

Fig. 3.1 Normal angiogram. The arterial phase (*top left*) is seen at 11 s following dye injection. The early arteriovenous phase (*top middle*) is seen at 14 s and is characterized by laminar flow in the veins. The late arteriovenous phase (*top right*) is seen at 16 s as the venular lumens fill with fluorescein. Maximal fluorescence is achieved at 25 s (*bottom right*). The recirculation phase (*bottom middle*) follows at 30 s as the kidneys remove fluorescein from circulation. The late phase (*bottom right*) is marked by extravasation of fluorescein from the choriocapillaris, which often silhouettes large choroidal vessels that are devoid of fluorescein

3

Table 3.2. Approximate time course

Seconds	Phase	Event
0	Initiation	Dye injection
10	Choroidal flush	Fluorescein reaches short posterior ciliary arteries
11–12	Arterial phase	Fluorescein reaches central retinal artery
13	Capillary phase	Capillaries are perfused
14	Arteriovenous phase	Laminar flow in veins
16	Venous phase	Lumen of veins fill
25	Maximal fluorescence	Perifoveal capillaries best imaged
30	Recirculation phase	Kidneys remove fluorescein from circulation and the concentration decreases
180–300	Late phase	Leakage, pooling, and staining of fluorescein are best appreciated

3.5 Interpretation of Fluorescein Angiography

Comparisons to the normal time sequence described earlier are an important basis in fluorescein angiography interpretation and provide insight to vascular abnormalities. Second, the anatomic considerations described earlier help one to localize the depth of lesions. A third important method for describing and interpreting fluorescein angiographic findings is classifying the lesions as *hypofluorescent* or *hyperfluorescent*, exhibiting either more or less fluorescence, respectively, in a given area than would be expected in a normal angiogram. *Autofluorescent* lesions, such as optic nerve head drusen, astrocytic hamartomas, and lipofuscinopathies, are covered in greater detail in the section on fundus autofluorescence (FAF) (Table 3.3).

3.5.1 Hypofluorescent Lesions

Lesions may be hypofluorescent for one of the two basic reasons. *Vascular filling defects* are obstructions in normal retinal and/or choroidal circulation that lead to a decrease in the amount of fluorescein, which reaches tissue, causing a reduction in intensity on angiography. Vascular filling defects must therefore arise from obstructions in the retinal circulation (arterial, capillary, or venous), the choroidal circulation (a vascular plexus), or circulation about the optic disc. The distribution, timing, and location of the vascular filling defect help to determine the aspect of circulation that is impaired. Common hypofluorescent patterns due to vascular filling defect include branch/central retinal artery/vein occlusion, (Fig. 3.2) capillary nonperfusion, and choroidal infarction.

Lesions may also be hypofluorescent due to *blocked fluorescence* if the material is present anterior to the perfused tissue, obstructing the fluorescent signal from reaching the camera. Common substances to block fluorescent signal include blood, melanin, fibrin, other pigments, and lipid. Examining which circulatory elements remain visible helps to localize the lesion depth. For example, if the superficial retinal vessels are obscured or blocked, the substance blocking fluorescence (i.e., blood or pigment) is typically located in the preretinal space. However, if all retinal vessels track over the area of blocked fluorescence, then the blocking lesion is located in the subretinal space (Fig. 3.3).

Table 3.3. Interpretation of fluorescein angiogram

Time sequence of angiogram
Anatomic location and depth of lesions
Angiographic description of lesions
Hypofluorescence
Vascular filling defect
Blocked fluorescence
Hyperfluorescence
Window defect
Vascular abnormality
Pooling
Staining
Leakage
Autofluorescence

3.5.2 Hyperfluorescent Lesions

Hyperfluorescence is typically due to *window defect* or fluid/circulatory abnormalities. The RPE blocks some amount of choroidal fluorescence. When an area of RPE is absent, such as with geographic atrophy, RPE tear, or previous laser treatment, less choroidal fluorescence is blocked leading to a relatively brighter signal (Fig. 3.4).

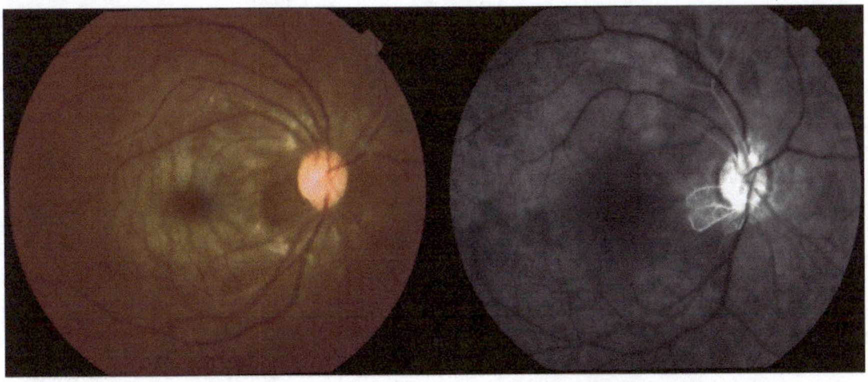

Fig. 3.2 Hypofluorescence: vascular filling defect. Illustration of central retinal artery occlusion (*left*) with characteristic *cherry red spot*. Note the lack of arterial filling in the angiogram (*right*) compared with the area of peripapillary sparing

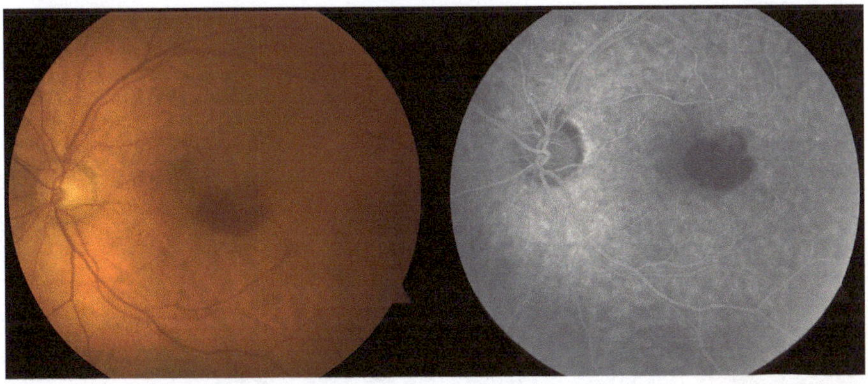

Fig. 3.3 Hypofluorescence: blocked fluorescence. Hemorrhage (*left*) secondary to exudative age-related macular degeneration. Note the blood blocks choroidal fluorescence but not retinal vascular fluorescence on angiography (*right*), indicating the location of the blood is in the subretinal space

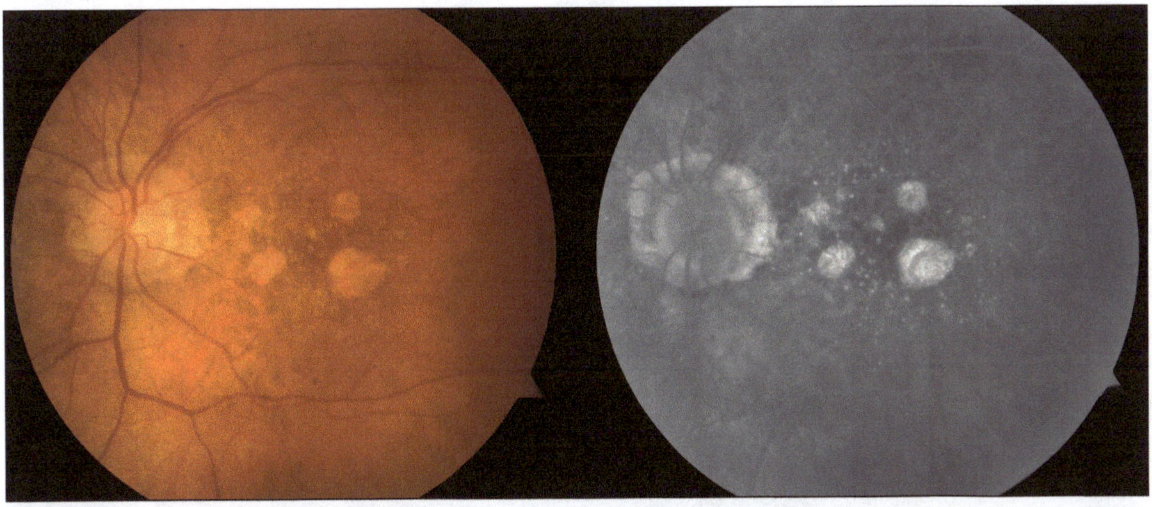

Fig. 3.4 Hyperfluorescence: window defect. Areas of geographic atrophy (*left*) secondary to nonexudative age-related macular degeneration. More choroidal fluorescence is transmitted in atrophic areas due to the lack of lipofuscin-containing retinal pigment epithelial cells

Hyperfluorescence can also be due to fluid and circulatory abnormalities. Retinal lesions that hyperfluoresce early in an angiogram include micro- and macro-aneurysms, neovascularization, arteriovenous abnormalities, and tumor vessels, among others. Choroidal lesions that hyperfluoresce early include choroidal neovascularization (CNV) and tumor vessels. Late in an angiogram, a number of different patterns may emerge:

Pooling is the accumulation of fluorescein in defined anatomic spaces characterized by defined margins that do not enlarge, such as underneath a pigment epithelial detachment (Fig. 3.5).

Staining is the accumulation of dye in tissue, such as the disk, sclera, and subretinal fibrosis, characterized by an increase in hyperfluorescence intensity without the expansion of borders (Fig. 3.6).

Leakage is the accumulation of dye from vascular abnormalities, characterized by an increase in hyperfluorescence intensity with the expansion of borders, such as that seen in CNV and macular edema (Fig. 3.7).

3.6 Fluorescein Angiography Today

The role of fluorescein angiography continues to evolve. Noninvasive imaging modalities such as optical coherence tomography (OCT) and FAF are playing an increasing role in the modern practice of retina. This is particularly noticeable in the management of macular degeneration. In the era of photodynamic therapy (PDT), fluorescein angiography was required for retreatment decisions [8]. However, as first-line therapy for macular degeneration has shifted toward anti-angiogenic drugs, retreatment decisions in a number of clinical protocols are guided primarily by the presence or absence of fluid as determined by OCT [9].

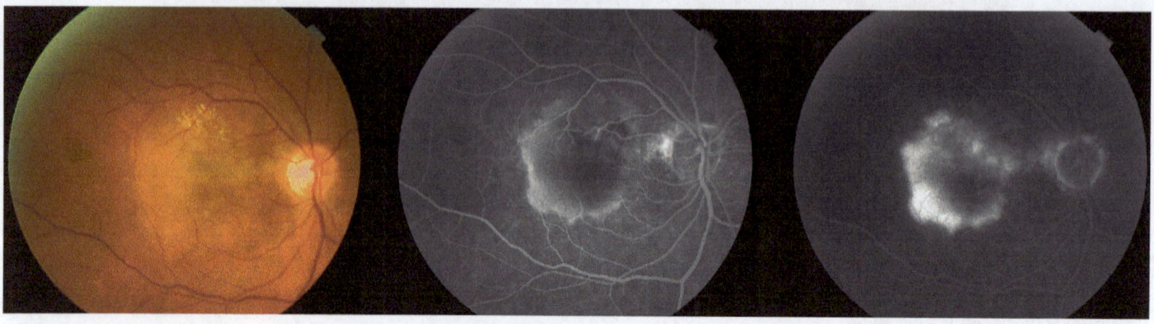

Fig. 3.5 Hyperfluorescence: pooling. Pigment epithelial detachment (*left*) in a patient with age-related macular degeneration. Fluorescein angiogram demonstrates the accumulation of dye in this anatomic space (*middle*), which becomes more intense in the late stage (*right*) without expanding borders. Note that there is a small area of leakage due to the underlying choroidal neovascularization at the superonasal aspect of the lesion

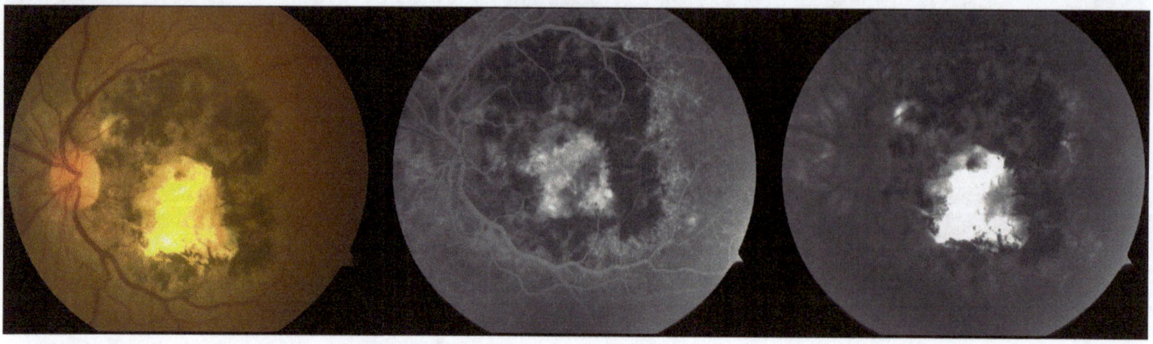

Fig. 3.6 Hyperfluorescence: staining. Patient with extensive disciform scarring (*left*) and hyperpigmentation. The disciform scar hyperfluoresces (*middle*) and late in the study stains (*right*) with an increase in intensity but no leakage beyond its borders

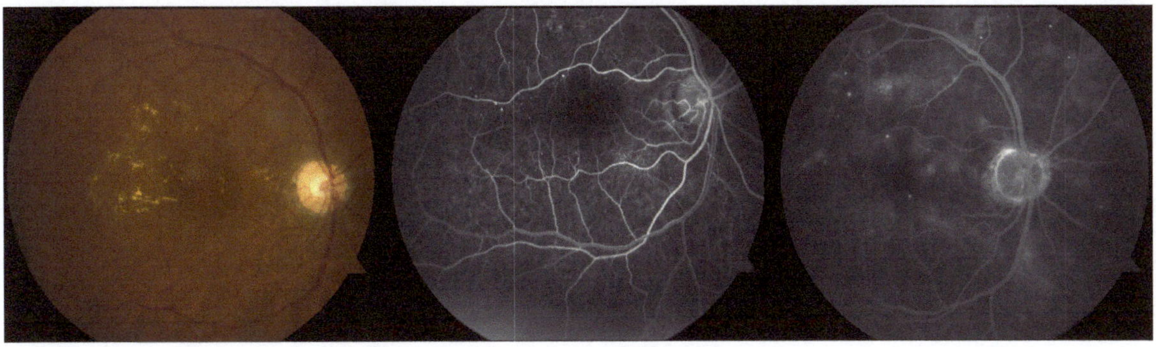

Fig. 3.7 Hyperfluorescence: leakage. Diabetic patients with clinically significant macular edema (*left*) evidenced by hard exudate and microaneurysms in the perifoveal area. During the early arteriovenous phase (*middle*), the microaneurysms hyperfluoresce. In the late phase of the study (*right*), fluorescein leakage is noted surrounding the microaneurysms

The digital photography revolution has quickly been adopted in angiography despite the initial resistance owing to the superior resolution and stereopsis afforded by traditional film systems [10]. Digital imaging systems possess a number of advantages over film-based systems. Photographers are provided instant feedback and can adjust photographic parameters to maximize image quality. Processing time is greatly reduced without the need for physicians to wait for film development. Image storage and transmission is simplified. Image processing software is readily applied to digital images, such as in the precise measurement of lesion dimension and area, automated montage formation, and a number of other applications.

There remains no doubt that fluorescein angiography will remain an indispensable tool for retina specialists in the diagnosis and management of a multitude of retinal disorders. Other imaging modalities provide complementary information for many conditions. Fluorescein angiography remains a mainstay of imaging for macular degeneration, retinovascular disease, inflammatory conditions, tumors, maculopathies, and peripheral retinopathies.

References

1. Berlman IB (1971) Handbook of fluorescence spectra of aromatic molecules, 2nd edn. Academic Press, New York
2. Novtny HR, Alvis DL (1961) A method of photographing fluorescence in circulating blood in the human retina. Circulation 24:28–86
3. Kwiterovich KA, Maguire MG, Murphy RP et al (1991) Frequency of adverse systemic reactions after fluorescein angiography: results of a prospective study. Ophthalmology 98:1139–1142
4. Kwan AS, Barry C, McAllister IL, Constable I (2006) Fluorescein angiography and adverse drug reactions revisited: the lions eye experience. Clin Experiment Ophthalmol 34(1):33–38
5. Olk RJ, Halperin LS, Soubrane G, Coscas G (1991) Fluorescein angiography – is it safe to use in a pregnant patient? Eur J Ophthalmol 1(2):103–106
6. Staurenghi G, Viola F, Mainster MA, Graham RD, Harrington PG (2005) Scanning laser ophthalmoscopy and angiography with a wide-field contact lens system. Arch Ophthalmol 123(2):244–252
7. Delaey C, Van De Voorde J (2000) Regulatory mechanisms in the retinal and choroidal circulation. Ophthalmic Res 32(6):249–256
8. Fine HF (2007) Photodynamic therapy in the anti-VEGF era. Br J Ophthalmol 91(6):707–718
9. Fung AE, Lalwani GA, Rosenfeld PJ, Dubovy SR, Michels S, Feuer WJ, Puliafito CA, Davis JL, Flynn HW Jr, Esquiabro M (2007) An optical coherence tomography-guided, variable dosing regimen with intravitreal ranibizumab (Lucentis) for neovascular age-related macular degeneration. Am J Ophthalmol 143(4):566–583
10. Yannuzzi LA, Ober MD, Slakter JS, Spaide RF, Fisher YL, Flower RW, Rosen R (2004) Ophthalmic fundus imaging: today and beyond. Am J Ophthalmol 137(3):511–524

Chapter 4

Wide-Field Imaging and Angiography

4

Thomas Friberg and Leanne Labriola

Core Messages

- Fundus imaging has become an integral part of the retinal examination.
- Several techniques of fundus imaging are available for clinicians and researchers.
- The scanning laser ophthalmoscope is an innovative system that is greatly improving fundus imaging because of the advantages it offers over traditional fundus photography.
- A specialized scanning laser ophthalmoscope is able to produce a picture of essentially the entire retina in a single image through a nonmydriatic pupil.
- Wide-field imaging and angiography can be used to diagnose disease, to aid in management decisions, and to follow the effectiveness of treatment for many retinal diseases.
- Wide-field angiography delineates a larger area of the retinal circulation than traditional fluorescein angiography.
- Expert analysis of wide-field images provides a reliable assessment of the patient's fundus and provides sufficient detail to enable the ophthalmologist to detect subtle pathological changes such as retinal tears, holes, and hemorrhages.
- Currently, the scanning-laser ophthalmoscope has been accepted as a supplement to a clinical retina examination but not as a replacement for it.
- Wide-field images are currently being validated as a screening tool for certain retinal pathologies such as diabetic retinopathy and retinal detachments.
- Wide-field imaging has special advantages in following the progression of certain choroidal diseases, specifically, large or peripheral nevi, tumors, and metastases.
- New techniques are being developed and pioneered that combine wide-field imaging with a scanning laser ophthalmoscope with different technologies, such as optical coherence tomography and indocyanine-green angiography that catapult this technology to an even higher level in delineating retinal pathology.

4.1 Introduction

Fundus imaging has become an integral part of ophthalmology practice. The improvements in our ability to view and document the posterior pole of the eye has increased our knowledge of ocular anatomy, sharpened our detection of pathological processes, developed our understanding of disease progression, enhanced our analysis of treatment efficacy, and broadened our research initiatives.

Today, a myriad of techniques for fundus imaging exist. Fundus photographs are still used, but the images are captured in digital quality. The first clinical use of digital images was reported by Friberg et al. in 1987. This paper outlined the advantages of digital images in clinical ophthalmology and demonstrated their impact in this field [1]. A second technique, intravenous dyes, can be used with optical filters to highlight the retinal or choroid circulation and to delineate pathological changes in these tissues. Another modality, echography, can be used to detect posterior pole lesions or retinal detachments using sound waves at specific frequencies. In addition, optical coherence tomography uses principles of interferometry to create cross-sectional analysis of the retina. Finally, scanning lasers use a raster pattern to reproduce fundus anatomy. The diversity of these techniques provides the ophthalmologist with a large inventory of tools that can be used individually or in combination to enhance the evaluation, diagnosis, and treatment of posterior pole pathology.

Summary for the Clinician

- Images of the posterior pole have greatly contributed to the field of medical retina.
- The ability to accurately document retinal anatomy with a standardized image has aided in the diagnosis, treatment, and management of ocular diseases.
- Today, several imaging options exist to aid the clinician.

4.2 History of Fundus Imaging

The first fundus photographs were obtained with standard film images captured in stereo-paired images. A standard picture displayed 20° of the posterior pole (Fig. 4.1). Contemporary digital fundus cameras can extend the angle of the posterior pole captured in a single photograph to 30 or 60° [1, 2]. Even with these cameras, documentation of the peripheral fundus was only possible with careful camera positioning and patient cooperation to print out several different angles of the posterior pole that would later be compiled into a montage of overlapping images. The investigators for the Early Treatment of Diabetic Retinopathy Study (EDTRS) popularized a protocol that was developed for imaging the peripheral retina in their study. This protocol consisted of seven standard photos that were placed in an overlapping collage, which collectively visualized 75° of the posterior pole [3]. However, this process is time-consuming and has limitations. The addition of a contact lens extended the angle of retina captured in a single photograph to 160° [2, 4]. Pediatric ophthalmologists can photograph 120° of the retina with a contact camera called the RetCam120, but the use of this camera requires either excellent patient cooperation with topical anesthetic or sedation to maintain adequate contact with the eye during image acquisition [5]. Today, a scanning laser ophthalmoscope (SLO) can capture 200° of the posterior pole, which is almost the entire posterior pole, in a single photograph [2, 3]. The prototype of this device is known as the Optos Panoramic 200 [Optos PLC, Dunfermline, Scotland, United Kingdom) [6, 7] and is currently at the forefront of ophthalmologic innovations.

Summary for the Clinician

- Advancements in technology have led to advancements in modalities for fundus imaging.
- Specialized scanning laser ophthalmoscopes surpass other posterior pole imaging system in their ability to capture a wide-field image of the posterior pole in a single image.

4.3 Wide-Field Images with a Scanning Laser Ophthalmoscope

The confocal scanning laser was first introduced to ophthalmology by Robert Webb in 1979 (Azad 2006), and Douglas Anderson used this imaging technique to create the wide-field Optos® system in 1999 after his son lost vision from a delay in the detection of a retinal detachment [7]. The Optos® is a scanning laser ophthalmoscope that uses a confocal laser system to obtain images of the fundus (Fig. 4.2). Confocal laser systems project light through a small aperture, or pinhole. This pinhole can filter a specific wavelength of light relative to the distance at which the pinhole is placed. Light traveling toward the

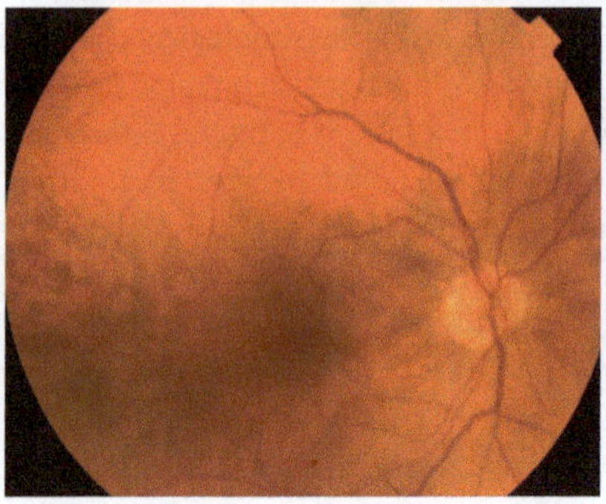

Fig. 4.1 Standard digital fundus photograph of the right eye showing the posterior pole

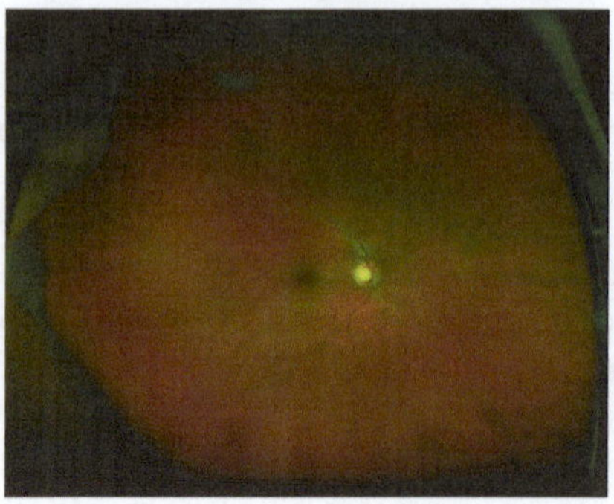

Fig. 4.2 Wide-field image of the posterior pole of a right eye produced by a specialized scanning laser ophthalmoscope

pinhole at different wavelengths from the one selected will be out of focus and will be filtered from the final image, because it cannot pass through the pinhole. Therefore, the light that does pass through the pinhole will be optically conjugate. These principles can be used to produce images that have depth-selectivity by altering the position of the pinhole. The image created by the Optos Panoramic 200® is referred to as the optomap® and is created by using a red laser with a wavelength of 633 nm with a green laser with a wavelength of 532 nm [7, 8]. The image requires an aperture of 2 mm to obtain the photograph [8]. The images are scanned in a raster pattern, from left to right and then top to bottom, and are obtained one pixel at a time. However, image acquisition is fast and each optomap® takes just 0.25 s to be completed [6]. Each collection of scans is called an optical section. The Optos® is unique within its class of scanning lasers, because it uses an elliptical mirror and two different focal points to obtain a large depth of focus [3, 9]. The main focal point is just posterior to the pupil, which is one of the key elements that enables the entire retina to be in focus, despite the differences in distance between each retina point and the mirror [6].

4.3.1 Fluorescein Angiography with a Scanning Laser Ophthalmoscope

Fluorescein angiography (FA) is a vital imaging tool for retinal specialist. The ability to delineate vascular pathology has drastically affected the practice of ophthalmology. Fluorescein angiography was first described by Novotny and Alvis in 1961 (Azad 2006). Fluorescein angiography has revealed the importance of maintaining adequate blood flow in the eye and the devastations of ischemic-induced conditions. Many retinal diseases cause alterations in blood flow within the retinal and choroid circulations. The ability to see and depict these pathological changes is the first step in recognizing the disease, which is important for accurate diagnosis and appropriate management decisions.

In addition to the replication of fundus photography, the scanning laser ophthalmoscope can be used to create angiographic images as depicted in Fig. 4.3 [10]. One of the lasers on the scanning laser ophthalmoscope can be replaced with a blue laser with a wavelength of 488 nm to capture the filtered light after fluorescein injection with circulation. A 500 nm barrier filter is placed in front of the machine [2]. The power of the laser is maintained at the same level. A fast recycling electronic flash is used [2, 6]. This technique has been labeled as the optomap®fa, when the Optos® system is used, and it is able to outline

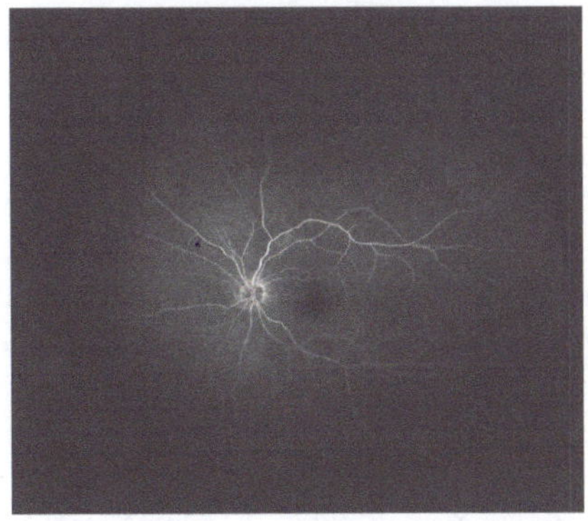

Fig. 4.3 Wide-field fluorescein angiography image produced by an optos scanning laser ophthalmoscope of the left eye

the retinal vasculature in much the same way as a standard fluorescein image on a digital photograph.

4.3.2 Advantages of Imaging with a Scanning Laser Ophthalmoscope

The novel scanning laser ophthalmoscope offers many advantages. The increased depth of focus allows the entire retina to be in focus in a single image in spite of the anatomical curved nature of the retina overcoming the limitations of standard photography, which is subject to peripheral blur from reflections and corneal astigmatic distortions [3]. Furthermore, unlike most posterior pole images, the entire 200° of posterior pole can be captured through a nonmydriatic pupil [6]. This reduces the number of photographs that need to be taken. It reduces both patient exposure to light and patient wait time, and increases patient tolerance. It also has enhanced features to increase the ease of picture acquisition for the photographer such as iris registration. Since the optomap® provides a digital image, it has many advantages over plain film. Digital images are easily captured and provide the photographer the ability to immediately view, edit, or recapture an image if there is poor quality. The images can be downloaded quickly, stored electronically, and reproduced on demand without degrading the image quality. These images can be transferred or shared with other professionals quickly through CDs or over the Internet, which allows for easy consultation or transfer of care.

In addition to these advantages, the Optos SLO is unique in its ability to capture the peripheral retina in less time and with less peripheral distortion when compared with the seven field montage images. The wide-field final image increases the amount of peripheral retina apparent in a single photograph by threefold when compared with standard contemporary photography.

Standard photographic images capture 3.3 disc diameters of the posterior pole in a single photograph, whereas the optomap® can display up to nine disc diameters [6]. Moreover, new features are being added to recent models of the Optos® to enable the technician to steer the machine during image acquisition to alter the patient's focus point and capture 100% of the peripheral retina [7]. Furthermore, the Optos® is advantageous when compared with prior fundus imaging techniques, because it is able to capture this wide view through a nonmydriatic pupil. In addition to obtaining a good image through a small pupil, the Optos® can overcome the challenges created by media opacities. The lasers are able to penetrate through haze created by the presence of cataracts, vitreous hemorrhage, or inflammation.

The wide-field FA also offers several unique advantages when compared with standard FA images with digital fundus photography and montage picture arrangement. Since this specialized SLO can capture almost the entire posterior pole in a single picture, it is able to show the effects of the fluorescein over the entire posterior pole within the same time frame. This not only allows peripheral pathology to be better seen and, therefore, studied with each image, but also allows simultaneous comparison of the macula with the peripheral retina during each angiographic phase. Furthermore, several studies are investigating the role of oral fluorescein with the scanning laser ophthalmoscope [11–14]. Since an SLO less light to capture a higher contrast image, the amount of intravascular dye from the oral administration of fluorescein is strong enough to delineate the intricate retinal circulation. Patients are given two ampules of 25% fluorescein (Fluorescite; Alcon Pharmaceuticals, Ft. Worth, Tx). The solution contains 1.0 g of sodium fluorescein mixed in 30 mL of pure orange juice for oral administration [13]. The ability to use an oral formulation of fluorescein over the traditional intravenous injection would offer many benefits, including decreased side effects of the fluorescein, elimination of transfusion problems, reduced technical assistance for administration of the dye, and increased patient comfort.

4.3.3 Disadvantages of Imaging with a Scanning Laser Ophthalmoscope

Despite numerous advantages, the system has its shortcomings. The machines have to be purchased individually and the cost of the scanning laser ophthalmoscope is higher when compared with digital cameras. The scanning laser ophthalmoscope uses red and green lasers to capture the images, which means that the colored fundus photographs produced by the scanning laser ophthalmoscope are actually reproductions created by the two lasers [3]. This can distort the true anatomical representation of the fundus. In addition, the use of the lasers can produce unusual color blotches where there is a mismatch between the red and green light used to produce the fundus image. Moreover, the Optos® creates such a wide-field image that the patient's eyelashes can actually interfere with the final image (Fig. 4.4). This has been termed "lash effect" and the interference of the lashes can block areas of peripheral retina and limit disease detection in those areas [3]. Efforts have been made to reduce this effect by using lid speculums; however, this decreases the efficiency of the examination as well as patient comfort during the examination.

Perhaps, the most significant limitation to the scanning laser ophthalmoscope image is its relative resolution. The raster pattern used by the scanning laser ophthalmoscope limits the temporal and spatial resolution of the images when compared with fundus camera pictures [15]. To capture a wide field of view, the resolution of the image is a trade-off. The Optos® system can produce images that are up to 3,000 × 3,000 pixels [3]; however, the final resolution is based on the overall resolution of the monitor on which the final image is displayed. For the wide image to be viewed on a standard monitor, the image is usually squeezed into the same number of pixels designed for the standard image; therefore, the resolution of the optomap® is decreased to one-seventh of that of the standard photo. However, efforts are underway to increase the resolution of the Optos® images. A new feature developed for Optos®, called, ResMax®, allows the technician to enhance the resolution of the image, even in the middle of image acquisition by scanning a smaller region of interest. The resolution of optomap® is 20 μm, but with ResMax® the resolution is 11 μm [7]. To counterbalance the decreased resolution, the Optos® relies on its high contrast. Even the prototype models of the Optos®

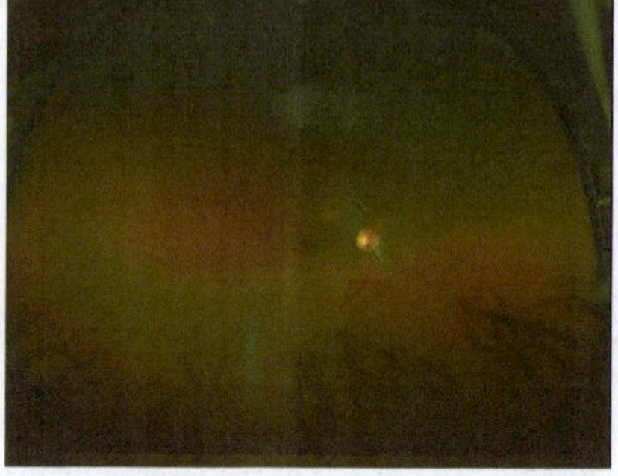

Fig. 4.4 Optos® fundus image. Note that the peripheral retina is blocked by the patient's eyelashes inferiorly. This is known as lash effect

offer a higher degree of contrast than digital images, which can aid in an accurate interpretation of the final image [6].

Summary for the Clinician

- The scanning laser ophthalmoscope image is created by using a red laser with a wavelength of 633 nm and with a green laser with a wavelength of 532 nm.
- The images are scanned in a raster pattern that takes 0.25 s to be completed.
- The wide-field image increases the amount of peripheral retina in a single photograph by threefold when compared with standard contemporary photography.
- The scanning laser ophthalmoscope can be altered to produce angiographic images with the use of fluorescein dye.
- Wide-field angiography allows simultaneous comparison of the macula with the peripheral retina during each angiographic phase.
- Scanning laser ophthalmoscope imaging can produce good-quality late phase angiographic images with the use of oral fluorescein instead of intravenous fluorescein.
- The main advantage of the scanning laser ophthalmoscope is its ability to capture almost the entire retina in a single image.
- The main disadvantage of the scanning laser ophthalmoscope is the decrease in resolution sacrificed for the increase in image field.

4.4 Clinical Use of Wide-Field Imaging

Overall, the advantages of the wide-field imaging have outweighed its recognized limitations. This device has already been implemented in many ophthalmology clinics and has already greatly impacted the way clinicians are able to diagnose, follow, and manage posterior pole diseases [16]. The Optos® system was approved by the Federal Drug Administration in February 1999 and became commercially available in January 2000 [17]. It has been estimated that there are currently 2,500 Optos® systems currently used in clinics throughout the United States [8]. The next section will highlight common diseases in which the Optos® contributed to overall patient management, and includes case reports as well as comparative studies between Optos® images and expert examination.

4.4.1 Wide-Field Imaging in Uveitis

The clinical examination of a patient with uveitis is particularly challenging since the disease process can create several obstacles that interfere with the proper visualization of the ocular anatomy. The anterior chamber or vitreous inflammation can prevent adequate slit lamp biomicroscopy of the fundus. Old inflammation can create posterior synechiae resulting in small pupil diameter and poor mydriasis even with topical cycloplegics. The patient's subjective photosensitivity makes the examination more challenging. In addition, tedious flash fundus photography can be particularly painful for the patient. The features of the scanning laser ophthalmoscope offer unique solution to overcome these obstacles. The Optos® is able to obtain wide-angled views in spite of small pupils. The laser is able to penetrate the haze from the aqueous or vitreous inflammation. The quick acquisition time, lower-level light, and single wide-field image make the Optos® ideal in the setting of uveitic patients.

Figure 4.5 illustrates a case of how scanning laser opthalmoscope image acquisition is beneficial in patients with active uveitis, in which posterior pathology needs to be visualized or documented. The photographs were taken of a new patient who previously lived in Vietnam and reported a long history of red, painful eyes with decreased vision. Clinical examination of the patient on that day was limited by the aqueous and vitreous cell from the active inflammation. The slit lamp pictures (Fig. 4.5a) illustrate the secluded pupils that developed from multiple bouts of iridocyclitis that resulted in the formation of posterior synechiae. The fundus photograph (Fig. 4.5b) shows the image obtained on this patient through the small pupil on the same day when the slit lamp pictures were taken. Figure 4.5c shows the extraordinary detail of the wide-field FA through the small pupil and anterior and posterior inflammation. In this case, the wide-field image and wide-field FA supplement the information gained through clinical examination. The pictures capture more of the posterior pole than is possible through the small pupil. In addition, these pictures assist in the management of the patient by documenting the key features of the fundus in order to be shared for consultation on the case. Because of the availability of the Optos® image, the consultant physician will not have to rely on verbal descriptions or drawings. The entire fundus is captured in the single wide-field image, which allows the consultant to have more information available to him or her to form a diagnosis or a treatment plan. This is extremely helpful in instances when direct patient examination is not possible by the consultant.

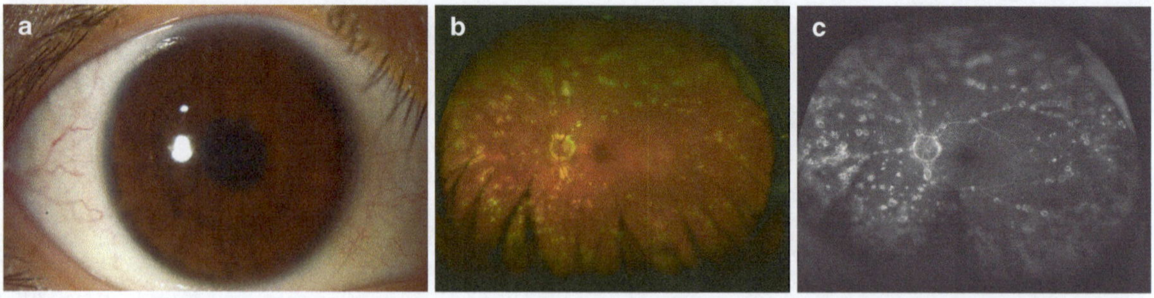

Fig. 4.5 (**a**) Slit lamp picture of a patient with seclusio pupillae from recurrent episodes of uveitis and the development of posterior synechiae. Careful inspection of the photograph reveals fibrin material in the anterior chamber in front of the lens, which makes the view to the posterior pole challenging with slit lamp biomicroscopy. (**b**) Optos® color image of the same patient depicting multiple chorioretinal punched out lesions in a perivascular distribution. (**c**) Wide-field angiography of the same patient. No evidence of active vasculitis

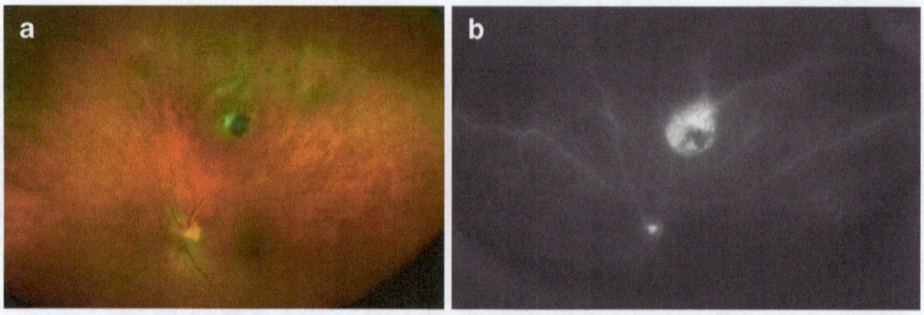

Fig. 4.6 (**a**) Optos® color fundus image of a left eye in a patient with a chorioretinal scar from infection with *toxoplasmosis gondii*. Retinal infiltrate is noted at the supranasal edge of the scar signifying reactivation of the infection. Adjacent shunt vessel is apparent as well as intraretinal hemorrhages, retinal edema, and acute optic disc edema. (**b**) Picture of a wide-field fluorescein angiography of the same patient in late frames that depicts minimal leakage of the lesion and extensive vasculitis

The next case is a patient who presented with an active chorioretinal lesion and disc edema from toxoplasmosis (Fig. 4.6a). Typically, these lesions are diagnosed based on clinical examination. The decision to treat is based on the clinical presentation. This patient had what appeared to be a small reactivation of an old chorioretinal scar from infection with *toxoplasmosis gondii*. Some ophthalmologists would favor the observation of such a lesion given its distal location when compared with the optic nerve. However, further workup, including a wide-field FA, revealed unexpected findings. Figure 4.6b shows extensive vasculitis seen around the lesion. After weighing the amount of inflammation on presentation, the decision was made to initiate medical treatment with the combination sulfamethozazole and trimethoprim. The patient's symptoms and visual acuity improved. The vasculitis and extent of inflammation associated with this toxoplasmosis lesion might have gone undetected without the wide-field FA image. This case illustrates the utility of the scanning laser ophthalmoscope system in diagnosis as well as management of patients.

A recent study from the Jules Stein Eye Institute supports the advantages of the wide-field imaging over standard digital photography because of its ability to outline the extent of peripheral pathology in addition to the ability to follow the effectiveness of treatment options [3]. The next case is of a patient diagnosed with intermediate uveitis. In intermediate uveitis or pars planitis, the peripheral examination is particularly important. Figure 4.7a–d illustrates the fundus of a patient with small vessel vasculitis seen on wide-field imaging and fluorescein angiography in both eyes. These lesions could have been missed on a traditional angiography, which currently photographs only 30–60° of the posterior pole [18, 19]; however, the optomap®fa was able to capture the entire area of vasculitis in great detail. Clinicians are realizing the utility of wide-field angiography for the detection of peripheral pathological changes such as in this example. Tsui et al. published a case report on six patients with active intermediate uveitis secondary to sarcoid each of who displayed peripheral periphlebitis that varied in

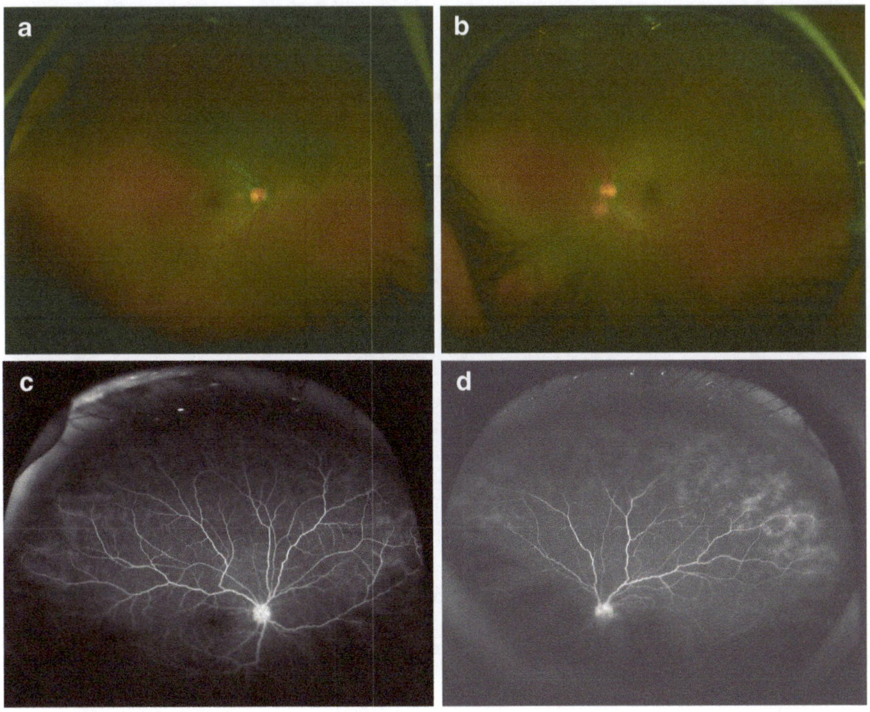

Fig. 4.7 (**a**) Color Optos® image of a right eye. Superiorly, there are small white subretinal infiltrates noted. (**b**) Color Optos® image with similar findings in the left eye. (**c**) Wide-field fluorescein angiography of the same patient, which shows peripheral vasculitis that is limited to the small vessels. (**d**) Wide-field fluorescein angiography of the left eye with similar findings when compared with the right eye

distribution and vessels affected in each case that was documented on wide-field angiography. Now, with the combination of the scanning laser ophthalmoscope with fluorescein angiography, our ability to study the peripheral vasculature has been improved. In the future, wide-field angiography can be used not only to help identify these lesions but also to classify different types of intermediate uveitis cases and to improve our understanding of the disease pathogenesis.

4.4.2 Wide-Field Imaging in Proliferative Retinopathies

Diabetic retinopathy is a well-known disease that causes proliferative changes that can damage the ocular structures. Diabetic Retinopathy is a leading cause of blindness in developed countries [6] and accountable for significant vision loss among working-age adults within the United States of America. The 2008 report from the Center for Disease Control states that there are an estimated 4.4 million individuals who suffer from diabetic retinopathy [20]. It is estimated that 50% of patients with Type 1 Diabetes Mellitus and 30% of patients with Type 2 Diabetes Mellitus will develop sight-threatening retinopathy in their lifetime [21]. Early detection of diabetic changes within the eye can lead to prompt treatment by an ophthalmologist and improved visual outcomes for the patient. The EDTRS study showed that early treatment could reduce an individual's risk of severe vision loss by 57% [22]. Current screening of diabetic retinopathy is inadequate since only 40–60% of people with diabetes receive annual examinations by a trained ophthalmologist [8]. Since changes from diabetic retinopathy affect the peripheral retina as well as the central retina, it is important to have high resolutions of both these areas to assess the disease state. Currently, the gold standard reference for the detection of diabetic retinopathy has been established by the EDTRS with stereo-photographs of seven standard fields taken for each patient through a dilated pupil [22–24]. Although this technique has been proven accurate and reproducible, it still remains labor-intensive for the patient and photographer [6]. Studies have focused on investigating alternative methods of screening for diabetic sensitivity. One group of researchers

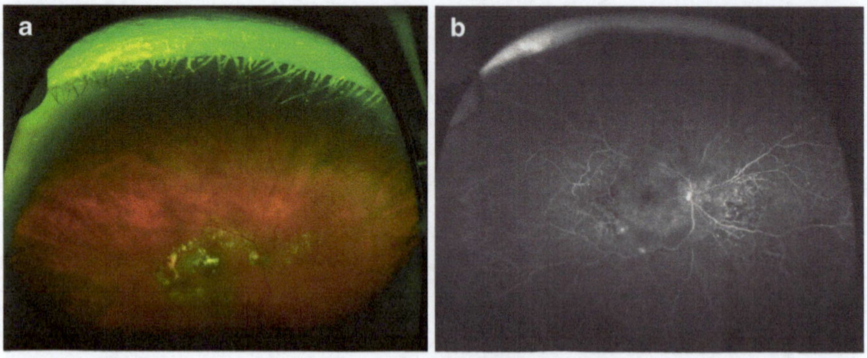

Fig. 4.8 (**a**) Optos® color image of a patient with intraretinal hemorrhages and venous dilation from diabetic retinopathy in addition to macular edema, microaneurysms, and exudates from diabetic macular edema. (**b**) Picture of a wide-field fluorescein angiography of the same patient, which shows apparent leakage from the microaneurysms in the macula and diffuse leakage that is developing into a petalloid pattern classic for cystic macular edema. Patches of hypofluoresence correspond with hemorrhages. Note the areas of capillary nonperfusion in the macula and peripheral retina as well as the neovascularization seen along the inferior arcade

showed that a two-field retinal image with a Topcon CRW6 nonmydriatic camera was equal to the seven-field images from the EDTRS report [25, 26]. However, the Topcon image does not have the ability to capture the entire retina. Other studies have shown that there is Level 1 evidence to support single image standard photography of the fundus for diabetic screening; however, a single photograph of the fundus that extends over a limited number of degrees cannot replace the clinical examination [24]. Theoretically, the Optos® should be ideal for diabetic screening since it is able to provide a single photograph of the entire retina through an undilated pupil. Friberg et al. performed a study to compare expert analysis of standard digital fundus photography with an Optos® generated retinal image to detect diabetic retinopathy [6]. The study showed that, as expected, the Optos® was able to identify more areas of retinal pathology, including neovascularization and retinal ischemia. However, the standard photographic method showed higher-quality images. Figure 4.8a shows a wide-field color fundus image and Fig. 4.8b shows a wide-field fluorescein angiography of a patient with diabetic maculopathy as well as diabetic retinopathy in the right eye.

Another study compared the analysis of an optomap® image with a clinical dilated examination for the detection of diabetic retinopathy by a retinal specialist. Fifty-one eyes were enrolled in the study and the results showed that the analysis of an optomap® is an accurate way of detecting diabetic retinopathy. The results for the detection of diabetic retinopathy reported above a stage of mild retinopathy had a sensitivity of 94% and a specificity of 100% [8]. The detection of clinically significant diabetic macular edema was also evaluated in this study and the optomap® analysis resulted in high sensitivity and specificity [8].

The advancements in the detection of diabetic retinopathy, especially in the peripheral retina, have suggested that wide-field imaging and angiography can not only help in the detection of diabetic lesions but also direct the treatment and management of such lesions [27]. This idea has led some researchers to develop new algorithms to locate the vascular leakage and ischemia to assist clinicians [28]. Such strategies are currently being reported in the literature. Reddy et al. define a new protocol for panretinal photocoagulation, which modifies the technique to only treat areas that show retinal nonperfusion on wide-field fluorescein imaging. This technique would result in less retinal area being treated; therefore, reducing the side effect from the laser at the same time as theoretically still achieving an adequate treatment effect [18]. The protocols in these reports still need to be validated, but each report offers a fresh look at treatment paradigms for diabetic retinopathy.

Other proliferative retinopathies include vein occlusions. Figure 4.9a shows an example of an Optos® image of a central retinal vein occlusion. Figure 4.9b shows the optomap®fa image of the same patient. This wide-field image can document the extent of pathological changes from the vein occlusion and can be used to monitor change in the amount of both hemorrhages and ischemic areas over time. Neovascularization can easily be identified on the optomap®; even if located in the far peripheral retina.

Figure 4.10a illustrates an example of an Optos® colored image of a branch retinal vein occlusion in the supratemporal arcade of the left eye. Although the

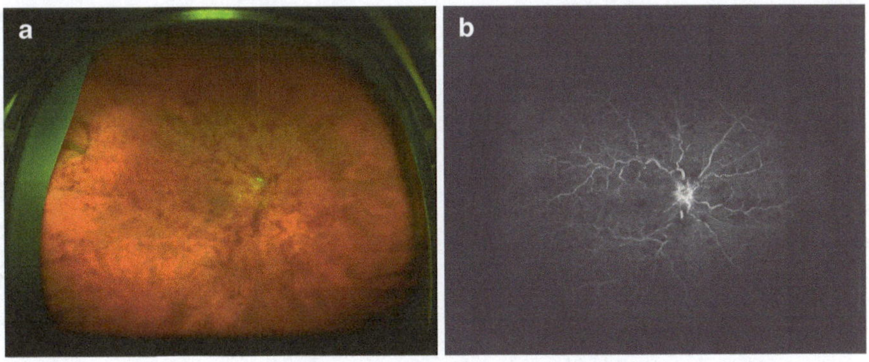

Fig. 4.9 (**a**) Color Optos® fundus image with hemorrhage in all four quadrants of the retina, venous dilation, and tortuosity as well as optic disc edema corresponding to a central retinal vein occlusion of the right eye. (The central bright circular reflection is artifact from the machine). (**b**) Wide-field fluorescein angiography of the same patient. The venous changes are more apparent. The areas of blockage correspond to retinal hemorrhages. The entire retina can be visualized for areas of nonperfusion or neovascularization

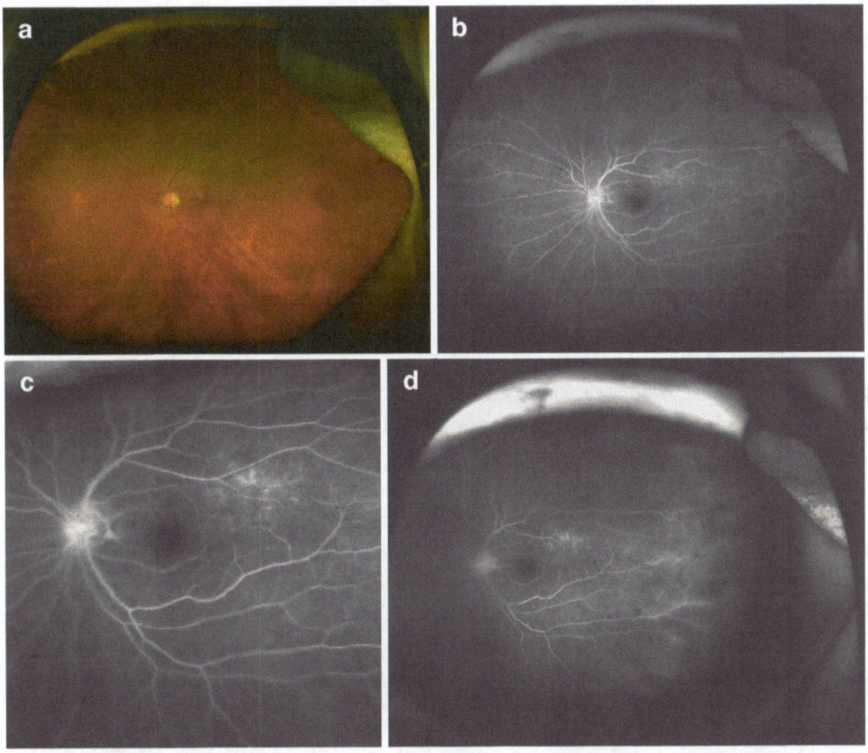

Fig. 4.10 (**a**) Color Optos® image of the left eye with attenuation of the retinal arterioles in the supratemporal quadrant, scattered retinal hemorrhages along the supratemporal arcade. There is an area of retinal hemorrhages in the superior macula.(**b**) Wide-field angiography of the same patient with areas of blockage from the retinal hemorrhages, leakage from the vessels in the superior macula, and early vasculitic changes in the peripheral vessels.(**c**) A magnified picture of (**b**) showing the capillary leakage creating macular edema. Note the resolution quality of the picture produced by the Optos® in spite of the magnification of the image. (**d**) Late frame of the angiography, which portrays extensive vasculitis and late fluorescein leakage in the macula

findings on the colored Optos® image are subtle, the patient's diagnosis was easily made clinically. Figure 4.10b is an example of a fluorescein angiography of the same patient. Figure 4.10c shows a close-up view; note how the resolution of the image is still acceptable even when the image is magnified. Figure 4.10d shows the late frames on fluorescein angiography with the scanning laser ophthalmoscope. Notice the peripheral ischemic changes and underlying vasculitis. These changes would have been missed with conventional imaging techniques. The presence of vasculitis in this setting initiated a thorough systemic work-up of the patient and the underlying cause of the patient's vein occlusion was revealed as secondary to systemic lupus erythematosus. The patient was referred to rheumatology for further systemic evaluation.

In addition, studies are analyzing the use of wide-field angiography in the detection of retinopathy of prematurity. The advantages of using wide-field imaging to supplement the pediatric retinal examination have already been identified with the invention of the RetCam 120. However, new studies with the scanning laser ophthalmoscope are going one step further by investigating the role of wide-field fluorescein angiography in this population. Azad et al. has shown that fluorescein can be safely injected in children and can be helpful in delineating the peripheral neovascularization seen in retinopathy of prematurity [29].

In the adult population in the United States, the main cause of vision loss if due to the formation of neovascular choroidal membranes that proliferate through Bruch's membrane and form disciform scars in the center macula. This is the pathological process of wet age-related macular degeneration [30]. Vision threatening lesions from this disease are located within the macula and can be easily photographed with standard fundus photography; however, wide-field images of these patients can reveal peripheral changes as well. These changes include extramacular drusen (Fig. 4.11) or peripheral reticular changes. The significance of these peripheral retinal changes is unknown and their presence is usually either disregarded or considered benign; however, perhaps some research largely suggests a correlation between these peripheral retinal findings and the prognosis of the disease.

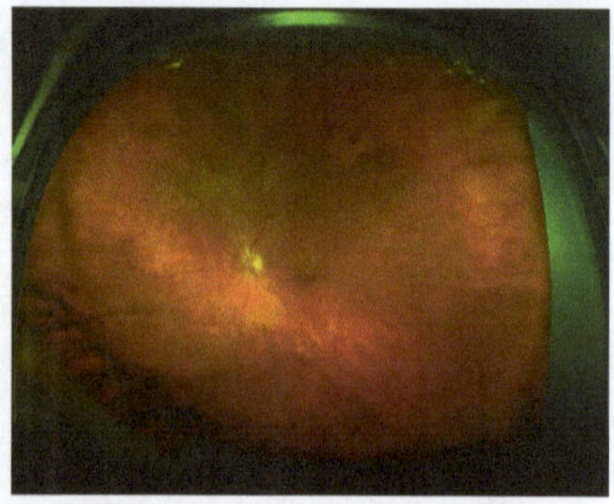

Fig. 4.11 Color Optos® retina image of the left eye with extramacular drusen

4.4.3 Wide-Field Imaging of Peripheral Retinal Lesions

The wide-field image has already provided advantages in supplementing a clinical fundus examination. The peripheral retina can be photographed more efficiently, and lesions can be defined more precisely, which has aided in diagnosis, management, and consultation with regard to the retinal diseases. This has been particularly beneficial regarding uncommon retinal pathology. Figure 4.12a, b shows an example of a chronic retinal detachment and subsequent macrocyst formation and peripheral neovascularization on wide-field imaging and angiography. The importance of these images in this setting has been published previously in a report by Labriola et al. [31], which illustrates how the wide-field image assisted in diagnosis, patient education, and the management of this patient. The detailed view of the peripheral retina was made possible by the unique features from the ultra-wide angle scanning laser ophthalmoscope.

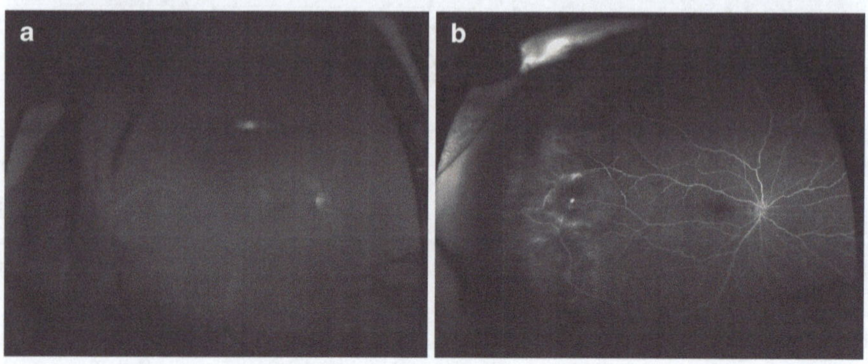

Fig. 4.12 (**a**) Color Optos® image of a chronic retinal detachment in the infratemporal quadrant with macrocyst formation and small adjacent retinal hemorrhages. (The central bright reflection above the optic nerve is artifact). (**b**) Wide-field fluorescein angiography of the same patient that shows discrete points of peripheral neovascularization adjacent to the retinal detachment and macrocyst

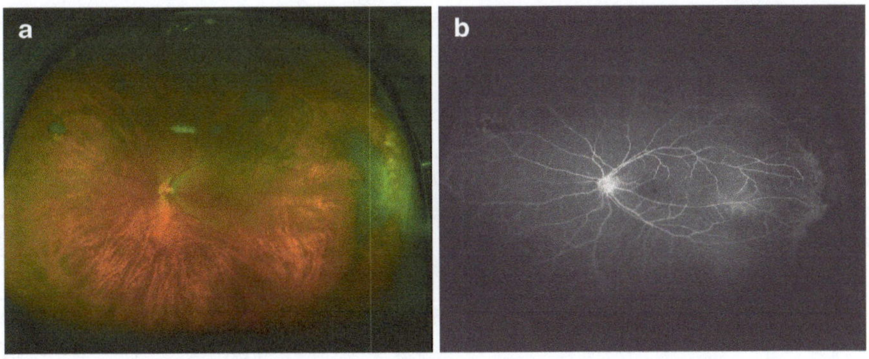

Fig. 4.13 (**a**) Color Optos® image of the left eye with operculated retinal tear in the supranasal quadrant. Note that the area of vascular abnormalities changes in the far temporal periphery. (The area of reflectance above the optic nerve is artifact). (**b**) Wide-field fluorescein angiography of the same patient. Note the temporal area of peripheral nonperfusion

Numerous case reports have been published illustrating how the wide-field imaging and angiography supplement the traditional clinical examination. However, some researchers suggest that the systems like the Optos® can serve not only as an additional step in the examination but instead as a replacement for it. Mackenzie et al. published a prospective study comparing an expert interpretation of an optomap® image with clinical examination [32]. Their research looked at the sensitivity and specificity of the optomap® in detecting peripheral lesions. Their design studies 93 eyes from 49 patients who consulted a retina specialist. Each patient received a dilated depressed examination by a retina specialist, after which a retinal image, obtained by a trained technician, was taken. The Optos® image was analyzed by one of the two masked retinal specialists and their results were recorded and compared with the results from the clinical examination. Of note is the fact that the Optos® image was obtained after pupillary dilation. Lesions anterior or posterior to the equator were classified separately. The results showed that for lesions that were determined to require treatment and were posterior to the equator, the Optos® had a sensitivity of 74% (95% CI 61–87%). For lesions that required treatment and were anterior to the equator, the sensitivity was 34% (95% CI 28–62%) [32]. This final result was lower than expected. One of the main reasons attributed to the lower sensitivity result was the lower resolution of the optomap® image, because it made it difficult to detect holes and tears, especially with anterior lesions where the resolution is most compromised. There were many limitations to this study. The study was performed at a retinal specialist office, which might create population bias since those patients might have had lesions that were more difficult to detect. In addition, the study only compared the interpretations of the optomap® between two specialists and their interpretations showed a high variability. It is very likely that interpretations of the optomap® among a larger groups of ophthalmologist would show different variability, especially if the interpretations were performed by nonretinal specialist [32]. To illustrate this case, Fig. 4.13a shows an optomap® image of a retinal hole that was an incidental finding during examination. Figure 4.13b shows an optomap®fa of the same patient. Interestingly, this patient has peripheral nonperfusion detected on the fluorescein angiographic image in the far periphery opposite from the retinal tear.

In addition to the peripheral retina tear detection, the scanning laser ophthalmoscope can play a role in following the progression of tears or detachments even after they are repaired. Anderson et al. published a case report, which showed that the ability of the Optos® to visualize the anterior retina makes it particularly valuable in documenting the extent of retinal detachments as well as in assisting with the postoperative examinations, which usually have to overcome the intravitreal gas bubble to view the retina to ensure that the surgery was successful [33].

4.4.4 Wide-Field Imaging of Choroidal Tumors

The ability to obtain an image of almost the entire retina in a single photograph is particularly beneficial when evaluating choroidal nevi, tumors, and metastases. Before wide-field images were possible, peripheral lesions would have to be carefully documented with fundus drawings or with detailed photographic montages. If the lesion is large, multiple images have to be taken to overcome the limitation of the small standard field image. Manipulation of the images when creating the montage could create distortions in alignment, magnification, or brightness between the pictures and the final result might be difficult to compare with future pictures. Furthermore, if the lesion is peripheral in location, it is even harder to document owing to the patient position required to capture that section of the posterior pole and the astigmatism that is usually induced from the cornea when the peripheral retina is photographed. Now, the wide-field image can replace the former methods and overcome the previous limitations to documenting choroidal lesions. When documenting lesions that change slowly over time or remain stable, such as a choroidal nevus, the single wide-field photograph of the posterior pole provides an invaluable asset. The small differences in size or shape that would be hard to discern from the comparison of hand drawings are more easily analyzed on the wide-field image. Additionally, the wide-field image offers a benefit in lesions that change quickly, such as cancerous lesions, since multiple follow-up examinations are needed. The quick single image decreases the time necessary to complete the workup for the patient as well as the physician. In theory, metastatic lesions can also be better followed with wide-field images since the entire retina is documented, the presence of new lesions or satellite lesions can more easily be identified, and not mistaken for previously seen lesions or missed entirely. Figure 4.14a shows a standard fundus photograph of the posterior pole. Figure 4.14b shows the nasal quadrant of this same patient, which captures a choroidal nevus that was missed on the standard photograph. Figure 4.14c shows the same patient with an Optos® wide-field image that captures the lesion and the posterior pole in its entirety. The advantage of the wide-field image in this previous case is evident from the pictures depicted in this figure. Recent reports have supported the Optos® as a superior method for documenting and following choroidal lesions for these reasons [34, 35].

Summary for the Clinician

- Wide-field imaging can help diagnosis, monitor, treat, and manage patients with a variety of retinal or choroidal pathologies including uveitis, proliferative retinopathies, and peripheral lesions or tumors.
- Wide-field imaging with the scanning laser ophthalmoscope is invaluable in patients with uveitis, because it can produce a high-quality image through small pupils, as well as aqueous and vitreous inflammation.
- The wide-field angiography can delineate peripheral retinal vasculature that is commonly affected in intermediate uveitis cases as well as posterior uveitis.
- The wide-field images can reveal pathology that may be missed with standard examination and imaging.
- Wide-field angiography is able to identify more areas of retinal pathology, including neovascularization and retinal ischemia in diabetic eye disease. Better quantification of retinal ischemia may lead to new algorithms of treatment.
- The wide-field image may be useful for screening retinal pathology, including diabetic changes as well as peripheral retinal tears.
- The wide-field angiography may soon become the standard for following peripheral or large posterior pole lesions, because it is able to document the entire borders of the lesions.

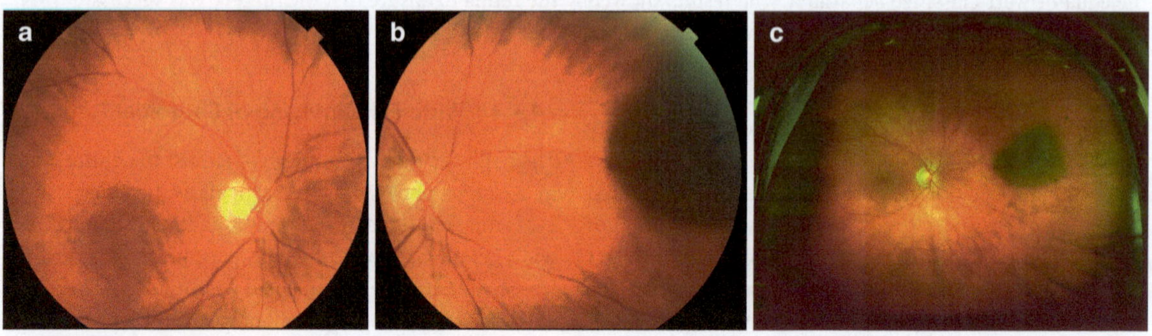

Fig. 4.14 (a) Standard fundus photograph of the posterior pole with digital camera. No pathology is seen in this image. (b) Standard fundus photograph of the posterior pole with digital camera of the same patient in (a) that shows a choroidal lesion in the nasal periphery. (c) Optos® color image of the same patient that shows the entire choroidal lesion as well as the posterior pole

4.5 Future Directions for Fundus Imaging

The principles of the scanning laser ophthalmoscope are being combined with other forms of ocular imaging. Current investigative efforts are looking at systems that combine a scanning laser ophthalmoscope with an optical coherence tomography retinal scan and with indocyanine green dye [36]. The images are taken by all three machines simultaneously to yield results that give precise anatomical location of posterior pole pathology and a detailed, accurate, and efficient way of documenting functional changes and real-time pathology in the eye.

In addition, future studies are analyzing the integration of a motion stabilizer that would identify specific areas on each image to better align the retinal anatomy and, therefore, increase image reproducibility. These stabilizers would adjust for motion artifact obtained during the raster image acquisition [37]. This technology will further advance the utility of the scanning laser ophthalmoscope in clinical practice.

Summary for the Clinician

- The unique design of the scanning laser ophthalmoscope enables it to be combined with other imaging modalities to provide even more information.

4.6 Conclusion

Overall, the scanning laser ophthalmoscope is an innovative invention that has found utility in many aspects of ophthalmology. Its unique features such as the ability to obtain wide-angle images of the fundus through a nonmydriatic pupil offer many advantages over other methods of fundus photography, and its design, resolution, and special features are still being developed and improved in newer models. Some ophthalmologists presently use the wide-field images to supplement their examination, or to assist with documentation or consultation. Research is underway to investigate if this image can replace a dilated examination to help with screening and to reach more patients in need of treatment who do not have a retinal specialist nearby. For now, the Optos® is not at the point where it can surpass the quality of an ophthalmologist's dilated examination; however, perhaps further improvements to the system will enable the optomap® to be used in many different ways at some point of time, such as in emergency departments for retinal screening of patients who present with floater and flashes of light and might be at the risk for retinal detachments, which was the idea behind the original creation of the Optos®.

References

1. Friberg TR, Rehkopf PG, Warnicki JW et al (1987) Use of directly acquired digital fundus and fluorescein angiographic images in the diagnosis of retinal disease. Retina 7:246–251
2. Manivannan A, Plskova J, Farrow A et al (2005) Ultra-wide-field fluorescein angiography of the ocular fundus. Am J Ophthalmol 140:525–527
3. Kaines A, Tsui I, Sarraf D et al (2009) The use of ultra wide field fluorescein angiography in evaluation and management of uveitis. Semin Ophthalmol 24:19–24
4. Spaide RF, Orlock DA, Herrmann-Delemazure B et al (1998) Wide-angle indocyanine green angiography. Retina 18:44–49
5. Lorenz B, Spasovska K, Elflein H et al (2009) Wide-field digital imaging based telemedicine for screening for acute retinopathy of prematurity (ROP). Six-year results of a multicentre field study. Graefes Arch Clin Exp Ophthalmol 247:1251–1262
6. Friberg TR, Gupta A, Yu J et al (2008) Ultrawide angle fluorescein angiographic imaging: a comparison to conventional digital acquisition systems. Ophthalmic Surg Lasers Imaging 39:304–311
7. Website Optos Company (2009) www.optos.com
8. Neubauer AS, Kernt M, Haritoglou C et al (2008) Nonmydriatic screening for diabetic retinopathy by ultra-widefield scanning laser ophthalmoscopy (Optomap). Graefes Arch Clin Exp Ophthalmol 246:229–235
9. Yang YS, Koh SI, Kim JD et al (1999) Wide-angle fluorescein angiographic scanning with high resolution using a scanning laser ophthalmoscope through a mirror image fixation target. Korean J Ophthalmol 13:92–99
10. Staurenghi G, Viola F, Mainster MA et al (2005) Scanning laser ophthalmoscopy and angiography with a wide-field contact lens system. Arch Ophthalmol 123:244–252
11. Argento CJ, Lopez Mato OR, Martinez-Cartier MD (2001) Oral fluorescein angiography with scanning laser ophthalmoscope. Int Ophthalmol 23:395–398
12. Azad RV, Baishya B, Pal N et al (2006) Comparative evaluation of oral fluorescein angiography using the confocal scanning laser ophthalmoscope and digital fundus camera

with intravenous fluorescein angiography using the digital fundus camera. Clin Experiment Ophthalmol 34:425–429
13. Garcia CR, Rivero ME, Bartsch DU et al (1999) Oral fluorescein angiography with the confocal scanning laser ophthalmoscope. Ophthalmology 106:1114–1118
14. Squirrell D, Dinakaran S, Dhingra S et al (2005) Oral fluorescein angiography with the scanning laser ophthalmoscope in diabetic retinopathy: a case controlled comparison with intravenous fluorescein angiography. Eye 19:411–417
15. Yannuzzi LA, Ober MD, Slakter JS, Spaide RF, Fisher YL, Flower RW, Rosen R (2004) Ophthalmic fundus imaging: today and beyond. Am J Ophthalmol 137:511–524
16. Friberg TR, Pandya A, Eller AW (2003) Non-mydriatic panoramic fundus imaging using a non-contact scanning laser-based system. Ophthalmic Surg Lasers Imaging 34:488–497
17. Chou B (2003) Limitations of the panoramic 200 optomap. Optom Vis Sci 80:671–672
18. Reddy S, Hu A, Schwartz SD (2009) Ultra wide field fluorescein angiography guided targeted retinal photocoagulation (TRP). Semin Ophthalmol 24:9–14
19. Tsui I, Kaines A, Schwartz S (2009) Patterns of periphlebitis in intermediate uveitis using ultra wide field fluorescein angiography. Semin Ophthalmol 24:29–33
20. Friedman D (2008) Diabetic retinopathy. In: Friedman D (ed) Vision problems in the U.S. Prevalence of adult vision impairment and age-related eye diseases in America. John Hopkins University, Baltimore, pp 26–36
21. Einarsdottir AB, Stefansson E (2009) Prevention of diabetic retinopathy. Lancet 373:1316–1318
22. EDTRS (1985) Photocoagulation therapy for diabetic eye disease. JAMA 254:3086
23. Group TDRR (1985) Photocoagulation therapy for diabetic eye disease. JAMA 254:3086
24. Williams GA, Scott IU, Haller JA et al (2004) Single-field fundus photography for diabetic retinopathy screening: a report by the American Academy of Ophthalmology. Ophthalmology 111:1055–1062
25. Ahmed J, Ward TP, Bursell SE et al (2006) The sensitivity and specificity of nonmydriatic digital stereoscopic retinal imaging in detecting diabetic retinopathy. Diabetes Care 29:2205–2209
26. Boucher MC, Gresset JA, Angioi K et al (2003) Effectiveness and safety of screening for diabetic retinopathy with two nonmydriatic digital images compared with the seven standard stereoscopic photographic fields. Can J Ophthalmol 38:557–568
27. Win PH, Young TA (2007) Optos panoramic200a fluorescein angiography for proliferative diabetic retinopathy with asteroid hyalosis. Semin Ophthalmol 22:67–69
28. Buchanan CR, Trucco E (2008) Contextual detection of diabetic pathology in wide-field retinal angiograms. Conf Proc IEEE Eng Med Biol Soc 2008:5437–5440
29. Azad R, Chandra P, Khan MA et al (2008) Role of intravenous fluorescein angiography in early detection and regression of retinopathy of prematurity. J Pediatr Ophthalmol Strabismus 45:36–39
30. Loewenstein A (2007) The significance of early detection of age-related macular degeneration: Richard & Hinda Rosenthal Foundation lecture, The Macula Society 29th annual meeting. Retina 27:873–878
31. Labriola LT, Brant AM, Eller AW (2009) Chronic retinal detachment with secondary retinal macrocyst and peripheral neovascularization. Semin Ophthalmol 24:2–4
32. Mackenzie PJ, Russell M, Ma PE et al (2007) Sensitivity and specificity of the optos optomap for detecting peripheral retinal lesions. Retina 27:1119–1124
33. Anderson L, Friberg TR, Singh J (2007) Ultrawide-angle retinal imaging and retinal detachment. Semin Ophthalmol 22:43–47
34. Coffee RE, Jain A, McCannel TA (2009) Ultra wide-field imaging of choroidal metastasis secondary to primary breast cancer. Semin Ophthalmol 24:34–36
35. Jain A, Shah SP, Tsui I et al (2009) The value of optos panoramic 200MA imaging for the monitoring of large suspicious choroidal lesions. Semin Ophthalmol 24:43–44
36. Rosen RB, Hathaway M, Rogers J et al (2009) Simultaneous OCT/SLO/ICG imaging. Invest Ophthalmol Vis Sci 50:851–860
37. Burns SA, Tumbar R, Elsner AE et al (2007) Large-field-of-view, modular, stabilized, adaptive-optics-based scanning laser ophthalmoscope. J Opt Soc Am A Opt Image Sci Vis 24:1313–1326

Chapter 5

Autofluorescence Imaging

5

Steffen Schmitz-Valckenberg, Monika Fleckenstein,
Richard Spaide, and Frank G Holz

Core Messages

- Fundus autofluorescence (FAF) imaging allows for noninvasive metabolic mapping of intrinsic retinal fluorophores in vivo.
- These fluorophores accumulate chiefly in the retinal pigment epithelium (RPE), but in certain pathological conditions they can also accumulate in the outer retina or subretinal space.
- Both the confocal scanning laser ophthalmoscope and the modified fundus camera permit to record FAF in the clinical setting; although, the composition of the detected autofluorescent signal may vary between both systems.
- FAF findings are useful for the identification of early disease stages and phenotyping. They may serve as disease markers and for monitoring disease progression.
- Several FAF findings topographically correlate with retinal dysfunction.
- For future applications, FAF imaging may be helpful in the development and assessment of new therapeutic strategies. The combination of FAF imaging with spectral-domain optical coherence tomography in one instrument is helpful to further investigate the origin of the FAF signal.

5.1 Introduction

The imaging of fundus autofluorescence (FAF) phenomena in vivo has been initially demonstrated during the early days of fluorescein angiography. Pre-injection fluorescence of optic disc drusen, optic disc hamartomas in tuberous sclerosis, and within lesions of Best vitelliform macular dystrophy have been reported at the time [1–4]. However, these observations were limited to a few patients with pathological accumulation of highly fluorescent material. In contrast, the naturally occurring intrinsic fluorescence of the ocular fundus is quite low in intensity, about two orders of magnitude lower than the background of a fluorescein angiogram at the most intense part of the dye transit. Absorption of excitation and emission light with partly additional generation of fluorescence by anatomical structures anterior to the retina further interferes with the detection of FAF. Hereby, the main barrier is the crystalline lens that has highly fluorescent characteristics in the short-wavelength range (excitation between 400–600 nm results in peak emission at ca. 520 nm [5]). With increasing age and particularly with the development of nuclear lens opacities, the fluorescence of the lens becomes even more prominent. Therefore, FAF imaging with a conventional fundus camera using the excitation and emission filters as applied for fluorescein angiography produces images with relatively low contrast and high background noise in young individuals. In the elderly, quality further drops and analysis of FAF distribution becomes practically impossible.

The era of FAF imaging as applied today has begun in 1995. Von Rückmann, Fitzke, and Bird described in their landmark paper the use of a confocal scanning laser ophthalmoscope for FAF imaging in a large number of patients [6]. Pioneering work on the spectral analysis of the origin of the autofluorescence signal was performed by Delori and co-workers in parallel [7]. In 2003, Spaide introduced a modified fundus camera (using longer wavelengths as originally applied) for FAF imaging and, recently, near-infrared autofluorescence imaging was described [8–10]. Various studies on FAF imaging have been performed in the meantime and, subsequently, this imaging technique is being increasingly used for research purposes. Today, FAF imaging is more widely used as a noninvasive clinical imaging tool in various retinal diseases.

5.2 What is Fundus Autofluorescence?

FAF imaging is an in vivo imaging method for metabolic mapping of naturally or pathologically occurring fluorophores of the ocular fundus. The dominant sources are fluorophores such as A2-E (N-retinyliden-N-retinylethanolamin) in lipofuscin granules, which accumulate in the postmitotic retinal pigment epithelium (RPE) as a by-product from the incomplete degradation of photoreceptor outer segments [7, 11, 12]. The topographic distribution of FAF intensities is altered in the presence of excessive accumulation or loss of lipofuscin/RPE cells. Additional intrinsic fluorophores may occur with the disease in various retinal layers or the subneurosensory space. Minor fluorophores such as collagen and elastin in choroidal blood vessel walls may become visible in the absence or atrophy of RPE cells. Bleaching phenomena and loss of photopigment may result in increased FAF by reduced absorbance of the excitation light. Finally, pathological alterations in the inner retina at the central macula, where the FAF signal is usually partially masked by luteal pigment (lutein and zeaxanthin), may result in apparent variations in FAF intensities.

Recording of FAF is relatively easily accomplished, requires little time, and is noninvasive. FAF signals are emitted across a broad spectrum ranging from 500 to 800 nm [7]. With the cSLO, excitation is usually induced in the blue range ($\lambda = 488$ nm), and an emission filter between 500 and 700 nm is used to detect emission of the autofluorescence signal [13]. Excitation when using the fundus camera is usually done in the green spectrum (535–580 nm) and emission is recorded in the yellow–orange spectrum (615–715 nm [according to the modifications by Spaide [14]]). Because of the difference in excitation and emission spectra, in addition to technical differences between the cSLO and the fundus camera, theoretical considerations would imply that the composition of the detected autofluorescent signal may vary between both systems. For example, the decreased FAF signal in the macula of healthy individuals that has been attributed mainly to the absorption of the excitation light by luteal pigment (peak absorbance at 460 nm, marked reduction > 510–540 nm) is much more prominent with the cSLO. In contrast, the fundus camera without the confocal optics makes this system somewhat more prone to light-scattering effects and generation of secondary reflectance, which may reach the detector and cannot be differentiated from the fluorescence signal.

5.3 Identification of Early Disease Stages

FAF imaging may allow for the identification of retinal diseases, when these are not otherwise evident. Metabolic changes at the level of the RPE/photoreceptor complex may not be visualized by funduscopy or other routine imaging techniques such as fluorescein angiography in early manifestations of macular and retinal dystrophies. This is particularly helpful in investigating patients with unknown visual loss or a positive familiar history of hereditary retinal diseases [15, 16]. Recently, it has been shown that FAF imaging reveals distinct abnormalities in idiopathic juxtafoveolar retinal telangiectasia type 2a (Fig. 5.1) [17]. Already, in early disease stage where only subtle dilation of parafoveal retinal blood vessels can be detected by fluorescein angiography, the FAF signal in the central macula is typically increased, which is thought to result from a depletion of luteal pigment in layers anterior to the RPE. In early dry age-related macular degeneration (AMD), alterations in the level of the RPE may become visible in areas that appear normal on funduscopy. Reticular drusen as a particular drusen phenotype is readily visible on FAF images.

5.4 Phenotyping

Alterations in FAF intensities at the outer retina in various retinal diseases are typically much more pronounced with structural or optical alterations seen with other imaging techniques. This helps in diagnosing hereditary retinal disorders such as Stargardt disease, vitelliform macular and pattern dystrophies, and may be used for correlation with specific genetic defects [16]. For example, well-defined flecks in Stargardt disease associated with a markedly increased FAF signal are more readily delineated on FAF images when compared with fundus photographs (Fig. 5.2) [18]. Furthermore, it has been demonstrated that distinct alterations can be detected in patients who had been diagnosed with AMD. Classification systems for FAF patterns both in early AMD and advanced atrophic AMD have been introduced [19, 20]. FAF findings in this context also help to distinguish AMD from late onset macular dystrophies mimicking age-related changes. Drusen in early-stage AMD usually (except of soft drusen) exhibits a normal or mildly increased FAF signal, whereas focal deposits not related to AMD (e.g., dominant drusen) are typically characterized by strong levels of increased FAF; although, they may not be distinguishable from AMD-related changes on fundus photography [16]. However, systematic investigations in this regard along with genotyping are lacking. In advanced atrophic AMD, i.e., in patients above 55 years of age and clinically diagnosed with AMD, the diffuse FAF pattern with peripheral punctuate spots (GPS) phenotype appears to be very similar to FAF changes typically observed in

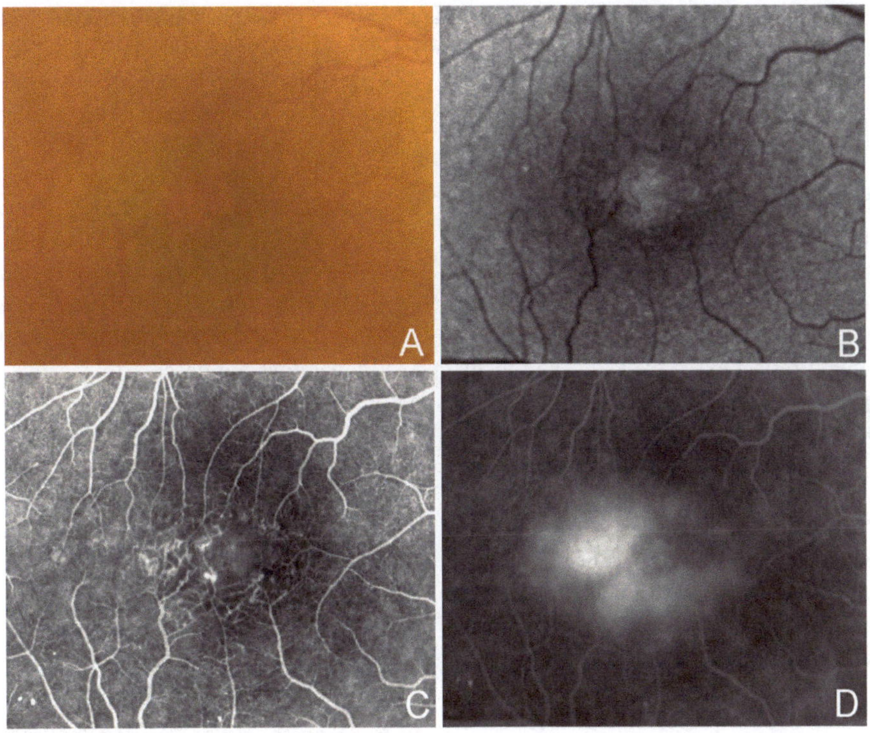

Fig. 5.1 Idiopathic juxtafoveolar telangiectasia Type 2a shown by fundus photography (**a**), fundus autofluorescence (FAF) (**b**), and early (**c**) and late-phase (**d**) fluorescein angiography. No obvious alterations are visible by fundus photography. Fluorescein angiography shows telangiectatic vessels in the parafovea and late-phase hyperfluorescence. FAF imaging reveals markedly increased levels of the central fovea as opposed to the typical decreased signal in normal subjects

young individuals with Stargardt disease, which is caused by biallelic mutations in the ABCA4 gene [19, 21]. Even the role of ABCA4 variants in AMD etiology is still controversial; preliminary data suggests that the GPS phenotype is associated with a single heterozygous mutation in the ABCA4 gene [22].

5.5 Disease Markers

Several lines of evidence suggest that excessive lipofuscin accumulation represents a common downstream pathogenetic pathway in various hereditary and complex retinal diseases [12, 23]. Clinical observations

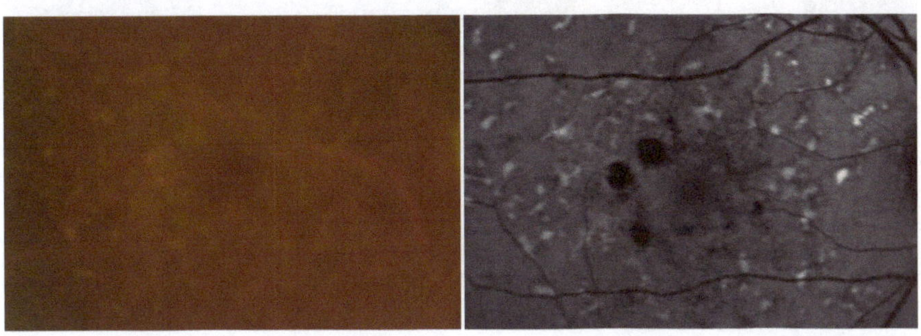

Fig. 5.2 In Stargardt macular dystrophy, the detection of fundus pathology is much better with FAF imaging when compared with that of fundus photography. Typically, autofluorescence imaging shows a central oval area of reduced signal surrounded by small disseminated spots of reduced and increased intensity. A central multifocal RPE atrophy is also present showing severely decreased FAF intensity. Yellowish appearing flecks on fundus photography correspond to punctuate spots with bright autofluorescence signal

indicate different degrees and extension of levels of increased FAF that do not or only poorly correlate with findings obtained by other imaging techniques (Fig. 5.3). These FAF changes that are far-off from visible alterations may suggest more widespread abnormalities and diseased retinal areas [24]. Focally increased FAF, and therefore, excessive RPE lipofuscin load, may indicate dysfunctioning RPE cells. Indeed, the pathophysiological role of abnormal FAF is underscored by recent longitudinal studies. For example, it has been demonstrated that areas with increased FAF signal, which might reflect excessive RPE LF built-up, precede the development of new areas or the enlargement of pre-existing atrophic patches in geographic atrophy secondary to AMD [25]. Furthermore, the extension of abnormal FAF as well as the previously introduced FAF pattern classification have an impact on atrophy enlargement rates over time, and may therefore serve as predictive determinants [26, 27]. The identification of high-risk characteristics, i.e., clinical biomarkers, for disease progression may be helpful not only for monitoring patients with advanced atrophic AMD, but also for performing clinical interventional trials with "fast progressers." In patients with choroidal neovascularization or in inflammatory diseases, FAF abnormalities typically extend beyond the angiographically visible alterations indicating a more widespread disease as well [24, 28–30]. Changes in the FAF signal may permit to estimate the extent of damage, diagnose sequella such as secondary CNV, learn more about the inflammatory process, and possibly anticipate future problems caused by the disease. One recent study indicates that FAF changes are better correlated with visual acuity than with the symptoms length and lesion size [30]. Although early CNV was typically manifested with patches of "continuous" or "normal" autofluorescence (corresponding to areas of hyperfluorescence on the comparative fluorescein angiograms), long-standing CNV exhibited more areas with decreased intensity. The latter observation was explained by photoreceptor loss and scar formation with increased melanin deposition. Of note, a decreased FAF signal does not necessarily mean irreversible retinal damage, as it might also be caused by subretinal fluid or hemorrhages. A possible predictive value of FAF imaging with regard to the determination of therapeutic success by anti-VEGF treatment has been demonstrated by Heimes and co-workers [31]. They demonstrate that, in particular, the development of visual acuity is less favorable in eyes with initially increased central FAF.

5.6 Monitoring of Disease Progression

Because of the absence of RPE lipofuscin, atrophic areas such as in atrophic AMD or Stargardt disease exhibit a markedly reduced signal. Such diseased areas and atrophic patches can be easily identified and, moreover, precisely quantified by customized image analysis software [32, 33]. This allows for noninvasive monitoring of atrophy progression over time (Fig. 5.4).

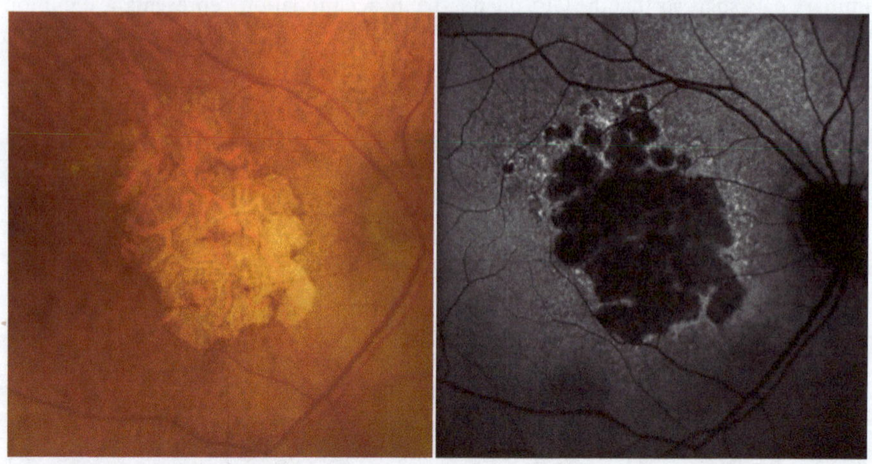

Fig. 5.3 In atrophic AMD, atrophy areas appear as sharply demarcated areas with depigmentation and enhanced visualization of deep choroidal vessels on fundus photograph (*left*). At the corresponding FAF image (*right*), atrophic patches are clearly delineated by decreased intensity and high contrast to nonatrophic retina. Surrounding atrophy, in the junctional zone of atrophy, levels of marked FAF intensity are observed, which are invisible on fundus photography. These abnormalities tend to precede atrophy over time and may serve as disease markers

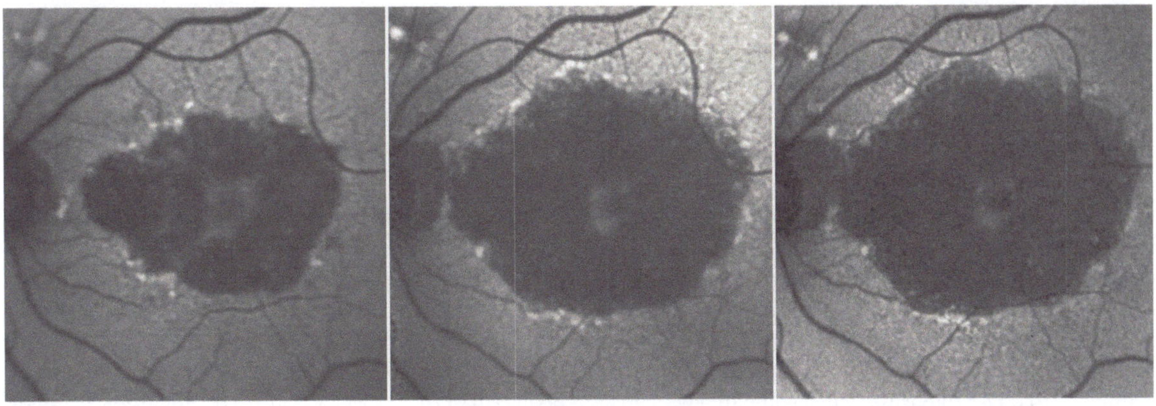

Fig. 5.4 Monitoring of atrophic progression over time with FAF imaging, showing the natural course of the disease over 5 years. Note, the preserved foveal island ("foveal sparing") in the center of the central atrophic patch, which becomes smaller during the review period

5.7 Disease Mapping

Central serous chorioretinopathy produces predictable changes in FAF imaging in relation to the chronicity of disease. Soon after the separation of the retina, an increase in autofluorescence is observed. This is associated with an increase in thickness of the photoreceptor outer segments layer by the OCT [34]. Over time, increasing atrophy occurs and the autofluorescence signal decreases. The visual acuity in eyes with central serous chorioretinopathy was found to be correlated with the normalized level of autofluorescence from the foveal region [34]. Autofluorescence photography provides a simple method of mapping the areas of involvement in central serous chorioretinopathy (Fig. 5.5). Although serous detachment can be determined with OCT, a montage image of the fundus can be obtained in a matter of seconds using autofluorescence imaging.

Pseudoxanthoma elasticum (PXE) is caused by a mutation in the ABCC6 gene; more than 300 distinct loss-of-function mutations representative of over 1,000 mutant alleles in ABCC6 have been found [35]. Many of the missense mutations occur at locations in the protein involving domain–domain interactions in the ABCC6 transporter [36]. Even heterozygotes can show disease manifestations [37]. FAF abnormalities are very common in PXE. Eyes of patients with PXE can have angioid streaks, peau d' orange, and drusen of the optic nerve, all of which have autofluorescence correlates. Eyes with PXE can show what has been termed a pattern dystrophy, this pigment patterning shows increased pigmentation and is associated with subretinal accumulations of the material [38]. Large areas of RPE atrophy can occur, even in areas not suspected to have RPE abnormalities, and were first documented with autofluorescence photography [39]. Choroidal neovascularization is a common secondary consequence and is readily visible during FAF imaging. All of these changes are readily visible using autofluorescence imaging as a screening tool.

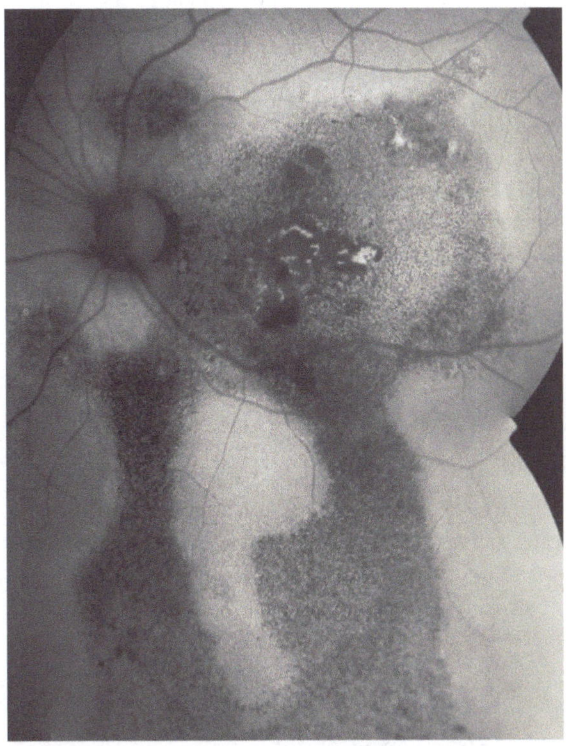

Fig. 5.5 Chronic central serous retinopathy as imaged by the modified fundus camera shows decreased FAF in the macula due to atrophy. Additional FAF abnormalities outside the central macula, including prominent descending tracts are visualized. Clinically, the patient has no signs of subretinal fluid

5.8 Functional Correlation

The relevance of alterations in FAF images can further be addressed by assessing corresponding retinal sensitivity. Severe damage to the RPE such as atrophy, melanin pigment migration, or fibrosis leading to compromised photoreceptor function as confirmed by microperimetry is topographically confined to decreased autofluorescence [40, 41]. In patients with geographic atrophy secondary to AMD, it has been shown that – in addition to the absence of retinal sensitivity over atrophic areas – retinal function is relatively and significantly reduced over areas with increased FAF intensities when compared with areas with normal background signal [40]. Localized functional impairment over areas with increased FAF has also been recently confirmed in patients with early AMD. Using fine matrix mapping, it has been demonstrated that rod function is more severely affected than cone function over areas with increased FAF in AMD patients [41]. These studies are in accordance with the observation of increased accumulation of autofluorescent material at the level of the RPE prior to cell death. As the normal photoreceptor function is dependent on normal RPE function, in particular with regard to the constant phagocytosis of shed distal outer segment stacks for photoreceptor cell renewal, a negative feedback mechanism has been proposed, whereby cells with lipofuscin-loaded secondary lysosomes would phagocytize less-shed POS, subsequently leading to impaired retinal sensitivity. This would also be in line with the experimental data showing that compounds of lipofuscin such as A2-E possess toxic properties and may interfere with normal RPE cell function via various molecular mechanisms including impairment of lysosomal function [23].

In patients with retinitis pigmentosa and cone dystrophies, parafoveal rings of increased FAF have been identified in the absence of funduscopically visible correlates, which tend to shrink or enlarge with disease progression, respectively (Fig. 5.6) [42, 43]. Interestingly, functional testing using microperimetry and electrophysiology indicates that these rings demarcate areas of preserved photoreceptor function. In retinitis pigmentosa, a gradient loss of sensitivity is present outside the arc of the ring with increasing eccentricity.

5.9 Future Applications for Therapeutic Interventions

In patients with advanced atrophic AMD, FAF imaging may also be helpful to develop and assess new emerging therapeutic strategies. Visual cycle modulators, which aim to target the detrimental accumulation of toxic by-products of the visual cycle in the RPE, appear as promising pharmaceutical agents to slow down the progression of atrophy. Fenretinide (*N*-[4-hydroxyphenyl] retinamide), an oral compound, has been shown to lower the production of toxic fluorophores in the RPE in a dose-dependent manner in the albino ABCA4$^{-/-}$ mice [44]. This vitamin A derivate acts by competing with serum retinol for the binding sites of retinal-binding protein and promotes renal clearance of retinol. The bioavailability of retinol for the RPE and photoreceptors is consequently reduced and less toxic retinoid by-products such as A2-E may be generated. A Phase II randomized, double-masked, placebo-controlled multicenter study, which aims to include over 200 GA patients, has been already initiated in the USA in 2006 (Sirion Therapeutics, Inc.; Tampa, FL; http://www.siriontherapeutics.com). The therapeutic concept of Fenretinide is not only underscored by previous FAF findings. To reduce the observational period in a slowly progressive disease, to minimize the sample size, and to better demonstrate possible treatment effects, the patient recruitment in this study involves the identification of high-risk features in this first large interventional trial in patients with geographic atrophy secondary to AMD.

In retinal dystrophies, FAF imaging may be used to assess the potential functional preservation of the outer retina, and would therefore serve as an implication for future treatment. In patients with Leber congenital amaurosis having vision reduced to light perception and undetectable ERGs, normal or minimally decreased FAF intensities have been reported [45]. This suggests that the RPE/photoreceptor complex is, at least in part, functionally and anatomically intact and would indicate that the photoreceptor function may still be rescuable.

Because of the increased sensitivity and improved signal-to-noise ratio, modern confocal scanning laser ophthalmoscopy allows – in addition to the well-known FAF with blue excitation light as described earlier – for the visualization of FAF phenomena by near-infrared light [8, 10]. Hereby, the so-called ICG-mode is used. Application in patients and case reports in animal models and donor eye suggest that near-infrared FAF detects fluorophores at the level of the RPE. Melanin has been postulated as the major candidate. However, no spectral analyses as for lipofuscin for blue light FAF have been reported.

The recent introduction of combined simultaneous spectral-domain optical coherence tomography (SD-OCT) with cSLO imaging in one instrument with real-time eye tracking that allows for the accurate orientation of OCT-scans and therefore for the 3D mapping of pathological changes at specific anatomic sites represents an important step forward to better investigate the origin of the FAF signal within the retina (Fig. 5.7) [46–50].

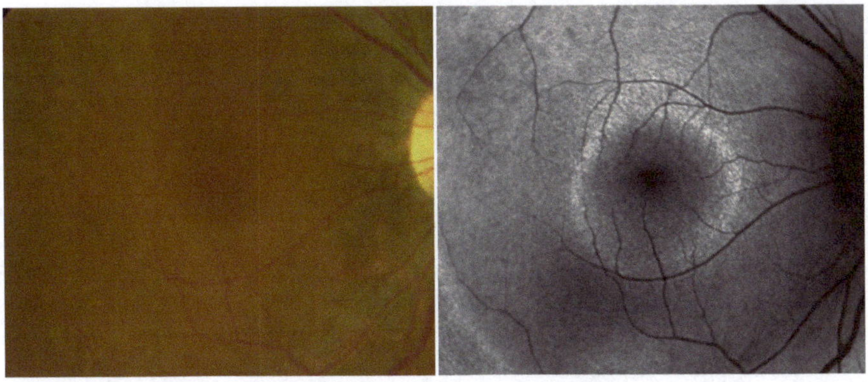

Fig. 5.6 This patient with retinitis pigmentosa shows a typical ring of increased autofluorescence in the parafovea, which is not visible on fundus photography. Functional testing reveals that this ring correlates with functional abnormalities and represent a demarcation line between normal and abnormal functional retina

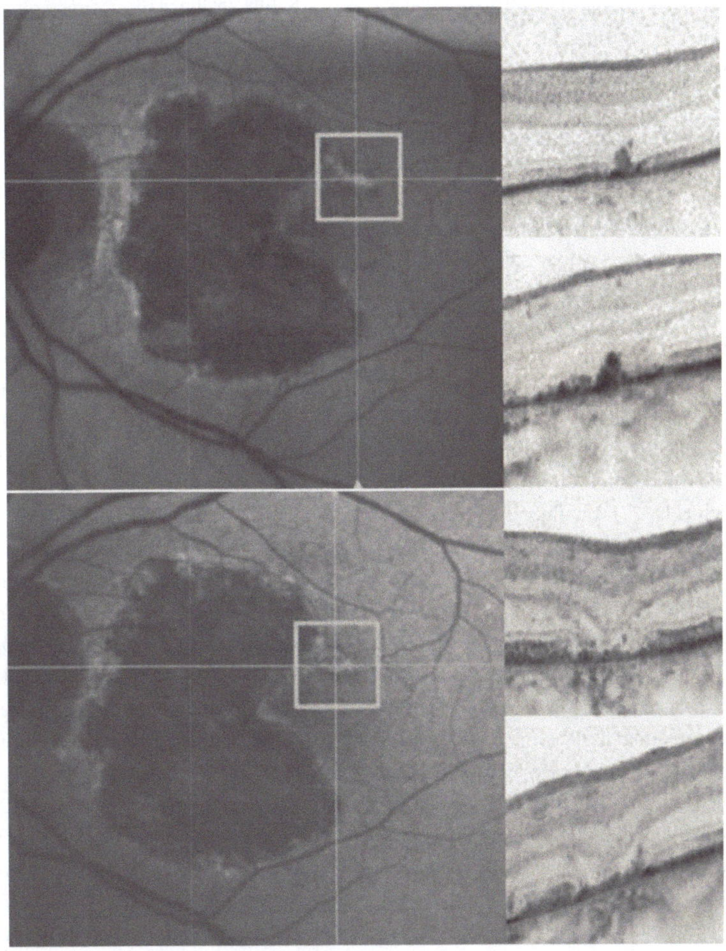

Fig. 5.7 Combined simultaneous confocal scanning laser ophthalmoscopy FAF and spectral-domain optical coherence (SD-OCT) imaging in a patient with geographic atrophy secondary to age-related macular degeneration allows for 3D assessment of pathological changes and also to better investigate the origin of the autofluorescence signal. The *white lines* mark the orientations of horizontal and vertical location of SD-OCT scans, respectively. The *rectangle* illustrates the section of OCT scans. The combined imaging suggests that deposition of the material in the outer retina causes an increase in autofluorescence signal at baseline (*top row*). After 1 year, the autofluorescence signal is decreased with concomitant development of incipient atrophy (*bottom row*)

Summaries for the Clinician

- FAF imaging provides information over and above conventional imaging techniques in various retinal disorders, and, thus adds to our armentarium to diagnose and manage patients.
- FAF imaging is a non time-consuming, easy to perform, and a noninvasive imaging method. Particularly in disorders of the outer retina, the application offers the opportunity to identify disease-related abnormalities and to determine the integrity of the RPE/photoreceptor complex.
- FAF imaging represents not just a technique to visualize structural changes, but actually allows for metabolic mapping and correlation with retinal function.
- Several studies have demonstrated its clinical relevance, while there are numerous promising future applications. In combination with other emerging technologies such as SD-OCT, FAF imaging may add to our understanding of retinal disease and management of patients.

References

1. Mustonen E, Nieminen H (1982) Optic disc drusen – a photographic study. I. Autofluorescence pictures and fluorescein angiography. Acta Ophthalmol (Copenh) 60:849–858
2. Neetens A, Burvenich H (1977) Autofluorescence of optic disc-drusen. Bull Soc Belge Ophtalmol 179:103–110
3. Schatz H, Burton TC, Yannuzzi LA, Rabb MF (1978) Preinjection fluorescence. Disc leak. In: Schatz H, Burton TC, Yannuzzi LA, Raab MF (eds) Preinjection fluorescence. Disc leak. C.V. Mosby, St Louis
4. Wessing A, Meyer-Schwickerath G (1968) Veränderungen der Papille. Papillenschwellung. In: Wessing A and G. M-S (eds) Veränderungen der Papille. Papillenschwellung. Georg Thieme Verlag, Stuttgart
5. Bessems GJ, Keizer E, Wollensak J, Hoenders HJ (1987) Non-tryptophan fluorescence of crystallins from normal and cataractous human lenses. Invest Ophthalmol Vis Sci 28:1157–1163
6. von Ruckmann A, Fitzke FW, Bird AC (1995) Distribution of fundus autofluorescence with a scanning laser ophthalmoscope. Br J Ophthalmol 79:407–412
7. Delori FC, Dorey CK, Staurenghi G et al (1995) In vivo fluorescence of the ocular fundus exhibits retinal pigment epithelium lipofuscin characteristics. Invest Ophthalmol Vis Sci 36:718–729
8. Keilhauer CN, Delori FC (2006) Near-infrared autofluores cence imaging of the fundus: visualization of ocular melanin. Invest Ophthalmol Vis Sci 47:3556–3564
9. Spaide RF (2003) Fundus autofluorescence and age-related macular degeneration. Ophthalmology 110:392–399
10. Weinberger AW, Lappas A, Kirschkamp T et al (2006) Fundus near infrared fluorescence correlates with fundus near infrared reflectance. Invest Ophthalmol Vis Sci 47:3098–3108
11. Holz FG, Schmitz-Valckenberg S, Spaide RF, Bird AC (2007) Atlas of fundus autofluorescence imaging. Springer, Berlin
12. Sparrow JR, Boulton M (2005) RPE lipofuscin and its role in retinal pathobiology. Exp Eye Res 80:595–606
13. Jorzik JJ, Bindewald A, Dithmar S, Holz FG (2005) Digital simultaneous fluorescein and indocyanine green angiography, autofluorescence, and red-free imaging with a solid-state laser-based confocal scanning laser ophthalmoscope. Retina 25:405–416
14. Spaide RF (2007) Autofluorescence Imaging with the fundus camera. In: Holz FG, Schmitz-Valckenberg S, Spaide RF, Bird AC (eds) Autofluorescence imaging with the fundus camera. Springer, Berlin
15. Poloschek CM, Hansen LL, Bach M (2007) Annular fundus autofluorescence abnormality in a case of macular dystrophy. Doc Ophthalmol
16. von Ruckmann A, Fitzke FW, Bird AC (1997) In vivo fundus autofluorescence in macular dystrophies. Arch Ophthalmol 115:609–615
17. Helb HM, Charbel Issa P, van der Vehn RL et al (2008) Abnormal macular pigment distribution in type 2 idiopathic macular telangiectasia. Retina 28:808–816
18. Lois N, Halfyard AS, Bird AC et al (2004) Fundus autofluorescence in Stargardt macular dystrophy-fundus flavimaculatus. Am J Ophthalmol 138:55–63
19. Bindewald A, Schmitz-Valckenberg S, Jorzik JJ et al (2005) Classification of abnormal fundus autofluorescence patterns in the junctional zone of geographic atrophy in patients with age related macular degeneration. Br J Ophthalmol 89:874–878
20. Bindewald A, Bird AC, Dandekar SS et al (2005) Classification of fundus autofluorescence patterns in early age-related macular disease. Invest Ophthalmol Vis Sci 46: 3309–3314
21. Allikmets R, Singh N, Sun H et al (1997) A photoreceptor cell-specific ATP-binding transporter gene (ABCR) is mutated in recessive Stargardt macular dystrophy. Nat Genet 15:236–246
22. Fleckenstein M, Fiebig BS, Fritsche L et al. (2009) A fundus autofluorescence phenotype in advanced dry AMD is associated with heterozygous mutations in the ABCA4 gene. EURETINA, Nice [abstract]
23. Bergmann M, Schutt F, Holz FG, Kopitz J (2004) Inhibition of the ATP-driven proton pump in RPE lysosomes by the major lipofuscin fluorophore A2-E may contribute to the pathogenesis of age-related macular degeneration. Faseb J 18:562–564

24. Dandekar SS, Jenkins SA, Peto T et al (2005) Autofluorescence imaging of choroidal neovascularization due to age-related macular degeneration. Arch Ophthalmol 123:1507–1513
25. Holz FG, Bellman C, Staudt S et al (2001) Fundus autofluorescence and development of geographic atrophy in age-related macular degeneration. Invest Ophthalmol Vis Sci 42:1051–1056
26. Holz FG, Bindewald-Wittich A, Fleckenstein M et al (2007) Progression of geographic atrophy and impact of fundus autofluorescence patterns in age-related macular degeneration. Am J Ophthalmol 143:463–472
27. Schmitz-Valckenberg S, Bindewald-Wittich A, Dolar-Szczasny J et al (2006) Correlation between the area of increased autofluorescence surrounding geographic atrophy and disease progression in patients with AMD. Invest Ophthalmol Vis Sci 47:2648–2654
28. Sawa M, Ober MD, Spaide RF (2006) Autofluorescence and retinal pigment epithelial atrophy after subretinal hemorrhage. Retina 26:119–120
29. Spaide R (2008) Autofluorescence from the outer retina and subretinal space: hypothesis and review. Retina 28:5–35
30. Vaclavik V, Vujosevic S, Dandekar SS et al (2007) Autofluorescence imaging in age-related macular degeneration complicated by choroidal neovascularization a prospective study. Ophthalmology
31. Heimes B, Lommatzsch A, Zeimer M et al (2008) Foveal RPE autofluorescence as a prognostic factor for anti-VEGF therapy in exudative AMD. Graefes Arch Clin Exp Ophthalmol 246:1229–1234
32. Deckert A, Schmitz-Valckenberg S, Jorzik J et al (2005) Automated analysis of digital fundus autofluorescence images of geographic atrophy in advanced age-related macular degeneration using confocal scanning laser ophthalmoscopy (cSLO). BMC Ophthalmol 5:8
33. Schmitz-Valckenberg S, Jorzik J, Unnebrink K, Holz FG (2002) Analysis of digital scanning laser ophthalmoscopy fundus autofluorescence images of geographic atrophy in advanced age-related macular degeneration. Graefes Arch Clin Exp Ophthalmol 240:73–78
34. Spaide RF, Klancnik JM Jr (2005) Fundus autofluorescence and central serous chorioretinopathy. Ophthalmology 112: 825–833
35. Li Q, Jiang Q, Pfendner E et al (2009) Pseudoxanthoma elasticum: clinical phenotypes, molecular genetics and putative pathomechanisms. Exp Dermatol 18:1–11
36. Fulop K, Barna L, Symmons O et al (2009) Clustering of disease-causing mutations on the domain-domain interfaces of ABCC6. Biochem Biophys Res Commun 379:706–709
37. Martin L, Maitre F, Bonicel P et al (2008) Heterozygosity for a single mutation in the ABCC6 gene may closely mimic PXE: consequences of this phenotype overlap for the definition of PXE. Arch Dermatol 144:301–306
38. Charbel Issa P, Finger RP, Holz FG, Scholl HP (2009) Multimodal imaging including spectral domain OCT and confocal near infrared reflectance for characterisation of outer retinal pathology in pseudoxanthoma elasticum. Invest Ophthalmol Vis Sci [epub ahead of print] Jul 24
39. Sawa M, Ober MD, Freund KB, Spaide RF (2006) Fundus autofluorescence in patients with pseudoxanthoma elasticum. Ophthalmology 113:814–820 e812
40. Schmitz-Valckenberg S, Bultmann S, Dreyhaupt J et al (2004) Fundus autofluorescence and fundus perimetry in the junctional zone of geographic atrophy in patients with age-related macular degeneration. Invest Ophthalmol Vis Sci 45:4470–4476
41. Scholl HP, Bellmann C, Dandekar SS et al (2004) Photopic and scotopic fine matrix mapping of retinal areas of increased fundus autofluorescence in patients with age-related maculopathy. Invest Ophthalmol Vis Sci 45:574–583
42. Robson AG, Saihan Z, Jenkins SA et al (2006) Functional characterisation and serial imaging of abnormal fundus autofluorescence in patients with retinitis pigmentosa and normal visual acuity. Br J Ophthalmol 90:472–479
43. Robson AG, Michaelides M, Saihan Z et al (2008) Functional characteristics of patients with retinal dystrophy that manifest abnormal parafoveal annuli of high density fundus autofluorescence; a review and update. Doc Ophthalmol 116:79–89
44. Radu RA, Han Y, Bui TV et al (2005) Reductions in serum vitamin A arrest accumulation of toxic retinal fluorophores: a potential therapy for treatment of lipofuscin-based retinal diseases. Invest Ophthalmol Vis Sci 46:4393–4401
45. Bellmann C, Neveu MM, Scholl HP et al (2004) Localized retinal electrophysiological and fundus autofluorescence imaging abnormalities in maternal inherited diabetes and deafness. Invest Ophthalmol Vis Sci 45:2355–2360
46. Drexler W, Morgner U, Ghanta RK et al (2001) Ultrahigh-resolution ophthalmic optical coherence tomography. Nat Med 7:502–507
47. Fleckenstein M, Charbel Issa P, Helb HM et al (2008) High-resolution spectral domain-OCT imaging in geographic atrophy associated with age-related macular degeneration. Invest Ophthalmol Vis Sci 49:4137–4144
48. Helb HM, Charbel Issa P, Fleckenstein M et al (2008) Clinical evaluation of simultaneous confocal scanning laser ophthalmoscopy imaging combined with high-resolution, spectral-domain optical coherence tomography. Ophthalmologica (in press)
49. Wojtkowski M, Bajraszewski T, Gorczynska I et al (2004) Ophthalmic imaging by spectral optical coherence tomography. Am J Ophthalmol 138:412–419
50. Wolf-Schnurrbusch UE, Enzmann V, Brinkmann CK, Wolf S (2008) Morphologic changes in patients with geographic atrophy assessed with a novel spectral OCT-SLO combination. Invest Ophthalmol Vis Sci 49:3095–3099

Chapter 6

Imaging the Macular Pigment

6

Tos T. J. M. Berendschot

Core Messages

- Macular pigment (MP) is composed of the stereo-isomers lutein and zeaxanthin. The absorption peaks at the center of the fovea and decreases rapidly with eccentricity. In the central 0–2.3 mm region, zeaxanthin predominates over lutein, whereas for eccentricities beyond this region, lutein is the major carotenoid. An exponentially decaying density as a function of eccentricity yields a good description of the spatial distribution. For some subjects, a Gaussian-like ring pattern has to be added around 0.7° eccentricity.
- There is a growing body of evidence in support of the view that MP protects against or ameliorates the clinical course of age-related macular degeneration (AMD), the most common cause of irreversible blindness in the industrialized world. There are some plausible arguments to assume that MP indeed exerts a protective effect in the retinal area. First of all, it acts as a blue light filter, thereby decreasing chances for photochemical light damage. In addition, MP is capable of scavenging free radicals. Finally, lutein is capable of suppressing inflammation.
- Humans are unable to synthesize lutein and zeaxanthin. Thus, the MP optical density (MPOD) depends on the dietary intake. It has been shown that MPOD can be increased by a dietary modification or by supplements in healthy subjects as well as in subjects with a diseased macula.
- There are several ways to determine the MPOD in the living human eye. The most widespread are the psychophysical techniques, where a subject adjusts color or luminosity, generally through a minimum flicker, or a minimum motion task. The second, more objective approach is through analysis of light returning from the retina. It relies either on spectral analysis, autofluorescence, or resonant Raman spectroscopy. In particular, the latter three are suited to obtain MPOD maps that show the spatial distribution of the MP with a high resolution.

6.1 Macular Pigment

6.1.1 Characteristics and Potential Functions

In primates, the fovea appears as a yellow spot, as already documented by Buzzi in 1782 [1].

Initially, the yellow color was thought to represent a retinal hole [2] or caused by postmortem changes [3, 4]. Later, studies showed that it is caused by the so-called macular pigment, which is concentrated in the central area of the retina along the axons of the cone photoreceptors (see Fig. 6.1) [5–7, 7]. The specific yellow color is caused by carotenoids [8], more in particular, the stereo-isomers lutein and zeaxanthin [9, 10] and the intermediate meso-zeaxanthin [11]. Figure 6.2 shows the extinction coefficient of lutein and zeaxanthin [12]. There are many potential functions attributed to the MP, like reducing the consequences of chromatic aberration [13–15], minimize stray light [16], preservation of visual sensitivity [17] in older subjects, and improving glare disability and photostress recovery [18, 19]. However, some argue that the presence of the MP in the fovea is merely the remains of an earlier form of color vision [20]. In 1994, Seddon et al. observed an inverse association

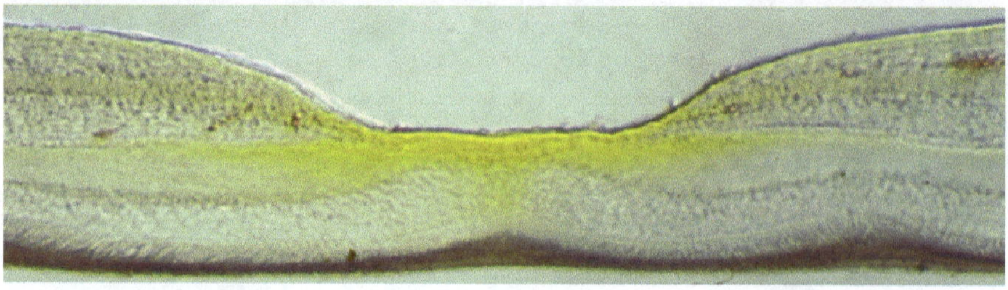

Fig. 6.1 Unstained retina. Courtesy by Dr. M. M. Snodderly

between a diet with a high content of the carotenoids lutein and zeaxanthin and the prevalence of AMD [21]. This pointed to even another potential role of MP, that is almost exclusively composed of these two carotenoids [9, 22], namely in preventing age related macular degeneration (AMD). AMD is a degenerative disease of the retina, and in the developed world, it is the leading cause of visual impairment in people 50 years and older [23–25]. AMD affects the macula that enables the central high-resolution visual acuity. Dysfunction of the macula results in the inability to see fine detail, read, and recognize faces. The disease has a great impact on the quality of life and leads to large negative financial and economic consequences [26–31]. The prevalence of AMD is likely to rise as a consequence of increasing longevity. Although new treatments have emerged, they are suitable only for the small proportion of people with neovascular AMD. No treatments are available for the geographic atrophy AMD. Therefore, it is very important to identify preventative factors for the development of AMD [32]. Apart from quitting smoking, MP that can be modified by diet could well be an easy target to decrease the susceptibility for AMD.

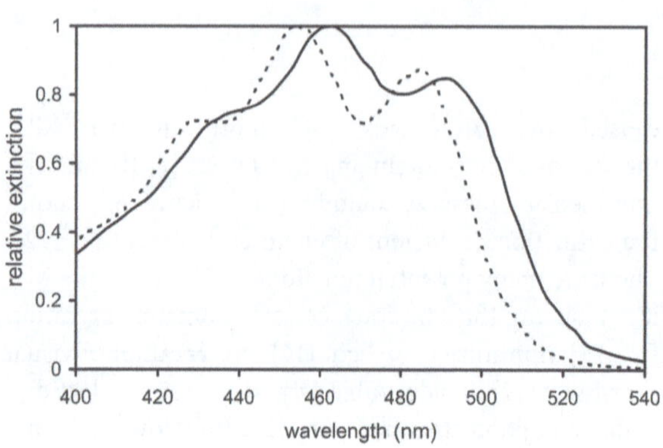

Fig. 6.2 Relative extinction coefficient of lutein (*dashed*) and zeaxanthin (*solid line*). The parallel slopes of the extinction spectra at the long wavelengths show a difference of about 10 nm

6.1.2 Macular Pigment and Age-Related Macular Degeneration

There are some plausible arguments to assume that MP, that is almost exclusively composed of these two carotenoids [9, 22], exerts a protective effect in the retinal area. First of all, it acts as a blue light filter, absorbing between 390 and 540 nm (see Fig. 6.2) [33–36], thereby decreasing the chances for photochemical light damage [37]. In addition, MP is capable of scavenging free radicals [38]. Finally, lutein is capable to suppress inflammation [39]. This is probably the reason that since Seddon's paper in 1994 [21], many papers that study the relation between lutein, zeaxanthin, and MP, on the one hand, and AMD, on the other hand, have been published [40–58]. Unfortunately, their results are ambiguous. In 2005, the Food and Drugs Administration reviewed intervention and observational studies that evaluated the role of lutein and zeaxanthin in reducing the risk of AMD [59]. At that time, the agency concluded that there was no credible evidence to support a health claim for lutein or zeaxanthin intake and the risk of AMD. A more detailed discussion of the above-mentioned characteristics and potential functions is beyond the scope of this chapter. This can be found in reviews by Davies and Moreland [22], Loane et al. [49], Nussbaum et al. [60], and Weale [20].

6.1.3 Spatial Distribution

MP is composed of the stereo-isomers lutein and zeaxanthin [9, 10] and the intermediate meso-zeaxanthin [11]. The absorption peaks at the center of the fovea and decreases rapidly with eccentricity. In the central 0–2.3 mm region, zeaxanthin predominates over lutein [9], whereas for eccentricities beyond this region, lutein is the major carotenoid. Figure 6.3 shows mean lutein and zeaxanthin profiles of 19 healthy individuals (13 women, 6 men, aged 26 ± 8 years) determined by spectral fundus reflectance [61]. The MPOD spatial distribution for a long time was assumed to decrease monotonously to very low values at an eccentricity of about

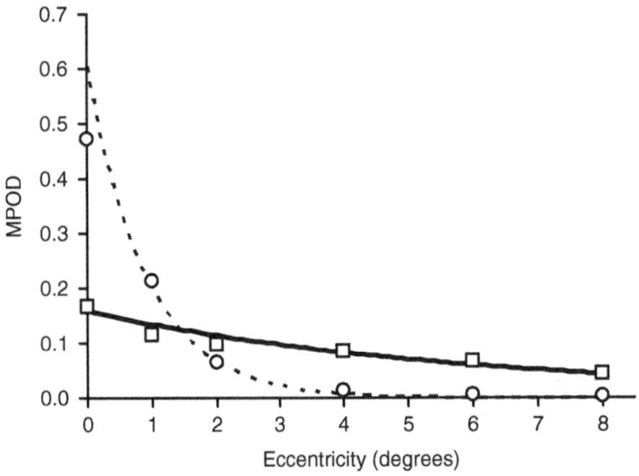

Fig. 6.3 Mean lutein (*circles*) and zeaxanthin profiles (*squares*) of 19 healthy individuals, 13 women, 6 men, aged 26 ± 8 years, determined by spectral fundus reflectance [136]. Lines are guides to the eye, based on an exponential decreasing function with eccentricity

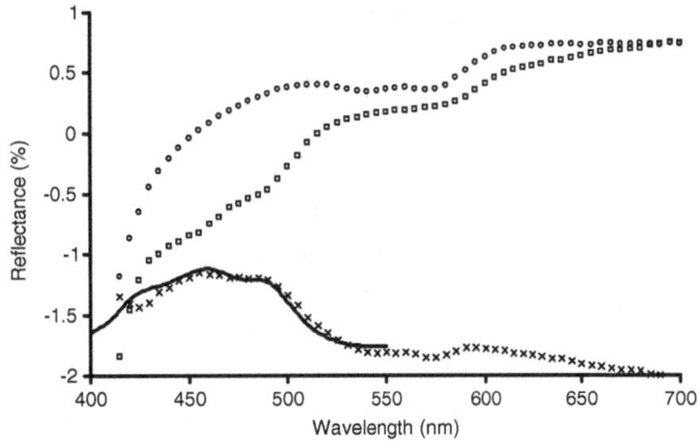

Fig. 6.4 Reflection spectra measured at the fovea (squares) and at a site temporal to the fovea (circles). At the bottom, the log-ratio spectrum is shown (crosses). The solid line is a best fit with macular pigment

10°. However, some doubts were already expressed in 1954 by Miles [62] when studying the so-called Maxwell's Spot [63]. He found an additional ring in 14 of the 19 subjects who were able to see this phenomenon. In 1984, Snodderly et al. [5, 64] measured MP profiles by two-wavelength micro-densitometry in squirrel, macaque, and cebus monkeys, and found a central peak with shoulders or flanking peaks around 0.8° eccentricity. The main peak was associated with MP along the receptor axons, whereas the shoulders followed the inner plexiform layer. However, both lutein and zeaxanthin reached their highest concentrations at the center of the fovea and declined monotonically with eccentricity. The discrepancy between these two findings were explained by variations in the orientation of the dichroic lutein and zeaxanthin as a function of eccentricity [12, 65]. Several authors studied the spatial distribution of the MP with a rather low resolution using the technique of heterochromatic flicker photometry (HFP, see below, see Fig. 6.4). Using this technique, Hammond et al. noted in 40% of their subjects small, but significant deviations from an exponential decreasing function with eccentricity between 0.5° and 1.0° that took the form of valleys or flanking peaks [66]. Recently, this has been quantified by other techniques having a high spatial resolution like autofluorescence and fundus reflectance (see below, see Fig 6.5). They all found a distinct ring pattern at a distance of about 0.7° of the fovea (see Fig. 6.5) [66–70]. Although not present in all subjects, in some of them, the ring had even larger optical density than the central peak [67]. A simple model with an exponentially decaying density as a function of eccentricity, in combination with a Gaussian distributed ring pattern yields a good description of the data. The peak MPOD as well as the prominence of the ring seems to be independent of age [67, 71, 72]. Further, the spatial profile of MPOD seems also to be related to an individual's foveal architecture. Liew et al. [73] and van der Veen et al. [74] found a positive correlation between foveal thickness and MPOD. However, Kanis et al. [75] and Nolan et al. [76] did not confirm these findings. The discrepancy in the findings may in part be due to a different measurement procedure, i.e., using the mean value of six radial OCT scans, instead of taking their minimal value [74]. Other biometric

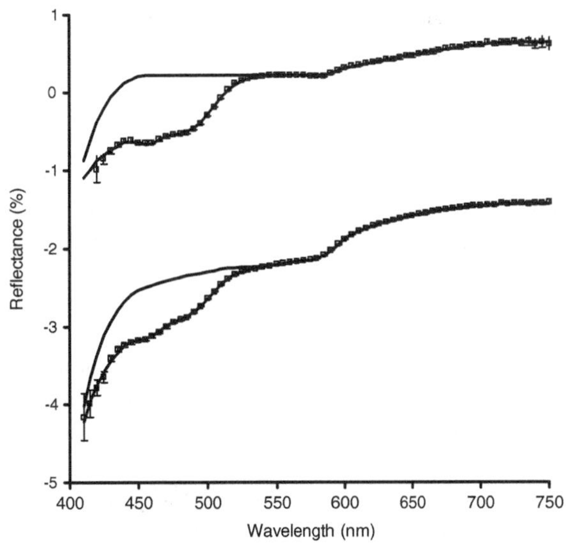

Fig. 6.5 Spectral distribution of the foveal reflection for a young subject (age 20, upper panel) and a middle-aged subject (age 55, middle panel). The squares represent measurements. The solid lines are model fits: one with all parameters optimized and another in which the macular pigment optical density (MPOD) is set to zero and with all other parameters identical as in the fit

parameters do not correlate with MPOD [77]. We have already mentioned that the MPOD can be modified by diet or supplementation (See also next section). Most of the modification studies mentioned earlier measured only the peak MPOD. A recent supplementation study in rhesus monkeys, however, stated that the increase in MPOD was substantially higher in the periphery than in the central fovea [78], which may or may not depend on the supplementation of lutein or zeaxanthin. The clinical relevance of this finding is still in debate.

In most of the retinal degenerations, the spatial profile of the MPOD resembles that of the healthy subjects (see Fig. 6.4). However, patients with macular telangiectasia type 2 have a distribution that seems to be unique for this disease, namely a reduction of MPOD within the central retina with a surrounding ring-like structure of preserved MPOD at about 6° eccentricity [79–81]. It may be due to an inability to accumulate MP in the central retina.

6.1.4 Modifying the Macular Pigment

Humans are unable to synthesize carotenoids, but make extensive use of them by transforming and transporting them to serve a variety of functions. Serum levels of lutein and zeaxanthin are therefore dependent upon the dietary intake. Serum levels associated with the normal diet are far below the maximal levels achieved by supplementation. The normal Western diet contains 1.3–3 mg/day of lutein and zeaxanthin combined [82]. The highest concentration of lutein is found in food sources with yellow color, such as corn and egg yolk. Dark, leafy green vegetables, such as spinach and kale, are also good sources of lutein. Orange peppers, followed by egg yolk, corn, and orange juice also serve as good sources for zeaxanthin [83–86]. In general, fruit and vegetables contain 7–10 times more lutein than zeaxanthin. Meso-zeaxanthin is virtually nonexistent in food sources originating from plants.

Lutein serum levels and the amount of MP correlate, in particular, in men [87–91]. It has further been shown that MP optical density (MPOD) can be increased by a dietary modification [82, 92–94] or by supplements [56, 78, 89, 95–106] in healthy subjects as well as in subjects with a diseased macula [107, 108]. Note that meso-zeaxanthin is primarily formed in the retina following conversion from lutein [11, 109]. Since MP may protect against AMD, this opens the road for an easy intervention.

6.1.5 MPOD and Age

The association between age and MPOD has been studied with all the different techniques to determine the MPOD (for details see below). Most studies that used heterochromatic flickerphotometry found no age effect: Werner et al. [110] ($n = 50$, aged 10–90 years), Hammond et al. [66] ($n = 10$, aged 21–63 years), Delori et al. [111] ($n = 159$, aged 16–80 years), Ciulla et al. [112] ($n = 280$, aged 18–50 years), Mellerio et al. [113] ($n = 124$, aged 18–84 years), and Ciulla and Hammond [72] ($n = 390$, aged 18–90). The latter study included even subjects with cataracts and AMD. Only Hammond et al. [114] ($n = 217$, aged 18–92 years) and Beatty et al. [40] ($n = 46$, aged 21–81 years) found a small decline in MPOD with age using HFP. Also Nolan et al. [115] ($n = 100$, aged 20–60) found a small decrease with age. However, after correction of body fat, the significance of the relationship persisted only in males.

In another study, Nolan et al. assessed MPOD every month for 24 consecutive months in four healthy subjects aged between 23 and 51 years. They concluded that fluctuations in serum concentrations of lutein and zeaxanthin, in the absence of dietary modification or supplementation, are associated with stable MP optical density [116]. Using color matching as another psychophysical technique, Davies et al. [117] ($n = 34$, aged 20–65 years) found no age effect either.

Delori et al., using fundus reflectance in 159 subjects, found a 17% higher MPOD for older subjects (aged 65–80) than for younger subjects, aged 15–30 years [111]. Analyzing the MP spatial distribution, Chen et al. found no change in the peak optical density in 54 subjects aged 20–84 years [118], and neither did Wüstemeyer et al. in 109 subjects. From Zagers et al.'s data of 38 subjects, where the directional reflectance method was used, there was no change in MPOD with age [119, 120]. Figure 6.6 shows MPOD as a function of age obtained in three different studies using fundus reflectance spectroscopy [121]. The upper panel shows data from a cross-sectional study on 376 volunteers aged 18–75 years [87]. There is no correlation with age ($r = 0.037$, $p = 0.47$). The middle panel depict data of 435 subjects, aged 55 and over taken from a random population-based study [42] showing a small, but significant increase with age ($r = 0.14$, $\beta = 0.004$, $p = 0.002$). No age effect was found in data on 138 healthy subjects aged 18–76 years presented in the lower panel ($r = 0.058$, $p = 0.50$).

Using autofluorescence, Delori et al. [111] found no relationship with age in 159 subjects, aged 16–80 years. Jahn et al. [122] found a weak negative correlation in AMD subjects ($n = 146$, aged 50–88 years). Berendschot and van Norren compared several techniques (reflectance spectroscopy, AF, HFP) in a study that was aimed at studying the age effect and found no such age effect.

High performance liquid chromatography (HPLC) has been employed to study age effects in donor eyes. Both, Bone et al. [9] ($n = 87$, range 3–95 years) and Handelman et al. [123] ($n = 16$, range 1 week–81 years)

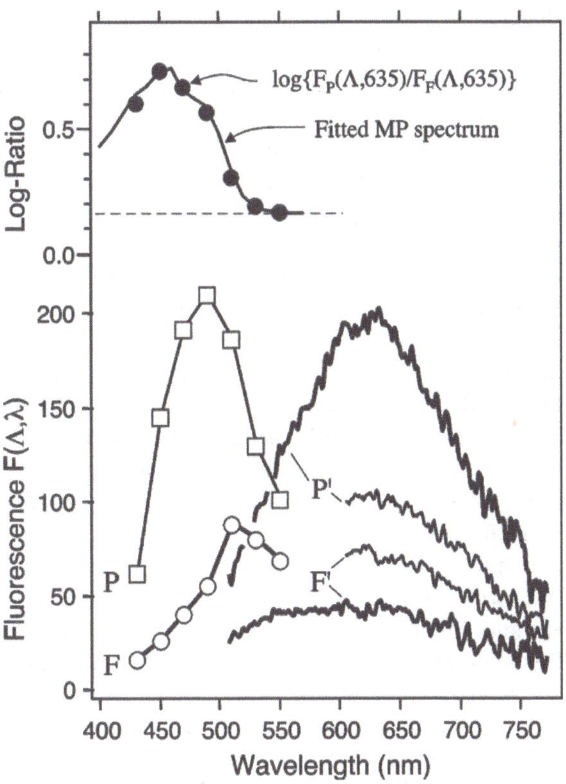

Fig. 6.6 Autofluorescence excitation spectra for the fovea (F, open circles) and for a site at 7° temporal to the fovea (P, open squares) in a 32-year old man. Excitation spectra represent the mean fluorescence intensity in 620–650 nm band as a function of the excitation wavelength λ (430, 450, 470, 490, 510, 530, and 550 nm); only emission spectra at the fovea (F′) and perifovea (P′) for both Λ = 470 nm (thick lines) and Λ = 550 nm (thin lines) excitation are shown for clarity. Fluorescence is expressed in nJnm^{-1}sr^{-1}/J. Top left: log-ratio spectrum of perifoveal to foveal fluorescence (filled circles) and fitted MP spectrum. Reprinted with permission of Archives of Biochemistry and Biophysics

found no age effect. Bone et al., in another study comparing donor eyes with and without AMD, found a slight increase with age in 56 donor eyes of healthy subjects, aged 58–98 years [43].

Studies using Raman spectroscopy initially showed a strong decrease with age [124–126]. This seemed strange in view of the results from all other methods. A number of possible causes like aberrations, scatter, and fixation were discussed extensively in eLetters and their replies [127–130]. In the end, the most important parameter seems to be pupil size. If eyes for which pupil diameter smaller than 7 mm are excluded, the age-related decline vanishes to nonsignificance [131]. Taken together, most studies found no age effect; a few found either a slight decrease or a slight increase. This makes us to conclude that the relationship between age and MPOD, if any, is marginal.

Summary for the Clinician

- The yellow spot, or macula lutea, in the center of the retina is caused by the presence of the so-called macula pigment (MP). Its absorption has its peak at the center of the fovea and decreases rapidly with eccentricity.
- The MP consists of the carotenoids lutein and zeaxanthin. In the central 0–2.3 mm region, zeaxanthin predominates over lutein, whereas for eccentricities beyond this region, lutein is the major carotenoid.
- Many benefits have been ascribed to the MP like reducing the consequences of chromatic aberration, minimize stray light, preservation of visual sensitivity, improving glare disability, and photostress recovery. However, from a clinical point of view, the most important is its possible role in the prevention of age-related macular degeneration.
- Plausible arguments to assume that MP indeed exerts a protective effect in the retinal area are:
  - MP acts as a blue light filter, thereby decreasing chances for photochemical light damage.
  - MP is capable of scavenging free radicals.
  - Lutein is capable of suppressing inflammation.
- The MP optical density (MPOD) seems to be independent of age, but can be increased by dietary modification or supplementation with lutein or zeaxanthin.

6.2 Measurement Techniques

There are several ways to determine the MPOD. The most widespread are the psychophysical techniques, where the subject adjusts color or luminosity, generally through a minimum flicker, or a minimum motion task [132–134]. The second, more objective approach is through analysis of light returning from the retina. It relies either on spectral analysis [121, 135], autofluorescence [136], or on Raman spectroscopy [124].

6.2.1 Heterochromatic Flickerphotometry

The most common method is heterochromatic flickerphotometry (HFP). Here, measurement of the MPOD is accomplished using a stimulus that alternates between a test wavelength that is absorbed by the MP (blue, around 460 nm) and a reference wavelength that is not absorbed (green, around 540 nm). Flicker observed by the subject is reduced to a null point by adjusting the intensity of the former, while viewing the stimulus centrally, and then peripherally, where the MP is assumed to be absent. A higher intensity of the blue component of the stimulus is needed under central viewing conditions owing to attenuation by the MP. The MPOD is then derived by taking the logarithm of the ratio between blue and green luminance measured centrally and peripherally. Bone et al. [137] noted that the luminosity function may differ between fovea and parafovea. Therefore, one should probably account for an additional (small) correction factor when determining MPOD with flicker-based methods. The psychophysical approach has the advantage of requiring no special measures like pupil dilatation or head fixation. However, a complete measurement is rather time consuming, and the task, in particular, when making a match in the peripheral retina, is not trivial. Nevertheless, it has been proven to be a reliable method [134, 138, 139], also in the elderly, if a proper setup and measurement protocol is employed [140].

6.2.2 Fundus reflectance

Using fundus reflectance spectroscopy, MPOD can be determined either through comparison of the reflection at the macular region and peripheral region, where the MPOD can be assumed to be negligible [111], or by a spectral analysis of the reflected light [121].

Figure 6.7 is an example of a comparison between a foveal and a peripheral site. At the bottom of the graph, the log ratio of these two spectra is drawn, clearly showing the macular pigment fingerprint. Using the known spectral absorption of the macular pigment, the solid line shows a best fit to this Log ratio spectrum to the MPOD on an offset. Figure 6.8 shows the spectral distribution of the foveal reflection for a young subject (age 20, upper panel) and a middle-aged subject (age 55, middle panel). Using known spectral characteristics of the different absorbers within the eye, the densities of the pigments and the percent reflectance at the interfaces were optimized to fit the measured data at all wavelengths. The solid lines in Fig. 6.8 result from this model analysis. Also shown is a model spectrum with the MPOD set to zero and all other parameters identical as in the fit. A big hurdle in fundus reflectance spectroscopy is the presence of stray-light may. Reflectance at the cornea and lens greatly exceed the reflectance of the fundus, due to the rather large changes in refractive indices [141]. In most of the experimental setups, this problem is alleviated by careful separation of entrance pupil and exit pupil. Although reflectance at the nerve fiber layer, in principle, may be rather high [142–144], in the fovea this layer is nearly absent, and its reflectance can be neglected. A final, small contribution to the stray light caused by vitreous backscatter and reflectance at the inner limiting membrane is hard to avoid. Rather low-mean MPOD compared with others found by Bour et al. [145], Wüstemeyer et al. [146], and Chen et al. [118] were probably caused by this pre-retinal

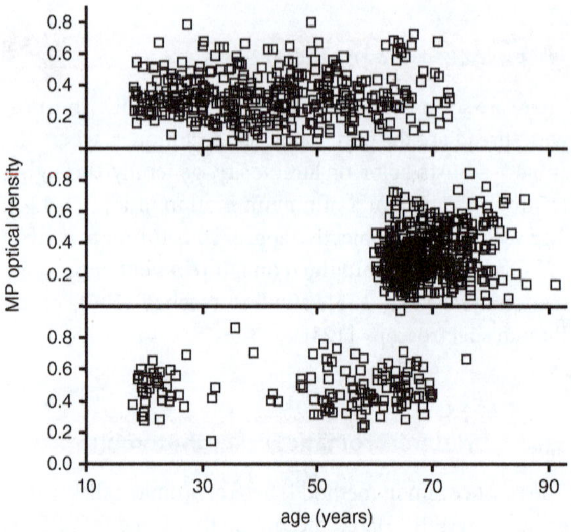

Fig. 6.7 Macular pigment optical density as a function of age obtained in three different studies using fundus reflectance spectroscopy. Reprinted with permission of Archives of Biochemistry and Biophysics

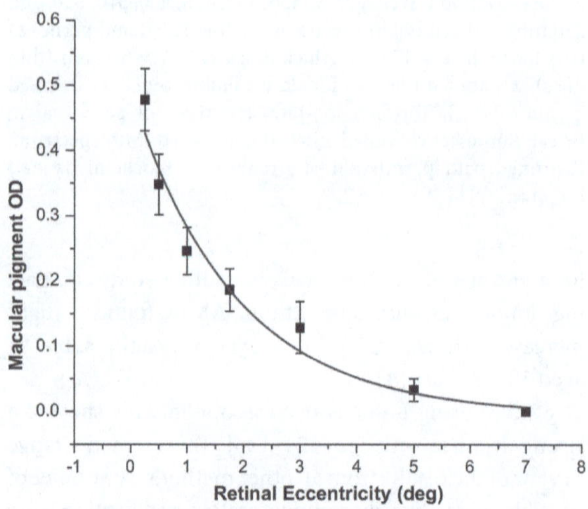

Fig. 6.8 Mean macular pigment optical density (MPOD) as a function of eccentricity for 19 patients with age related macular degeneration (AMD), determined with heterochromatic flicker-photometry (HFP). At 7° eccentricity MP is assumed to be absent. This point is taken as a reference. The smooth line is a least-squares fit with an exponential decaying function with eccentricity. Error bars represent standard error of the mean. Reprinted with permission of Experimental Eye Research

and intra-retinal scatter. Delori et al. also had some remaining stray light that could explain his somewhat lower MPOD results. The use of the model analysis described earlier has the advantage that stray light can be incorporated. An elegant way to fully circumvent the latter sources of stray light is to only use the directional component of the reflected light [147, 148], since it will not show a directional dependence. Another advantage of the spectral analysis, compared with the comparison method and also with psychophysical methods, is the absence of a reference spectrum at a peripheral retinal location. The spatial extent of the macular pigment may exceed the 6° or even 8° eccentricity commonly used, which leads to an underestimate of the MPOD if these sites are used as a zero reference. For a detailed discussion on the spectral analysis, see van de Kraats et al. [149, 150]. Most setups for fundus reflectance require pupil dilation. However, the Macular Pigment Reflectometer can do without it [151]. A very recent improvement has been the ability to measure in vivo lutein and zeaxanthin separately [61], based on the fact that between 500 and 520 nm the parallel slopes of the extinction spectra of lutein and zeaxanthin differ about 10 nm (see Fig. 6.2).

6.2.3 Autofluorescence

Noninvasive measurement of the optical density of the human macular pigment by the autofluorescence (AF) method takes advantage of the fluorescence of lipofuscin in the human retinal pigment epithelium (RPE) cells [111]. Fundus AF is dominated by the AF of lipofuscin that accumulates throughout life in the RPE, as a result of phagocytosis of the photoreceptors' outer membranes [152]. The AF is emitted in the 520–800 nm spectral range and can be excited in the 400 and 590 nm spectral range [153]. This excitation range is broader than the absorption range of MP [6, 34], which makes it possible to excite lipofuscin without substantial absorption by MP. Thus, measuring the intensity of fluorescence above 550 nm, where macular pigment has essentially zero absorption, and stimulating the fluorescence with two wavelengths, one well absorbed by macular pigment and the other minimally absorbed by macular pigment, provides a single-pass measurement of the macular pigment optical density [136]. Figure 6.9 shows AF excitation spectra for the fovea and for a site at 7° temporal to the fovea and the MPOD spectrum, determined by the log-ratio of perifoveal to foveal AF.

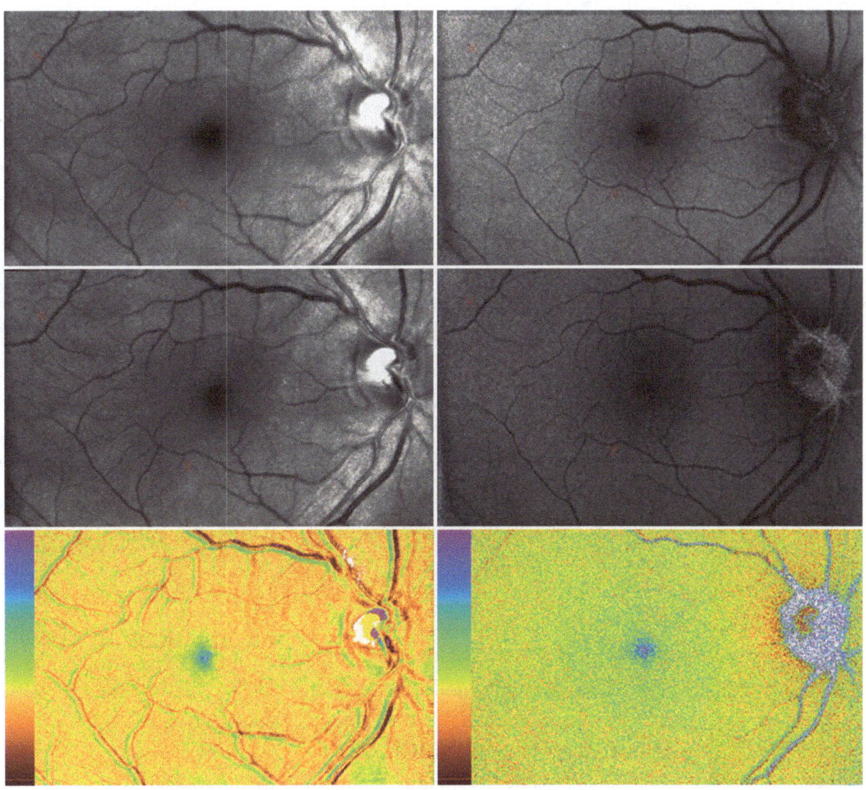

Fig. 6.9 Reflectance (left) and autofluorescence maps (right) at a wavelength of 488 nm (top) and 514 nm (middle). The lower images show the corresponding color coded macular pigment optical density (MPOD) maps. Reprinted with permission of Investigative Ophthalmology and Visual Science

6.2.4 Raman spectroscopy

Elastic scattering of light, i.e., the scattered ray has the same wavelength as the incoming ray, is very common. However, in some cases, in addition a small portion of the incident light is scattered inelastically, i.e., at longer or shorter wavelengths. This process is known as Raman scattering [154]. The light frequency shifts correspond to the vibrational energies of the molecules at which the light scatters. It can be used to obtain specific optical fingerprint spectrum of molecules. In general, Raman spectroscopy in biological systems yields quite complex spectra because of the wide variety of chemical compounds present. Moreover, these spectral peaks tend to be of weak intensity, because only a small proportion of the scattered light is Raman shifted. However, under certain situations when the incident light overlaps with a molecule's major absorption band, if the molecule is Raman active, and if there is no interfering fluorescence, the Raman signals can be resonantly enhanced by many orders of magnitude. In particular, carotenoids have intense absorption bands in the blue/green wavelength range that result in large resonant enhancements [124]. Fortunately, no other biological molecules found in significant concentrations in human ocular tissues exhibit similar resonant enhancement with blue laser excitation. This makes the in vivo carotenoid Raman spectra remarkably free from confounding responses. Bernstein et al. have shown that this technique can be used to measure the MP in vivo in the human eye [155–157]. Although there were some concerns about this technique [127–130, 158, 159], it seems to give reliable results that compare well with HFP, provided a proper protocol is used [131].

6.2.5 How do different techniques compare

All techniques have been shown to correlate well. However, correlation analyses only reveal the strength of relation between techniques but they do not necessarily reveal agreement in an absolute sense. In fact, it is unlikely that different methods will agree quantitatively, since they use different principles and probe different retinal areas. Indeed, systematic, but explainable differences between different methods are observed [71, 102, 111, 131, 134, 160–163]. For instance, optical technique probes a retinal area and provides MPOD estimates averaged over this particular area. Further, because of its spatial peakedness, the size of the retinal field probed has a major effect. This contrasts with HFP, in which subjects make their judgment as to the absence/presence of flicker at the edge of the flickering target. As a result in HFP, MPOD will be biased toward lower values [110, 111, 164–166].

Summary for the Clinician

- There are psychophysical and optical techniques to determine the MPOD, which give reliable results.
- The most widespread are the psychophysical techniques, where the subject adjusts color or luminosity, generally through a minimum flicker task. The advantage of these approaches is that there is no need for pupil dilation. A disadvantage is that they are rather time consuming, and the task, in particular, when making a match in the peripheral retina, is not trivial.
- There are several optical approaches to obtain the MPOD. They all rely on the analysis of light returning from the retina, either on spectral analysis, autofluorescence (AF), or on Raman spectroscopy. The advantage of these techniques is their more objective approach and measuring time. A disadvantage for some setups (but not all) is that they require pupil dilation. Moreover, not all are commercially available.
- All the techniques have been shown to correlate well. However, they do not reveal agreement in an absolute sense. Since different methods probe the MP differently, systematic, but explainable differences are observed. Therefore, in longitudinal studies an individual should stick to one and the same method.
- For all methods, a proper setup and protocol should be used to avoid measurement errors like the use of improper frequencies in heterochromatic flicker photometry, or the influence of stray light in reflectance spectroscopy or the influence of pupil width in resonant Raman spectroscopy.

6.3 Imaging

All techniques described earlier started off to have MPOD estimates over a well-defined retinal area. In most of the cases, this has been 1° field. To measure the spatial extent of the MP, setups have been developed for imaging a wider area and with a finer spatial resolution.

6.3.1 Heterochromatic Flickerphotometry

Using HFP it is time-consuming to measure the full spatial distribution of the MP. The reason for this is twofold. First, the stimulus, i.e., the target that the subjects have to reduce to a null point, needs a finite size. Second, as already mentioned, the method is rather time-consuming (about 30 min for 6 eccentricities [167]). This may be a limiting factor for both large epidemiological trials and a clinical setting. Nevertheless, some studies have been presented with a low spatial solution. Hammond et al. were the first to study the spatial profile by HFP in normal subjects at 0, 0.5, 1, 2, 3, and 4° and a reference point at 5.5° [66]. Stringham et al. measured patients with intermediate stages of age-related macular degeneration (AMD) [167]. Patients with visual acuity as poor as 20/80 were included. MPOD was measured at 15′, 30′, 1°, 1.5°, 3°, and 5° along the horizontal meridian and a reference location at 7° eccentricity (see Fig. 6.4). Spatial profiles of MPOD were similar to those that have been measured with HFP in subjects without retinal disease. Nolan et al. measured MPOD at eccentricities of 0.25, 0.5, 1, 1.75, 3, and 5° along the horizontal meridian relative to a reference location at 7° eccentricity and looked for correlations with foveal architecture (see above) [76].

6.3.2 Fundus Reflectance

The technique of comparing the reflection at the macular region and at a peripheral region can be exploited to obtain MPOD maps. The most common method is the use of a Scanning Laser Ophthalmoscope (SLO) with 488 and 514 nm Argon laser wavelengths to obtain fundus reflectance maps [67, 81, 95, 121, 146, 168, 169]. Since the lens and the macular pigment are the only absorbers in this wavelength region, digital subtraction at these two wavelengths of log reflectance can provide density maps of the sum of both absorbers. MPOD is assumed to be negligible at a peripheral site. If this site is used to provide an estimate for the lens density, the mean MPOD at the fovea can be calculated [95, 168]. Figure 6.10 shows an example of these maps and the resulting MPOD map. Using this technique, the MPOD spatial can be imaged easily and with a high resolution. It allowed the quantification of a ring-like structure on top of the decreasing function with eccentricity as discussed earlier (see Fig. 6.5) [67]. A confocal setup, like the SLO is necessary to obtain reliable results. Attempts to use a fundus camera yielded rather low MPOD values, probably due to stray light [118, 145].

6.3.3 Autofluorescence

The most widespread method to obtain a detailed MPOD is using AF, probably because of the availability of commercial devices to do so. Like in fundus reflectance, here AF maps are made at different wavelengths, and a MPOD map is created by digital subtraction of the two log AF maps. Because of the low signal-to-noise ratio in AF maps, in general, several AF images are averaged, whereas in reflectance image a single image suffices. However, image registration algorithms are well developed and images can be aligned easily. Using this approach, a high spatial resolution can be achieved and many studies have been published, both in normal subjects and in patients with different diseases of the retina.[7, 67, 70, 71, 73, 81, 108, 146]. Figure 6.10 shows an example of autofluorescence maps at 488 and 514 nm and the resulting MPOD map. The AF image at 488 nm is substantially brighter than the one at 514 nm. The AF method uses the intrinsic fluorescence of the lipofuscin with its absorption peak at 490 nm. This makes the 488 nm more efficient than the 514 nm excitation. Further, in this particular setup, the filters to capture the AF had a cut-off wavelength of 510 nm for the blue excitation and a cut-off wavelength for the green excitation. As a result, more fluorescence was captured from

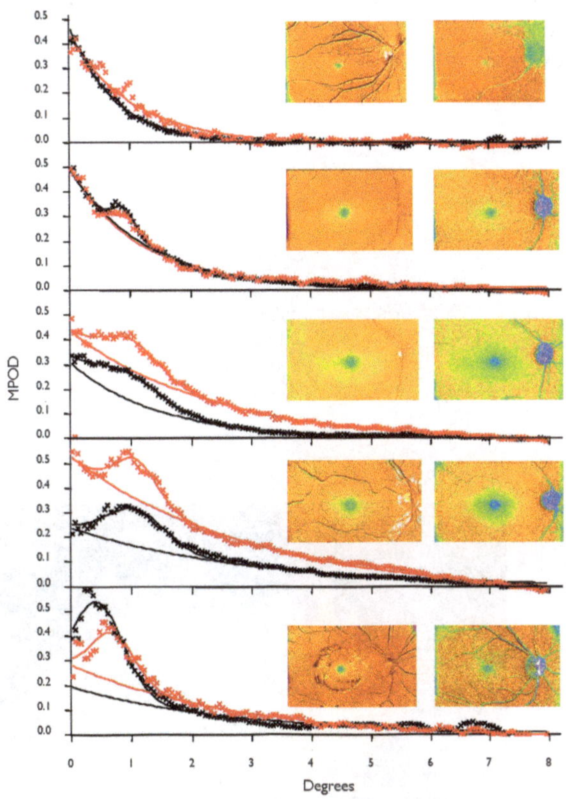

Fig. 6.10 Macular pigment optical density (MPOD) as a function of eccentricity from reflectance (black) and autofluorescence (red) maps. MPOD maps obtained from reflectance (left) and autofluorescence (right) are shown as insets. The MPOD distribution was assumed to be circularly symmetric and MPOD was determined as a function of eccentricity by calculating for each pixel the distance to the peak. Solid lines: results of a model fits. Reprinted with permission of Investigative Ophthalmology and Visual Science

the 488 nm excitation than from the 514 excitation. Finally, the voltage of the photomultiplier tube may differ between the two wavelengths. All these phenomena may result in an apparent difference in gain between the 488 and 514 nm maps. However, MPOD maps are obtained by digital subtraction at two wavelengths of log AF, which implies only an offset in the MPOD map. Analyzing the MPOD maps, it is assumed that the MPOD essentially vanishes at 8°; thus, at this point the optical density is defined to be zero. Figure 6.5 shows MPOD as a function of eccentricity obtained from AF maps by Berendschot et al. [67] showing the same ring-like structure as in those obtained from reflectance maps. Similar MPOD maps from AF images were obtained independently by Delori et al. [180] and Wolf-Schnurrbusch et al. [181].

Some studies only measured AF maps at 488 nm, without a reference measurement at a wavelength that is not absorbed by the MP [70, 174, 182,]. Here, the observed MPOD map may be diluted by varying lipofuscin and melanin concentrations as a function of eccentricity, the exact shape of which is unknown. It makes these results difficult to interpret [183].

6.3.4 Raman spectroscopy

Resonant Raman spectroscopy has also become available in imaging mode [125], even without the need of pupil dilation [184]. Using laser excitation of lutein and zeaxanthin at 488 nm, and sequential camera detection of light emitted back from the retina at the strongest Raman peak position and at an off-peak position, resonant Raman maps of MP are determined (See Fig. 6.11). The resolution of these maps allows the determination of fine structures like the rings seen by fundus reflectance and AF maps (see Fig. 6.12) [184].

Summary for the Clinician

- Both psychophysical and optical techniques can be used to map the spatial distribution of the MP. Psychophysical techniques are rather time-consuming in measuring the MPOD spatial profile, and still have a rather low resolution (about 30 min for 6 eccentricities only). Optical techniques are more suited since they can produce MPOD maps with a high resolution within minutes.

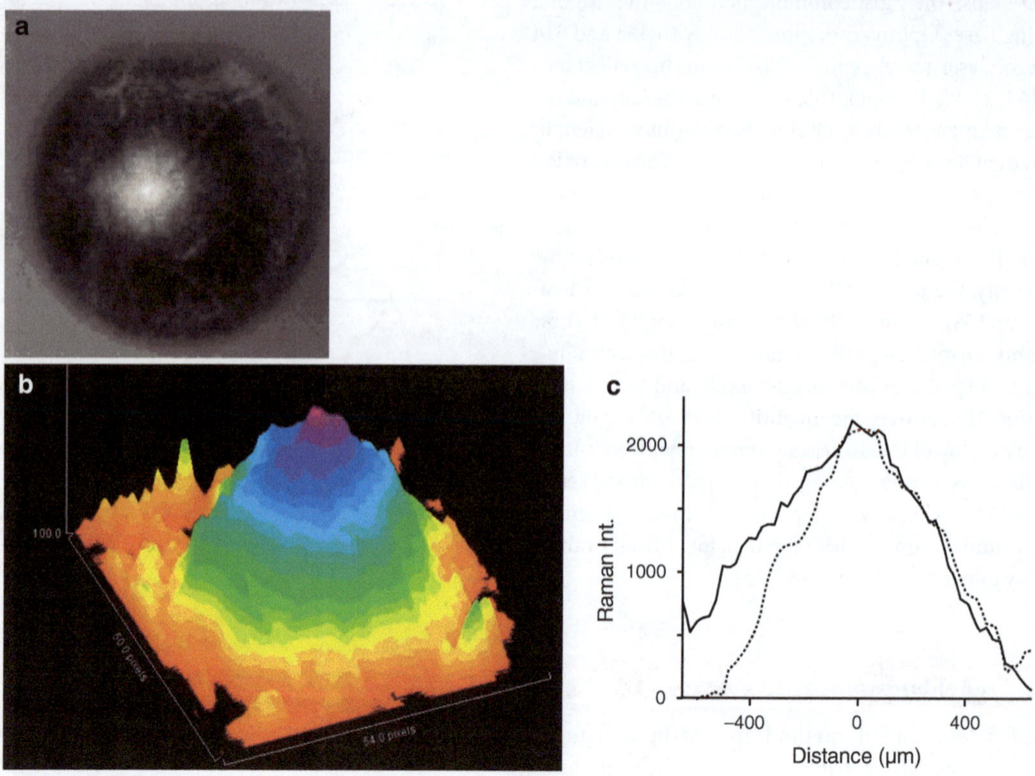

Fig. 6.11 Spatial distribution of the MP determined by resonant Raman imaging. (**a**) Gray-scale image obtained after subtraction of fluorescence background from pixel intensity map containing Raman response and superimposed fluorescence background. (**b**) Pseudocolor-scaled, three-dimensional representation of gray-scale image. (**c**) Line plots along nasal–temporal (*solid curve*) and inferior–superior meridians (*dashed curve*), both running through the center of the MP distribution. Reprinted with permission from the *Journal of the Optical Society of America A*

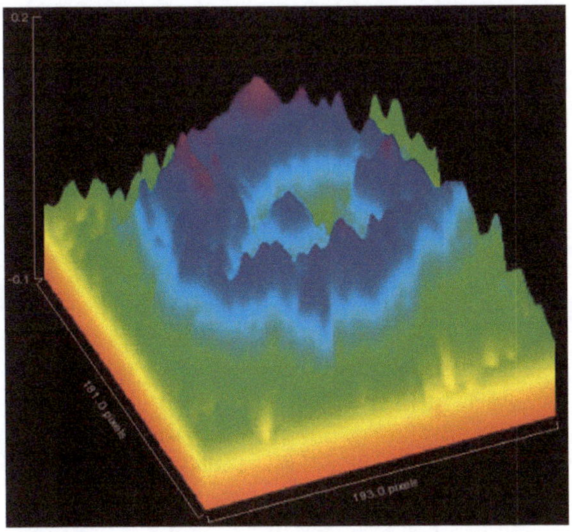

Fig. 6.12 MP map determined by resonant Raman imaging showing a ring-like distribution with central spike. Reprinted with permission from the *Journal of the Optical Society of America A*

References

1. Buzzi F (1782) Nuovo sperienze fatte sull' occhio umano. Opuscoli scelti di Milano 5:87
2. Soemmering S (1799) De Foramine Centralis limbo luteo cincto retinae humane. Soc Reg Sic Goetting 13:3
3. Gullstrand F (1906) Die farbe der Macula centralis retinae. Graefes Arch Clin Exp Ophthalmol 62:1–72
4. Nordenson JW (1958) Neue Argumente zur der Frage der Makulafarbe. Graefes Arch Clin Exp Ophthalmol 160:43–46
5. Snodderly DM, Auran JD, Delori FC (1984) The macular pigment. II. Spatial distribution in primate retinas. Invest Ophthalmol Vis Sci 25:674–685
6. Snodderly DM, Brown PK, Delori FC, Auran JD (1984) The macular pigment. I. Absorbance spectra, localization, and discrimination from other yellow pigments in primate retinas. Invest Ophthalmol Vis Sci 25:660–673
7. Trieschmann M, van Kuijk FJ, Alexander R, Hermans P, Luthert P, Bird AC, Pauleikhoff D (2008) Macular pigment in the human retina: histological evaluation of localization and distribution. Eye 22:132–137
8. Wald G (1945) Human vision and the spectrum. Science 101:653–658
9. Bone RA, Landrum JT, Fernandez L, Tarsis SL (1988) Analysis of the macular pigment by HPLC: retinal distribution and age study. Invest Ophthalmol Vis Sci 29: 843–849
10. Bone RA, Landrum JT, Tarsis SL (1985) Preliminary identification of the human macular pigment. Vision Res 25:1531–1535
11. Bone RA, Landrum JT, Hime GW, Cains A, Zamor J (1993) Stereochemistry of the human macular carotenoids. Invest Ophthalmol Vis Sci 34:2033–2040
12. Handelman GJ, Snodderly DM, Krinsky NI, Russett MD, Adler AJ (1991) Biological control of primate macular pigment. Biochemical and densitometric studies. Invest Ophthalmol Vis Sci 32:257–267
13. Engles M, Wooten B, Hammond B (2007) Macular pigment: a test of the acuity hypothesis. Invest Ophthalmol Vis Sci 48:2922–2931
14. McLellan JS, Marcos S, Prieto PM, Burns SA (2002) Imperfect optics may be the eye's defence against chromatic blur. Nature 417:174–176
15. Schultze M (1866) Zur Anatomie und Physiologie der Retina. Arch Mickrosk Anat 2:165–286
16. Wooten BR, Hammond BR (2002) Macular pigment: influences on visual acuity and visibility. Prog Retin Eye Res 21:225–240
17. Hammond BR, Wooten BR, Snodderly DM (1998) Preservation of visual sensitivity of older subjects: association with macular pigment density. Invest Ophthalmol Vis Sci 39:397–406
18. Stringham JM, Hammond BR Jr (2007) The glare hypothesis of macular pigment function. Optom Vis Sci 84:859–864
19. Stringham JM, Hammond BR (2008) Macular pigment and visual performance under glare conditions. Optom Vis Sci 85:82–88
20. Weale RA (2007) Guest editorial: notes on the macular pigment. Ophthalmic Physiol Opt 27:1–10
21. Seddon JM, Ajani UA, Sperduto RD, Hiller R, Blair N, Burton TC, Farber MD, Gragoudas ES, Haller J, Miller DT; Eye Disease Case-Control Study Group (1994) Dietary carotenoids, vitamins A, C, and E, and advanced age-related macular degeneration. JAMA 272:1413–1420
22. Davies NP, Morland AB (2004) Macular pigments: their characteristics and putative role. Prog Retin Eye Res 23:533–559
23. Attebo K, Mitchell P, Smith W (1996) Visual acuity and the causes of visual loss in Australia. The Blue Mountains Eye Study. Ophthalmology 103:357–364
24. Klaver CC, Wolfs RC, Vingerling JR, Hofman A, de Jong PTVM (1998) Age-specific prevalence and causes of blindness and visual impairment in an older population: the Rotterdam Study. Arch Ophthalmol 116:653–658
25. Tielsch JM, Javitt JC, Coleman A, Katz J, Sommer A (1995) The prevalence of blindness and visual impairment among nursing home residents in Baltimore. N Engl J Med 332:1205–1209
26. Bandello F, Lafuma A, Berdeaux G (2007) Public health impact of neovascular age-related macular degeneration treatments extrapolated from visual acuity. Invest Ophthalmol Vis Sci 48:96–103
27. Covert D, Berdeaux G, Mitchell J, Bradley C, Barnes R (2007) Quality of life and health economic assessments of age-related macular degeneration. Surv Ophthalmol 52: S20–S25

28. Cruess A, Zlateva G, Xu X, Rochon S (2007) Burden of illness of neovascular age-related macular degeneration in Canada. Can J Ophthalmol 42
29. Gupta OP, Brown GC, Brown MM (2007) Age-related macular degeneration: the costs to society and the patient. [Miscellaneous]. Curr Opin Ophthalmol 18:201–205
30. Marback RF, Maia Junior OD, Morais FB, Takahashi WY (2007) Quality of life in patients with age-related macular degeneration with monocular and binocular legal blindness. Clinics 62:573–578
31. Soubrane G, Cruess A, Lotery A, Pauleikhoff D, Mones J, Xu X, Zlateva G, Buggage R, Conlon J, Goss TF (2007) Burden and health care resource utilization in neovascular age-related macular degeneration: findings of a multicountry study. Arch Ophthalmol 125:1249–1254
32. Evans JR (2007) Primary prevention of age related macular degeneration. BMJ 335:729
33. Bone RA, Landrum JT, Cains A (1992) Optical density spectra of the macular pigment in vivo and in vitro. Vision Res 32:105–110
34. DeMarco P, Pokorny J, Smith VC (1992) Full-spectrum cone sensitivity functions for X-chromosome-linked anomalous trichromats. J Opt Soc Am A 9:1465–1476
35. Sharpe LT, Stockman A, Knau H, Jägle H (1998) Macular pigment densities derived from central and peripheral spectral sensitivity differences. Vision Res 38:3233–3239
36. Vos JJ (1972) Literature review of human macular absorption in the visible and its consequence for the cone receptor primaries. Report Institute for Perception TNO 17
37. Landrum JT, Bone RA, Kilburn MD (1997) The macular pigment: a possible role in protection from age-related macular degeneration. Adv Pharmacol 38:537–556
38. Khachik F, Bernstein PS, Garland DL (1997) Identification of lutein and zeaxanthin oxidation products in human and monkey retinas. Invest Ophthalmol Vis Sci 38:1802–1811
39. Izumi-Nagai K, Nagai N, Ohgami K, Satofuka S, Ozawa Y, Tsubota K, Umezawa K, Ohno S, Oike Y, Ishida S (2007) Macular pigment lutein is antiinflammatory in preventing choroidal neovascularization. Arterioscler Thromb Vasc Biol 27:2555–2562
40. Beatty S, Murray IJ, Henson DB, Carden D, Koh H, Boulton ME (2001) Macular pigment and risk for age-related macular degeneration in subjects from a Northern European population. Invest Ophthalmol Vis Sci 42: 439–446
41. Beatty S, Stevenson M, Nolan JM, Woodside J, Chakravarthy U; The CARMA Study Group (2009) Longitudinal relationships between macular pigment and serum lutein in patients enrolled in the CARMA Clinical Trial (carotenoids and co-antioxidants in age-related maculopathy). Invest Ophthalmol Vis Sci 50:1719
42. Berendschot TTJM, Willemse-Assink JJM, Bastiaanse M, de Jong PTVM, van Norren D (2002) Macular pigment and melanin in age-related maculopathy in a general population. Invest Ophthalmol Vis Sci 43:1928–1932
43. Bone RA, Landrum JT, Mayne ST, Gomez CM, Tibor SE, Twaroska EE (2001) Macular pigment in donor eyes with and without AMD: a case-control study. Invest Ophthalmol Vis Sci 42:235–240
44. Carpentier S, Knaus M, Suh M (2009) Associations between lutein, zeaxanthin, and age-related macular degeneration: an overview. Crit Rev Food Sci Nutr 49:313–326
45. Cho E, Seddon JM, Rosner B, Willett WC, Hankinson SE (2004) Prospective study of intake of fruits, vegetables, vitamins, and carotenoids and risk of age-related maculopathy. Arch Ophthalmol 122:883–892
46. Chong EWT, Wong TY, Kreis AJ, Simpson JA, Guymer RH (2007) Dietary antioxidants and primary prevention of age related macular degeneration: systematic review and meta-analysis. BMJ 335:755–763
47. Delcourt C, Carriere I, Delage M, Barberger-Gateau P, Schalch W; The Pola Study Group (2006) Plasma lutein and zeaxanthin and other carotenoids as modifiable risk factors for age-related maculopathy and cataract: The POLA Study. Invest Ophthalmol Vis Sci 47:2329–2335
48. Gale CR, Hall NF, Phillips DI, Martyn CN (2003) Lutein and zeaxanthin status and risk of age-related macular degeneration. Invest Ophthalmol Vis Sci 44:2461–2465
49. Loane E, Kelliher C, Beatty S, Nolan JM (2008) The rationale and evidence base for a protective role of macular pigment in age-related maculopathy. Br J Ophthalmol 92:1163–1168
50. Mares-Perlman JA (1999) Too soon for lutein supplements. Am J Clin Nutr 70:431–432
51. Mares-Perlman JA, Millen AE, Ficek TL, Hankinson SE (2002) The body of evidence to support a protective role for lutein and zeaxanthin in delaying chronic disease. Overview. J Nutr 132:518S–524S
52. Mozaffarieh M, Sacu S, Wedrich A (2003) The role of the carotenoids, lutein and zeaxanthin, in protecting against age-related macular degeneration: a review based on controversial evidence. Nutrition J 2:20
53. Nolan JM, Stack J, O' Donovan O, Loane E, Beatty S (2007) Risk factors for age-related maculopathy are associated with a relative lack of macular pigment. Exp Eye Res 84: 61–74
54. O'Connell ED, Nolan JM, Stack J, Greenberg D, Kyle J, Maddock L, Beatty S (2008) Diet and risk factors for age-related maculopathy. Am J Clin Nutr 87:712–722
55. Richer S, Stiles W, Statkute L, Pulido J, Franskowski J, Rudy D, Pei K, Tsipusrky M, Nyland J (2004) Double-masked, placebo-controlled, randomized trial of lutein and antioxidant supplementation in the intervention of atrophic age-related macular degeneration: the Veterans LAST study (Lutein Antioxidant Supplementation Trial). Optometry 75:216–230

56. Richer S, Devenport J, Lang JC (2007) LAST II: Differential temporal responses of macular pigment optical density in patients with atrophic age-related macular degeneration to dietary supplementation with xanthophylls. Optometry 78:213–219
57. Snellen EL, Verbeek AL, Van Den Hoogen GW, Cruysberg JR, Hoyng CB (2002) Neovascular age-related macular degeneration and its relationship to antioxidant intake. Acta Ophthalmol Scand 80:368–371
58. Tsika CI, Kontadakis G, Makridaki M, Plainis S, Moschandreas J, Pallikaris IG, Tsilimbaris MK (2009) Assessment of macular pigment optical density in patients with unilateral wet Amd. Invest Ophthalmol Vis Sci 50:1720
59. Trumbo PR, Ellwood KC (2006) Lutein and zeaxanthin intakes and risk of age-related macular degeneration and cataracts: an evaluation using the Food and Drug Administration's evidence-based review system for health claims. Am J Clin Nutr 84:971–974
60. Nussbaum JJ, Pruett RC, Delori FC (1981) Historic perspectives. Macular yellow pigment. The first 200 years. Retina 1:296–310
61. van de Kraats J, Kanis MJ, Genders SW, van Norren D (2008) Lutein and zeaxanthin measured separately in the living human retina with fundus reflectometry. Invest Ophthalmol Vis Sci 49:5568–5573
62. Miles WR (1954) Comparison of functional and structural areas in human fovea. I. Method of entoptic plotting. J Neurophysiol 17:22–38
63. Maxwell JC (1856) On the unequal sensibility of the formanen centrale to light of different colours. Rep Brit Ass Adv Sci 2:12
64. Snodderly DM, Handelman GJ, Adler AJ (1991) Distribution of individual macular pigment carotenoids in central retina of macaque and squirrel monkeys. Invest Ophthalmol Vis Sci 32:268–279
65. Bone RA, Landrum JT (1983) Dichroism of lutein: a possible basis for Haidinger's brushes. Appl Opt 22:775–776
66. Hammond BR, Wooten BR, Snodderly DM (1997) Individual variations in the spatial profile of human macular pigment. J Opt Soc Am A 14:1187–1196
67. Berendschot TTJM, van Norren D (2006) Macular pigment shows ringlike structures. Invest Ophthalmol Vis Sci 47:709–714
68. Delori FC, Goger DG, Keilhauer C, Salvetti P, Staurenghi G (2006) Bimodal spatial distribution of macular: evidence of a gender relationship. J Opt Soc Am 23:521–538
69. Kirby ML, Galea M, Loane E, Stack J, Beatty S, Nolan JM (2009) Foveal anatomic associations with the secondary peak and the slope of the macular pigment spatial profile. Invest Ophthalmol Vis Sci 50:1383–1391
70. Trieschmann M, Spital G, Lommatzsch A, van Kuijk E, Fitzke F, Bird AC, Pauleikhoff D (2003) Macular pigment: quantitative analysis on autofluorescence images. Graefes Arch Clin Exp Ophthalmol 241:1006–1012
71. Berendschot TTJM, van Norren D (2005) On the age dependency of the macular pigment optical density. Exp Eye Res 81:602–609
72. Ciulla TA, Hammond JR (2004) Macular pigment density and aging, assessed in the normal elderly and those with cataracts and age-related macular degeneration. Am J Ophthalmol 138:582–587
73. Liew SH, Gilbert CE, Spector TD, Mellerio J, van Kuijk FJ, Beatty S, Fitzke F, Marshall J, Hammond CJ (2006) Central retinal thickness is positively correlated with macular pigment optical density. Exp Eye Res 82:915–920
74. van der Veen RLP, Ostendorf S, Hendrikse F, Berendschot TTJM (2009) Macular pigment optical density relates to foveal thickness. Eur J Ophthalmol 19:836–841
75. Kanis MJ, Berendschot TTJM, van Norren D (2007) Interocular agreement in melanin and macular pigment optical density. Exp Eye Res 84:934–938
76. Nolan JM, Stringham JM, Beatty S, Snodderly DM (2008) Spatial profile of macular pigment and its relationship to foveal architecture. Invest Ophthalmol Vis Sci 49:2134–2142
77. Neelam K, Nolan J, Loane E, Stack J, O'Donovan O, Au Eong KG, Beatty S (2006) Macular pigment and ocular biometry. Vision Res 46:2149–2156
78. Neuringer M, Sandstrom MM, Johnson EJ, Snodderly DM (2004) Nutritional manipulation of primate retinas, i: effects of lutein or zeaxanthin supplements on serum and macular pigment in xanthophyll-free rhesus monkeys. Invest Ophthalmol Vis Sci 45:3234–3243
79. Charbel Issa P, Berendschot TTJM, Staurenghi G, Holz FG, Scholl HP (2008) Confocal blue reflectance imaging in type 2 idiopathic macular telangiectasia. Invest Ophthalmol Vis Sci 49:1172–1177
80. Charbel Issa P, van der Veen RLP, Stijfs A, Holz FG, Scholl HPN, Berendschot TTJM (2009) Quantification of reduced macular pigment optical density in the central retina in macular telangiectasia type 2. Exp Eye Res 89: 25–31
81. Helb HM, Charbel Issa P, van der Veen RLP, Berendschot TTJM, Scholl HP, Holz FG (2008) Abnormal macular pigment distribution in type 2 idiopathic macular telangiectasia. Retina 28:808–816
82. Hammond BR, Johnson EJ, Russell RM, Krinsky NI, Yeum KJ, Edwards RB, Snodderly DM (1997) Dietary modification of human macular pigment density. Invest Ophthalmol Vis Sci 38:1795–1801
83. Granado F, Olmedilla B, Herrero C, Perez-Sacristan B, Blanco I, Blazquez S (2006) Bioavailability of carotenoids and tocopherols from broccoli: in vivo and in vitro assessment. Exp Biol Med 231:1733–1738
84. Maiani G, Periago Caston MJ, Catasta G, Toti E, Cambrodon IG, Bysted A, Granado-Lorencio F, Olmedilla-Alonso B,

Knuthsen P, Valoti M, Bohm V, Mayer-Miebach E, Behsnilian D, Schlemmer U (2009) Carotenoids: actual knowledge on food sources, intakes, stability and bioavailability and their protective role in humans. Mol Nutr Food Res 53:S194–S218
85. Sommerburg O, Keunen JEE, Bird AC, Van Kuijk FJGM (1998) Fruits and vegetables that are sources for lutein and zeaxanthin: the macular pigment in human eyes. Br J Ophthalmol 82:907–910
86. Thurnham DI (2007) Macular zeaxanthins and lutein ? a review of dietary sources and bioavailability and some relationships with macular pigment optical density and age-related macular disease. Nutr Res Rev 20:163–179
87. Broekmans WMR, Berendschot TTJM, Klöpping WA, de Vries AJ, Goldbohm RA, Tijssen CC, Karplus M, van Poppel G (2002) Macular pigment density in relation to serum and adipose tissue concentrations of lutein and serum concentrations of zeaxanthin. Am J Clin Nutr 76: 595–603
88. Johnson EJ, Hammond BR, Yeum KJ, Qin J, Wang XD, Castaneda C, Snodderly DM, Russell RM (2000) Relation among serum and tissue concentrations of lutein and zeaxanthin and macular pigment density. Am J Clin Nutr 71:1555–1562
89. Johnson EJ, Neuringer M, Russell RM, Schalch W, Snodderly DM (2005) Nutritional manipulation of primate retinas, III: effects of lutein or zeaxanthin supplementation on adipose tissue and retina of xanthophyll-free monkeys. Invest Ophthalmol Vis Sci 46:692–702
90. Landrum JT, Bone RA, Chen Y, Herrero C, Llerena CM, Twarowska E (1999) Carotenoids in the human retina. Pure Appl Chem 71:2237–2244
91. Loane E, Beatty S, Nolan JM (2009) The relationship between lutein, zeaxanthin, serum lipoproteins and macular pigment optical density. Invest Ophthalmol Vis Sci 50:1710
92. Burke JD, Curran-Celentano J, Wenzel AJ (2005) Diet and serum carotenoid concentrations affect macular pigment optical density in adults 45 years and older. J Nutr 135:1208–1214
93. Chung HY, Rasmussen HM, Johnson EJ (2004) Lutein bioavailability is higher from lutein-enriched eggs than from supplements and spinach in men. J Nutr 134:1887–1893
94. Wenzel AJ, Gerweck C, Barbato D, Nicolosi RJ, Handelman GJ, Curran-Celentano J (2006) A 12-wk egg intervention increases serum zeaxanthin and macular pigment optical density in women. J Nutr 136:2568–2573
95. Berendschot TTJM, Goldbohm RA, Klöpping WA, van de Kraats J, van Norel J, van Norren D (2000) Influence of lutein supplementation on macular pigment, assessed with two objective techniques. Invest Ophthalmol Vis Sci 41:3322–3326
96. Bhosale P, Zhao dY, Bernstein PS (2007) HPLC measurement of ocular carotenoid levels in human donor eyes in the lutein supplementation era. Invest Ophthalmol Vis Sci 48:543–549
97. Bone RA, Landrum JT, Cao Y, Howard AN, varez-Calderon F (2007) Macular pigment response to a supplement containing meso-zeaxanthin, lutein and zeaxanthin. Nutr Metab (Lond) 4:12
98. Bone RA, Landrum JT, Guerra LH, Ruiz CA (2003) Lutein and zeaxanthin dietary supplements raise macular pigment density and serum concentrations of these carotenoids in humans. J Nutr 133:992–998
99. Johnson EJ, Chung HY, Caldarella SM, Snodderly DM (2008) The influence of supplemental lutein and docosahexaenoic acid on serum, lipoproteins, and macular pigmentation. Am J Clin Nutr 87:1521–1529
100. Köpcke W, Schalch W; LUXEA-Study Group (2005) Changes in macular pigment optical density following repeated dosing with lutein, zeaxanthin, or their combination in healthy volunteers – results of the LUXEA-study. Invest Ophthalmol Vis Sci 46:1768
101. Landrum JT, Bone RA, Joa H, Kilburn MD, Moore LL, Sprague KE (1997) A one year study of the macular pigment: the effect of 140 days of a lutein supplement. Exp Eye Res 65:57–62
102. Rougier MB, Delyfer MN, Korobelnik JF (2008) [Measuring macular pigment in vivo]. J Fr Ophtalmol 31: 445–453
103. Schalch W, Cohn W, Barker FM, Kopcke W, Mellerio J, Bird AC, Robson AG, Fitzke FF, van Kuijk FJ (2007) Xanthophyll accumulation in the human retina during supplementation with lutein or zeaxanthin – the LUXEA (LUtein Xanthophyll Eye Accumulation) study. Arch Biochem Biophys 458:128–135
104. Snodderly DM, Chung HC, Caldarella SM, Johnson EJ (2005) The influence of supplemental lutein and docosahexaenoic acid on their serum levels and on macular pigment. Invest Ophthalmol Vis Sci 46:1766
105. Tanito M, Obana A, Okazaki S, Ohira A, Gellermann W (2009) Change of macular pigment density quantified with resonance Raman spectrophotometry and autofluorescence imaging in normal subjects supplemented with oral lutein or zeaxanthin. Invest Ophthalmol Vis Sci 50:1716
106. Zeimer M, Hense HW, Heimes B, Austermann U, Fobker M, Pauleikhoff D (2009) [The macular pigment: short- and intermediate-term changes of macular pigment optical density following supplementation with lutein and zeaxanthin and co-antioxidants. The LUNA Study]. Ophthalmologe 106:29–36
107. Koh HH, Murray IJ, Nolan D, Carden D, Feather J, Beatty S (2004) Plasma and macular responses to lutein

supplement in subjects with and without age-related maculopathy: a pilot study. Exp Eye Res 79:21–27
108. Trieschmann M, Beatty S, Nolan JM, Hense HW, Heimes B, Austermann U, Fobker M, Pauleikhoff D (2007) Changes in macular pigment optical density and serum concentrations of its constituent carotenoids following supplemental lutein and zeaxanthin: the LUNA study. Exp Eye Res 84:718–728
109. Bone RA, Landrum JT, Friedes LM, Gomez CM, Kilburn MD, Menendez E, Vidal I, Wang W (1997) Distribution of lutein and zeaxanthin stereoisomers in the human retina. Exp Eye Res 64:211–218
110. Werner JS, Donnelly SK, Kliegl R (1987) Aging and human macular pigment density. Appended with translations from the work of Max Schultze and Ewald Hering. Vision Res 27:257–268
111. Delori FC, Goger DG, Hammond BR, Snodderly DM, Burns SA (2001) Macular pigment density measured by autofluorescence spectrometry: comparison with reflectometry and heterochromatic flicker photometry. J Opt Soc Am A 18:1212–1230
112. Ciulla TA, Curran-Celentano J, Cooper DA, Hammond BR, Danis RP, Pratt LM, Riccardi KA, Filloon TG (2001) Macular pigment optical density in a midwestern sample. Ophthalmology 108:730–737
113. Mellerio J, Ahmadi-Lari S, van Kuijk F, Pauleikhoff D, Bird A, Marshall J (2002) A portable instrument for measuring macular pigment with central fixation. Curr Eye Res 25:37–47
114. Hammond BR, Caruso-Avery M (2000) Macular pigment optical density in a Southwestern sample. Invest Ophthalmol Vis Sci 41:1492–1497
115. Nolan J, O'Donovan O, Kavanagh H, Stack J, Harrison M, Muldoon A, Mellerio J, Beatty S (2004) Macular pigment and percentage of body fat. Invest Ophthalmol Vis Sci 45:3940–3950
116. Nolan JM, Stack J, Mellerio J, Godhinio M, O'Donovan O, Neelam K, Beatty S (2006) Monthly consistency of macular pigment optical density and serum concentrations of lutein and zeaxanthin. Curr Eye Res 31:199–213
117. Davies NP, Morland AB (2002) Color matching in diabetes: optical density of the crystalline lens and macular pigments. Invest Ophthalmol Vis Sci 43:281–289
118. Chen SF, Chang WuJC (2001) The spatial distribution of macular pigment in humans. Curr Eye Res 23:422–434
119. Zagers NPA (2004) Foveal reflection analyzer. On the spectral and directional reflectance of the retina. Utrecht University
120. Zagers NPA, van Norren D (2003) Photoreceptors act as spectrally flat reflectors. Invest Ophthalmol Vis Sci 44:2873
121. Berendschot TTJM, van Norren D (2004) Objective determination of the macular pigment optical density using fundus reflectance spectroscopy. Arch Biochem Biophys 430:149–155
122. Jahn C, Wüstemeyer H, Brinkmann C, Trautmann S, Mößner A, Wolf S (2005) Macular pigment density in age-related maculopathy. Graefes Arch Clin Exp Ophthalmol 243:222–227
123. Handelman GJ, Dratz EA, Reay CC, van Kuijk JG (1988) Carotenoids in the human macula and whole retina. Invest Ophthalmol Vis Sci 29:850–855
124. Bernstein PS, Zhao DY, Sharifzadeh M, Ermakov IV, Gellermann W (2004) Resonance Raman measurement of macular carotenoids in the living human eye. Arch Biochem Biophys 430:163–169
125. Gellermann W, Bernstein PS (2004) Noninvasive detection of macular pigments in the human eye. J Biomed Opt 9:75–78
126. Gellermann W, Ermakov IV, Ermakova MR, McClane RW, Zhao DY, Bernstein PS (2002) In vivo resonant Raman measurement of macular carotenoid pigments in the young and the aging human retina. J Opt Soc Am A 19:1172–1186
127. Bernstein PS, Gellermann W (2003) Author response: assessment of the Raman method of measuring human macular pigment. Invest Ophthalmol Vis Sci [serial online] Available at http://www.iovs.org/cgi/eletters?lookup = by_date&days = 9999#74. 15 Aug 2003
128. Bernstein PS, Gellermann W (2003) Author response: assessment of the Raman method of measuring human macular pigment (II). Invest Ophthalmol Vis Sci [serial online] Available at http://www.iovs.org/cgi/eletters?lookup = by_date&days = 9999#94. 30 Dec 2003
129. Wooten BR, Hammond BR (2003) Assessment of the Raman method of measuring human macular pigment. Invest Ophthalmol Vis Sci [serial online] Available at http://www.iovs.org/cgi/eletters?lookup = by_date&days = 9999#73:August 15, 2003
130. Wooten BR, Hammond BR (2003) Assessment of the Raman method of measuring human macular pigment (II). Invest Ophthalmol Vis Sci [serial online] Available at http://www.iovs.org/cgi/eletters?lookup = by_date&days = 9999#92:December 30, 2003
131. Neelam K, O'Gorman N, Nolan J, O'Donovan O, Wong HB, Eong KGA, Beatty S (2005) Measurement of macular pigment: Raman spectroscopy versus heterochromatic Flicker photometry. Invest Ophthalmol Vis Sci 46: 1023–1032
132. Bone RA, Landrum JT (2004) Heterochromatic flicker photometry. Arch Biochem Biophys 430:137–142
133. Moreland JD (2004) Macular pigment assessment by motion photometry. Arch Biochem Biophys 430:143–148
134. van der Veen RLP, Berendschot TTJM, Hendrikse F, Carden D, Makridaki M, Murray IJ (2009) A new desktop instrument for measuring macular pigment optical density

based on a novel technique for setting flicker thresholds. Ophthalmic Physiol Opt 29:127–137
135. Berendschot TTJM, de Lint PJ, Norren D (2003) Fundus reflectance-historical and present ideas. Prog Retin Eye Res 22:171–200
136. Delori FC (2004) Autofluorescence method to measure macular pigment optical densities fluorometry and autofluorescence imaging. Arch Biochem Biophys 430:156–162
137. Bone RA, Landrum JT, Adams M, Gibert JC (2007) Validity of macular pigment optical density measurements by heterochromatic flicker photometry. Invest Ophthalmol Vis Sci 48:2131
138. Gallaher KT, Mura M, Todd WA, Harris TL, Kenyon E, Harris T, Johnson KC, Satterfield S, Kritchevsky SB, Iannaccone A (2007) Estimation of macular pigment optical density in the elderly: Test-retest variability and effect of optical blur in pseudophakic subjects. Vision Res 47:1253–1259
139. Snodderly DM, Mares JA, Wooten BR, Oxton L, Gruber M, Ficek T (2004) Macular pigment measurement by heterochromatic Flicker photometry in older subjects: The Carotenoids and Age-Related Eye Disease Study. Invest Ophthalmol Vis Sci 45:531–538
140. Hagen S, Krebs I, Glittenberg C, Binder S (2009) Repeated measures of macular pigment optical density to test reproducibility of heterochromatic flicker photometry. Acta Ophthalmol (in press)
141. Liou HL, Brennan NA (1997) Anatomically accurate, finite model eye for optical modeling. J Opt Soc Am A 14:1684–1695
142. Knighton RW, Baverez C, Bhattacharya A (1992) The directional reflectance of the retinal nerve fiber layer of the toad. Invest Ophthalmol Vis Sci 33:2603–2611
143. Knighton RW, Huang XR (1999) Directional and spectral reflectance of the rat retinal nerve fiber layer. Invest Ophthalmol Vis Sci 40:639–647
144. Knighton RW, Jacobson SG, Kemp CM (1989) The spectral reflectance of the nerve fiber layer of the macaque retina. Invest Ophthalmol Vis Sci 30:2392–2402
145. Bour LJ, Koo L, Delori FC, Apkarian P, Fulton AB (2002) Fundus photography for measurement of macular pigment density distribution in children. Invest Ophthalmol Vis Sci 43:1450–1455
146. Wüstemeyer H, Mößner A, Jahn C, Wolf S (2003) Macular pigment density in healthy subjects quantified with a modified confocal scanning laser ophthalmoscope. Graefes Arch Clin Exp Ophthalmol 241:647–651
147. Gorrand JM, Bacin F, Doly M (2009) Directionality of foveal cones and macular pigment optical density. Invest Ophthalmol Vis Sci 50:1713
148. Zagers NPA, van ND (2004) Absorption of the eye lens and macular pigment derived from the reflectance of cone photoreceptors. J Opt Soc Am A Opt Image Sci Vis 21:2257–2268
149. van de Kraats J, Berendschot TTJM, van Norren D (1996) The pathways of light measured in fundus reflectometry. Vision Res 36:2229–2247
150. van de Kraats J, van Norren D (2008) Directional and nondirectional spectral reflection from the human fovea. J Biomed Opt 13:024010
151. van de Kraats J, Berendschot TTJM, Valen S, van Norren D (2006) Fast assessment of the central macular pigment density with natural pupil using the macular pigment reflectometer. J Biomed Opt 11:064031–064037
152. Delori FC, Dorey CK, Staurenghi G, Arend O, Goger DG, Weiter JJ (1995) In vivo fluorescence of the ocular fundus exhibits retinal pigment epithelium lipofuscin characteristics. Invest Ophthalmol Vis Sci 36:718–729
153. Delori FC (1994) Spectrophotometer for noninvasive measurement of intrinsic fluorescence and reflectance of the ocular fundus. Appl Opt 33:7439–7452
154. Raman CV, Krishnan KS (1928) A new type of secondary radiation. Nature 121:501–502
155. Bernstein PS, Yoshida MD, Katz NB, McClane RW, Gellermann W (1998) Raman detection of macular carotenoid pigments in intact human retina. Invest Ophthalmol Vis Sci 39:2003–2011
156. Zhao DY, Ermakov IV, Ermakova MR, McClane RW, Gellermann W, Wintch SW, Gregori NZ, Bernstein PS (2001) Resonance Raman spectroscopic measurement of macular carotenoids in normal and age-related macular degeneration subjects. Invest Ophthalmol Vis Sci 42: S126
157. Zhao DY, Wintch SW, Ermakov IV, Gellermann W, Bernstein PS (2003) Resonance Raman measurement of macular carotenoids in retinal, choroidal, and macular dystrophies. Arch Ophthalmol 121:967–972
158. Hogg RE, Anderson RS, Stevenson MR, Zlatkova MB, Chakravarthy U (2007) In vivo macular pigment measurements: a comparison of resonance Raman spectroscopy and heterochromatic flicker photometry. Br J Ophthalmol 91:485–490
159. Hogg RE, Zlatkova MB, Chakravarthy U, Anderson RS (2007) Investigation of the effect of simulated lens yellowing, transparency loss and refractive error on in vivo resonance Raman spectroscopy. Ophthalmic Physiol Opt 27: 225–231
160. Hammond BR, Wooten BR, Smollon B (2005) Assessment of the validity of in vivo methods of measuring human macular pigment optical density. Optom Vis Sci 82: 387–404
161. Loane E, Stack J, Beatty S, Nolan JM (2007) Measurement of macular pigment optical density using two different heterochromatic flicker photometers. Curr Eye Res 32: 555–564
162. Trieschmann M, Heimes B, Hense HW, Pauleikhoff D (2006) Macular pigment optical density measurement in

autofluorescence imaging: comparison of one- and two-wavelength methods. Graefes Arch Clin Exp Ophthalmol 244:1565–1574
163. Wolf S (2006) Macular pigment measurements: which method should we use? Graefes Arch Clin Exp Ophthalmol 1–3
164. Berendschot TT, van der Veen RLP, Makridaki M, Carden D, Murray IJ (2009) A comparison of psychophysical and optical methods for determining the spatial profile of macular pigment. Invest Ophthalmol Vis Sci 50:1725
165. Bone RA, Landrum JT, Gibert JC (2004) Macular pigment and the edge hypothesis of flicker photometry. Vision Res 44:3045–3051
166. Smollon WE, Wooten BR, Hammond BR (2005) Stimulus edge effects when measuring macular pigment using heterochromatic Flicker photometry. Invest Ophthalmol Vis Sci 46:4569
167. Stringham JM, Hammond BR, Nolan JM, Wooten BR, Mammen A, Smollon W, Snodderly DM (2008) The utility of using customized heterochromatic flicker photometry (cHFP) to measure macular pigment in patients with age-related macular degeneration. Exp Eye Res 87: 445–453
168. Elsner AE, Burns SA, Delori FC, Webb RH (1990) Quantitative reflectometry with the SLO. In: Naseman JE, Burk ROW (eds) Laser scanning ophthalmoscopy and tomography. Quintessenz-Verlag, Munich, pp 109–121
169. Ossewaarde-Van Norel J, van den Biesen PR, van de Kraats J, Berendschot TTJM, van Norren D (2002) Comparison of fluorescence of sodium fluorescein in retinal angiography with measurements in vitro. J Biom Optics 7:190–198
170. Brinkmann CK, Rothenbuehler SP, Wolf-Schnurrbusch UEK, Wolf S (2009) Enhancement of Macular Pigment by Oral Lutein Supplementation Study (EMPOLS): first results. Invest Ophthalmol Vis Sci 50:1708
171. Jahn C, Wüstemeyer H, Brinkmann C, Trautmann S, Moessner A, Wolf S (2005) Macular pigment density in age-related maculopathy. Graefes Arch Clin Exp Ophthalmol 243:222–227
172. Liew SHM, Gilbert CE, Spector TD, Mellerio J, Marshall J, van Kuijk FJ, Beatty S, Fitzke F, Hammond CJ (2005) Heritability of macular pigment: a twin study. Invest Ophthalmol Vis Sci 46:4430–4436
173. Robson AG, Harding G, Van Kuijk FJGM, Pauleikhoff D, Holder GE, Bird AC, Fitzke F, Moreland JD (2005) Comparison of fundus autofluorescence and minimum-motion measurements of macular pigment distribution profiles derived from identical retinal areas. Perception 34:1027–1032
174. Robson AG, Moreland JD, Pauleikhoff D, Morrissey T, Holder GE, Fitzke FW, Bird C, Van Kuijk FJGM (2003) Macular pigment density and distribution: comparison of fundus autofluorescence with minimum motion photometry. Vision Res 43:1765–1775
175. Trieschmann M, Heimes B, Hense HW, Pauleikhoff D (2006) Macular pigment optical density measurement in autofluorescence imaging: comparison of one- and two-wavelength methods. Graefes Arch Clin Exp Ophthalmol 244:1565–1574
176. Van Kuijk EF, Moreland JD, Robson AG, Pauleikhoff D, Morrissey T, Holder GE, Fitzke FW, Bird AC (2003) In vivo evidence for reduced autofluorescence efficiency at the fovea: implications for assessment of macular pigment. Invest Ophthalmol Vis Sci 44:U691
177. Van Kuijk EF, Robson AG, Pauleikhoff D, Harding G, Holder GE, Fitzke FW, Bird AC, Moreland JD (2004) Longitudinal studies of macular pigment distribution profiles assessed by minimum motion photometry and fundus autofluorescence. Invest Ophthalmol Vis Sci 45:U532
178. Wolf-Schnurrbusch UE, Wolf S, Volker D, Brinkmann C, Rothenbuehler SP, Delori FC (2009) Spatial distribution of macular pigment and its relation to the fovea size. Invest Ophthalmol Vis Sci 50:1724
179. Wüstemeyer H, Jahn C, Nestler A, Barth T, Wolf S (2002) A new instrument for the quantification of macular pigment density: first results in patients with AMD and healthy subjects. Graefes Arch Clin Exp Ophthalmol 240: 666–671
180. Delori FC, Goger DG, Keilhauer C, Salvetti P, Staurenghi G (2006) Bimodal spatial distribution of macular pigment: evidence of a gender relationship. J Opt Soc Am A Opt Image Sci Vis 23:521–538
181. Wolf-Schnurrbusch UEK, Roosli N, Weyermann E, Heldner MR, Hohne K, Wolf S (2007) Ethnic differences in macular pigment density and distribution. Invest Ophthalmol Vis Sci 48:3783–3787
182. Sharifzadeh M, Bernstein PS, Gellermann W (2006) Nonmydriatic fluorescence-based quantitative imaging of human macular pigment distributions. J Opt Soc Am A Opt Image Sci Vis 23:2373–2387
183. Trieschmann M, Heimes B, Hense HW, Pauleikhoff D (2006) Macular pigment optical density measurement in autofluorescence imaging: comparison of one- and two-wavelength methods. Graefes Arch Clin Exp Ophthalmol 244:1565–1574
184. Sharifzadeh M, Zhao DY, Bernstein PS, Gellermann W (2008) Resonance Raman imaging of macular pigment distributions in the human retina. J Opt Soc Am A Opt Image Sci Vis 25:947–957

Chapter 7

Near-Infrared Autofluorescence Imaging

7

Claudia N. Keilhauer and François C. Delori

Core Messages

- Fluorescence excitation of near-infrared autofluorescence (NIR-AF) is achieved with a laser diode at ~787 nm and the detection filter >800 nm.
- NIR-AF is 60–100 times less intense than the autofluorescence excited with short wavelength autofluorescence (SW-AF).
- NIR-AF results in large part from the fluorescence of melanin or compounds closely associated with melanin.
- The center of the macula exhibits high NIR-AF, corresponding to the high amounts of melanin in the central RPE.
- The NIR-AF image is influenced by ocular pigmentation since part of the signal is derived from choroidal melanin.
- NIR-AF may be useful in studying the biological changes associated with degradation, redistribution, or oxidation of melanin such as age-related macular degeneration (AMD).

7.1 Introduction

Autofluorescence (AF) imaging is playing an increasingly important role in the diagnosis of age-related macular degeneration (AMD) and retinal dystrophies. AF is most often generated with short-wavelength excitation (SW-AF) using a confocal Scanning Laser Ophthalmoscope (SLO) [1]. With this imaging mode, the signal is dominated by RPE lipofuscin [2].

AF imaging can also be obtained by near-infrared (NIR) excitation. AF excited in the near-infrared at 805 nm (NIR-AF) was first reported by Piccolino et al. using a nonconfocal video-imaging system as part of an investigation of possible pseudo-fluorescence in indocyanine green (ICG) angiography [3]. AF images with NIR excitation can also be obtained using a confocal SLO (HRAc or HRA2, Heidelberg Engineering) [4, 5].

NIR-AF images are acquired using the same laser and filters as used for ICG angiography (excitation: 787 ± 2 nm; detection above 800 nm). A weak fluorescent signal is produced that is 60–100 times less intense than that obtained in SW-AF imaging. Eighteen successive frames are generally aligned and averaged to improve the signal-to-noise ratio. All images presented here have been histogram-stretched.

7.2 Origin of Near-Infrared Autofluorescence

Several imaging studies [4–6] have suggested that the NIR-AF from the fundus emanates in large part from melanin in the RPE and in the choroid (Fig. 7.1). Furthermore, in ex vivo mouse retinas, Gibbs and colleagues [7] have recently shown that NIR-AF emanates from melanosomes in the RPE and choroid, and that the purified melanosomes emit the same fluorescence. Melanin has a broad absorption spectrum spanning the UV, visible, and NIR part of the spectrum; its absorption decreases monotonically with wavelength [8]. A weak melanin AF can be elicited using different excitation wavelengths throughout the spectrum [9–12].

The most striking feature in a NIR-AF image of the normal fundus is an area of high NIR-AF that is centered on the fovea (Fig. 7.2) that results from the higher amount of RPE melanin in the fovea, because the RPE cells are taller and narrower [13, 14]. In SW-AF images, this area exhibit increased absorption by RPE melanin, resulting in a darker area surrounding the central location of the macular pigment (Fig. 7.2).

Choroidal melanin also contributes to the NIR-AF signal. In subjects with brown irides, and thus a large amount of choroidal melanin, there is a relatively stronger

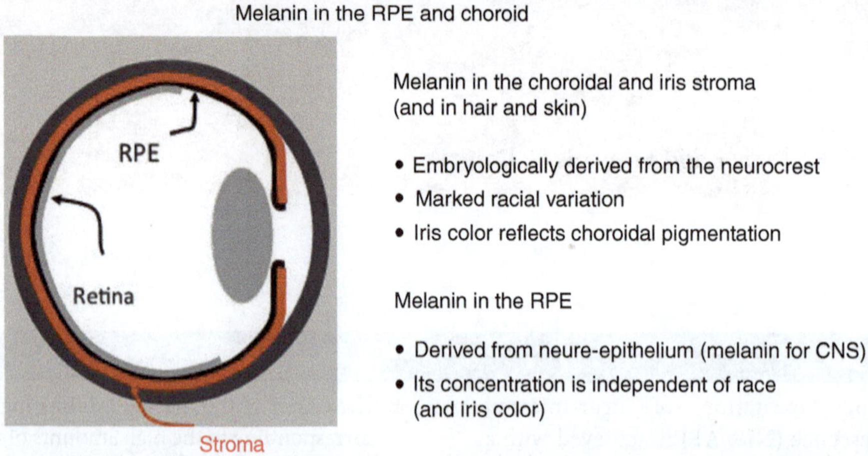

Fig. 7.1 Distribution of ocular melanin within the eye. There are two different sources of melanin: *red* melanin in the choroidal and iris stroma and *black* melanin in the RPE

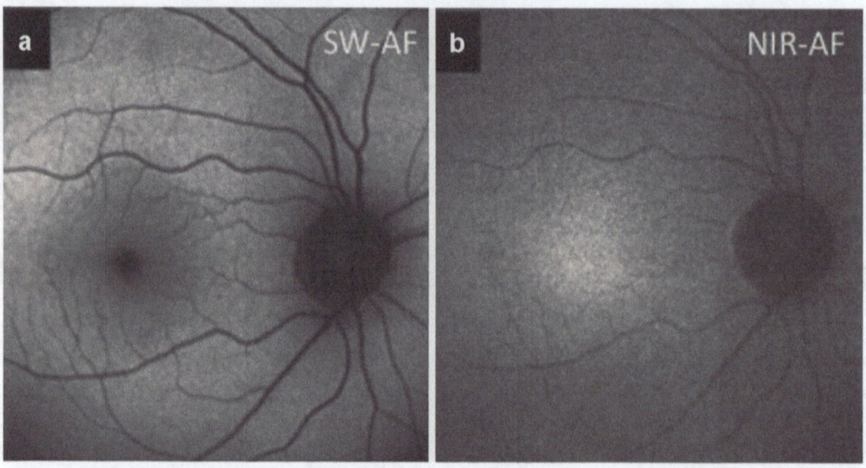

Fig. 7.2 AF images from a 44-year-old female with normal retinal status. **(a)** SW-AF image; excitation wavelength 488 nm; **(b)** NIR-AF image; excitation wavelength 787 nm. The color of the iris reflects the pigmentation of the choroid. Optic disc and the retinal vessels appear as darker structures in both imaging modes. The NIR-AF image shows an area of high IR fluorescence, which corresponds to the area of higher melanin pigmentation in the SW-AF images, extending outside the densest MP distribution

signal from the choroid. This results in the lowering of the contrast of RPE features including the central zone of high NIR-AF (Fig. 7.3).

Increasing age also lowers the contrast between the central area of high NIR-AF and the perifovea (Fig. 7.3) [4]. This could result from the decrease, by more than 50% over a lifetime, in the number of RPE melanin granules [15]with a resulting decrease in RPE fluorescence or from an increase in the contribution of choroidal melanin AF resulting from the increase in the light transmission of the RPE.

At the fovea, a small, localized depression can be identified in some normal subjects (Fig. 7.4) [4]. The origin of this local depression is largely unknown. Focal depigmentation of foveal RPE may account for this observation such as in cases of incipient ARM, where other signs as drusen are not yet visible. On the other hand, it may be the result of reduced photo-oxidation of RPE melanin, secondary to the protection from short-wavelength light by the densest part of the MP distribution. The observation shows that NIR-AF imaging is useful to study retinal alterations in the fovea, contrary to SW-AF imaging where the macular pigment generally masks such details.

Other secondary signals could contribute to the NIR-AF, but little is known about the NIR-AF properties

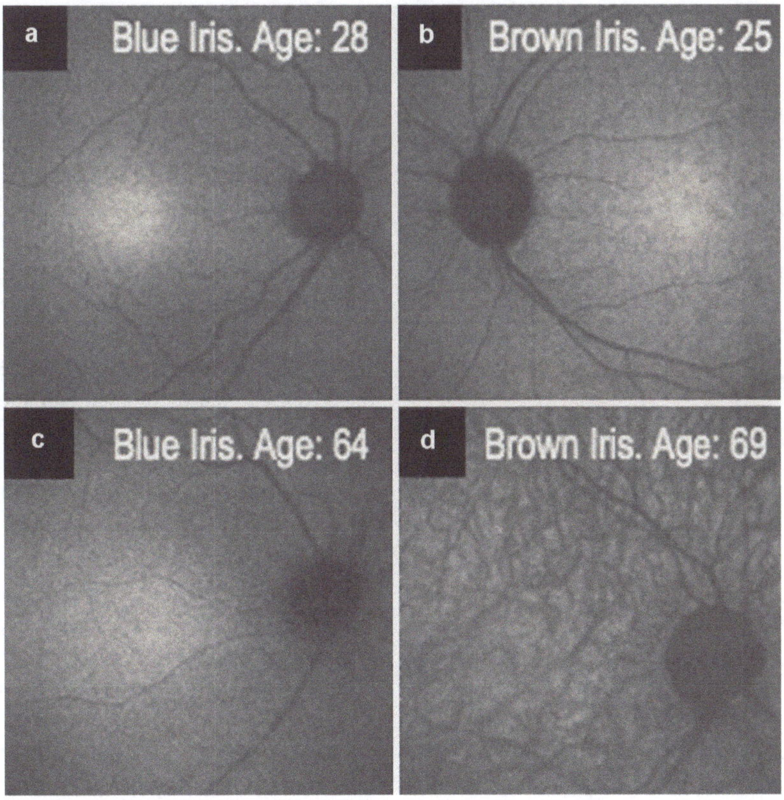

Fig. 7.3 NIR-AF images from subjects with light irides (**a** and **c**), and from subjects with dark irides (**b** and **d**). The color of the iris reflects the pigmentation of the choroid. The contrast of the bright central area is higher in young (**a** and **b**) than in old subjects (**c** and **d**), and also higher in subjects with light irides

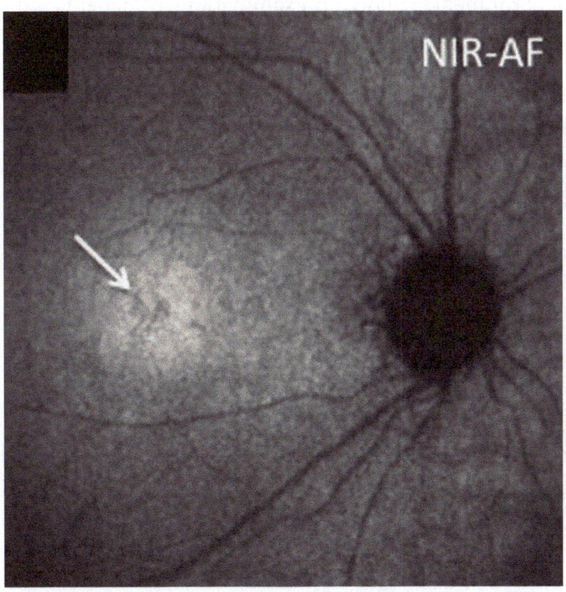

Fig. 7.4 NIR-AF image from a 47-year-old female with normal retinal status (*green iris color*). A focal reduction in NIR-AF is observed near the fovea (*arrow*). The color of the iris reflects the pigmentation of the choroid

of most ocular tissues. Porphyrin AF may contribute to NIR-AF from melanomas and lesions that contain degradation products of hemoglobin [5]. It should be stressed that the NIR-AF signal is very weak, often showing only a few gray levels above the zero gray level in the original image before histogram-stretching. The edges of the optic disc are close to this zero gray level (no AF), although they may appear dark gray in most images [4]. Imperfections in the barrier filter characteristics may result in some filter leakage (pseudo-fluorescence), particularly from structures with high reflectivity in confocal NIR images (hyperpigmentation) [5].

7.3 RPE Melanin: Role and Aging

Melanin has been attributed to protect the eye against several ocular diseases, including uveal melanoma and AMD. It acts as a powerful light-absorber that protects RPE lipofuscin from chronic light exposure, minimizes backscattered light toward the photoreceptors, dissipates absorbed energy into heat, binds many chemicals and heavy metal ions, scavenges free-radicals [16], and acts as a weak antioxidant [13, 17].

Oxidative or lysosomal degradation of RPE melanin with age reduces light absorption and may lower its capability of protecting the RPE [13, 18–20]. With age, degraded melanin granules tend to merge with lipofuscin in a complex granule called melanolipofuscin [21]. These granules contribute SW-AF [22], but whether these are also responsible for part of the NIR-AF is yet unknown.

7.4 Clinical Cases

More recently, the NIR-AF imaging mode has been used to study age-related, toxic, and hereditary macular diseases [5, 6, 23–28]. Here, we introduce selected examples.

7.4.1 Age-Related Macular Degeneration

AMD is a complex disease that is both genetically and environmentally influenced. This common blinding disorder is characterized by the degeneration of retinal pigment epithelial (RPE) cells at the central posterior pole. Accumulation of lipofuscin in RPE-cells accompanies the process of aging, and may play a role in the pathogenesis of AMD. Age-related changes of melanin granules in the RPE (degradation, oxidation, and formation of melanolipofuscin) may also contribute to the development of AMD.

Geographic atrophy (GA) represents the atrophic late-stage complication of AMD. Degeneration of RPE-cells usually starts at the perifovea often sparing the central fovea until late stages. Histologically, the marginal zone of the atrophy exhibits enlarged RPE-cells filled with accumulations of lipofuscin or melanolipofuscin [29].

SW-AF imaging is widely used for the diagnosis and follow-up examination of GA. The absence of lipofuscin and melanin-laden RPE cells within the zone of atrophy cause markedly decreased SW-AF, in sharp contrast to the higher SW-AF of the degenerating RPE in the marginal zone and the relatively unaffected surrounding of the atrophy. Similarly, the NIR-AF signal is also lower in the zone of atrophy compared with the surrounding intact RPE (Fig. 7.5). A relatively stronger NIR-AF signal from inside the atrophy in darkly pigmented patients compared with subjects with light ocular pigmentation results in a lower contrast of the GA in subjects with dark irides [4].

Choroidal vessels are often visible as darker structures within the area of atrophic RPE. Melanin is two to three times more abundant in the outer than in the inner choroid [14], and this contributes to the visibility of absorbing choroidal vessels seen against the bright AF from the outer choroid. Areas of high NIR-AF are often observed at the edge of the GA. These areas correspond to spots of hyperpigmentation in the color image and often correspond only marginally to spots of high SW-AF. Interestingly, the atrophy size is measured slightly larger on NIR-AF images compared with SW-AF images [26]. This might have resulted from the loss of melanin in degenerating RPE cells that are still loaded with lipofuscin and melanolipofuscin or from the reduction of the efficiency of melanin AF secondary to the changes in its environment. Follow-up examinations of patients with GA with both NIR-AF and SW-AF imaging could be

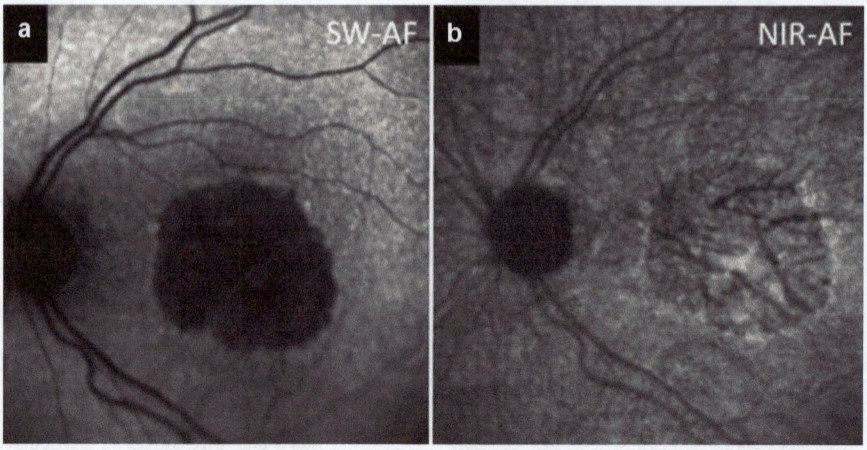

Fig. 7.5 AF images from a 84-year-old female patient with geographic atrophy (*brown iris*). The area of atrophic RPE is clearly delineated on SW-AF (**a**). The NIR-AF image (**b**) shows a much lower contrast of the atrophy to the surrounding. In darkly pigmented subjects (high NIR-AF signal from the deep choroidal layers), the choroidal vessel structure within and outside the area of atrophy is clearly visible

useful to study the biological changes associated with the development of GA.

7.4.2 Retinal Dystrophies

7.4.2.1 Stargardt's Disease

Stargardt's disease (STGD) is a common autosomal recessive maculopathy of early and young-adult onset, characterized by progressive loss of central vision and the appearance of yellowish flecks at the level of the retinal pigment epithelium (RPE) at the posterior pole. Later atrophy of the retinal pigment epithelium causes severe loss of central visual acuity.

Comparing the SW- and NIR-AF mode in patients with STGD, it is obvious that the distribution of NIR-AF does not correspond to the distribution of SW-AF [6, 24, 25, 28]. In early STGD, flecks that exhibit high SW-AF may also reveal high NIR-AF (Fig. 7.6). Histopathologic studies found condensation of apicalized melanin granules within RPE cells that are engorged with lipofuscin [30]. In more advanced disease stages (Fig. 7.6), flecks may still exhibit high SW-AF, but the NIR-AF image reveals more extended areas of degeneration and atrophy. Loss or degradation of RPE-melanin as RPE-cells accumulate excessive amounts of lipofuscin may be responsible for the low NIR-AF intensity. As RPE cell atrophy develops, low SW-AF and low NIR-AF are observed as in GA. Possible sequence of events in STGD is depicted in Fig. 7.7. As for SW-AF, NIR-AF may also serve as a marker for disease progression in STGD.

7.4.2.2 Best's Disease

Best's disease (BD) refers to a vitelliform dystrophy of the central retina with autosomal dominant inheritance but with variable penetrance and expressivity. The disease is characterized by large, yellow, yolk-like lesions of the central posterior pole, which usually appear during childhood. Later, the vitelliform cyst may disrupt and RPE atrophy causes central vision loss.

The lack of correspondence of NIR-AF and SW-AF distributions is particularly evident for the vitelliform lesion (Fig. 7.8) [25, 28]. NIR-AF is low at the site of high SW-AF accumulations of yellow lipofuscin-like material. At the edge of the lesion, a rim of high NIR-AF is often observed.

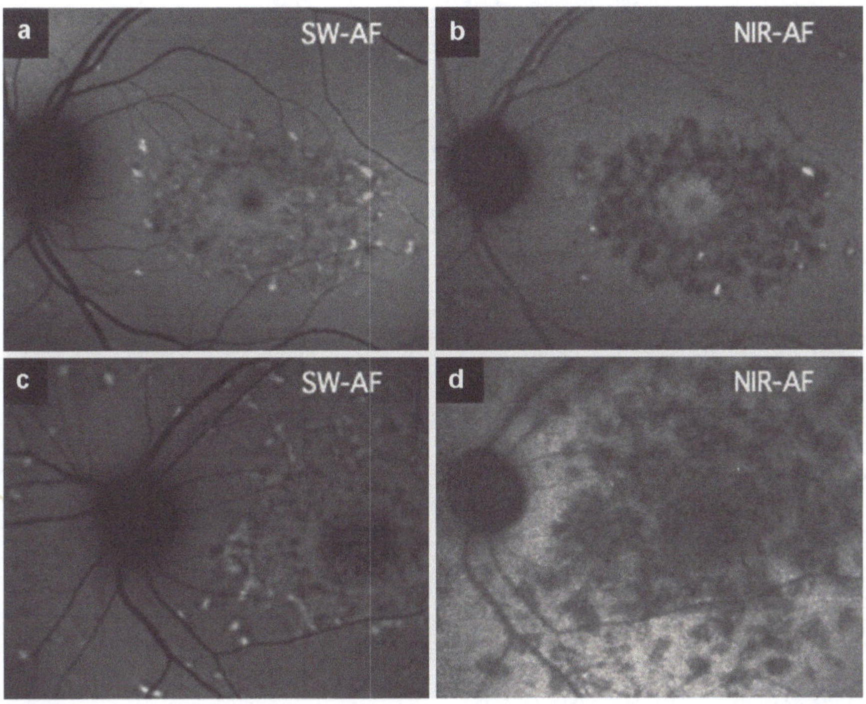

Fig. 7.6 SW-AF images (**a** and **c**) and NIR-AF images (**b** and **d**) from two patients with Stargardt's disease (STGD). Images (**a** and **b**) are from a 26-year-old female patient with early disease and preserved fovea, whereas images (**c** and **d**) are from a 42-year-old male patient with more advanced pathology. The SW-AF images show typical STGD-flecks with predominantly high AF intensity (lipofuscin). The NIR-AF images are dominated by areas of low NIR-AF (loss of melanin?), although a few flecks still show high AF early in the disease (**b**). The pathology appears much more extended in NIR-AF than in SW-AF

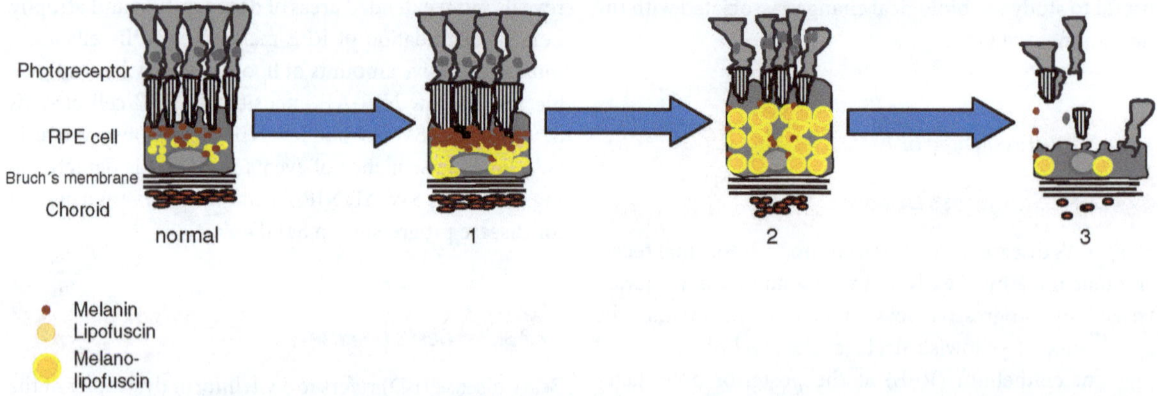

Fig. 7.7 Possible sequence of events in STGD. (*1*) Accumulation of lipofuscin within RPE cells and apicalization of melanin (flecks of high SW-AF and high NIR-AF); (*2*) accumulation of lipofuscin with enlargement of RPE-cells and loss or displacement of melanin (flecks dominated by high SW-AF and low NIR-AF); (*3*) RPE-cell death (low SW-AF and low NIR-AF)

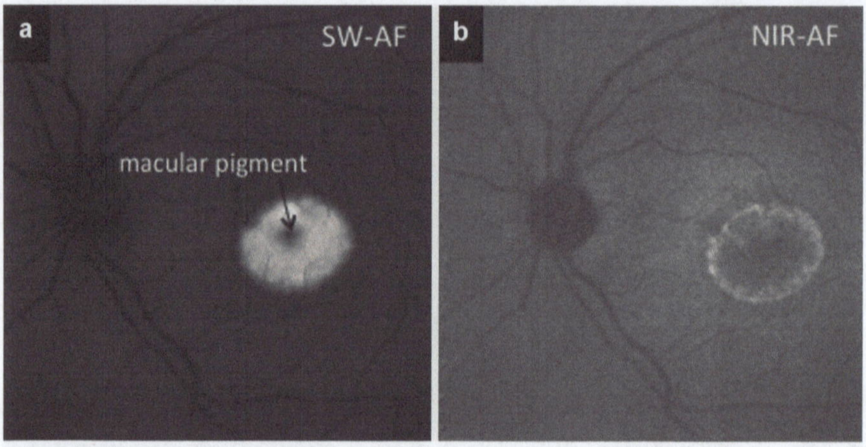

Fig. 7.8 AF images from a 31-year-old male patient with dominant Best's macular dystrophy. The egg-yolk stage is characterized by high SW-AF (**a**) and relatively low NIR-AF (**b**). The vitelliform lesion shows high SW-AF throughout the lesion but reduced SW-AF in its center due to blue light absorption of macular pigment

Histologic examinations [31] have shown that the vitelliform materials consisting of outer segment debris and debris from RPE cell disruption were lying anterior to the RPE. The material in the subretinal space had the cytochemical properties of lipofuscin. The RPE beneath the vitelliform material was flattened and revealed signs of atrophy. The RPE immediately adjacent to the central lesion consisted of several cell layers stacked on top of one another. These cells were nearly entirely filled with lipofuscin and melanolipofuscin granules.

Attenuation or atrophy of RPE-cells beneath the vitelliform cyst, as observed by histology, may explain the loss of NIR-AF at the central posterior pole. At the edge of the lesion, several layers of RPE cells that are filled with lipofuscin and melanolipofuscin may cause the rim of high NIR-AF. Later in the course of the disorder, degeneration of RPE cells leads to well-circumscribed areas of low SW-AF and low NIR-AF.

7.4.2.3 Retinitis Pigmentosa

Retinitis pigmentosa (RP) is a group of inherited retinal diseases characterized by early nyctalopia, progressive loss of photoreceptor function, and pigment deposition within the retina. Primary degeneration occurs in the

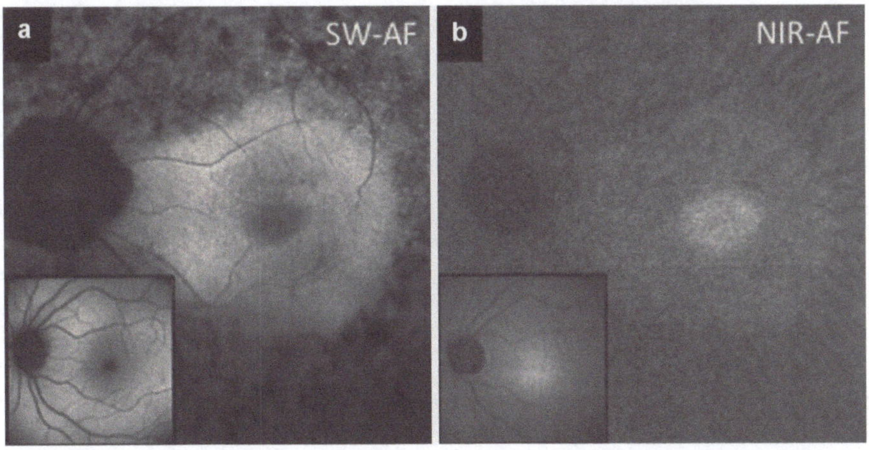

Fig. 7.9 AF images from 53-year-old male patient with advanced RP with concentric contraction of visual fields. The SW-AF image (**a**) shows degeneration of peripheral RPE indicated by low levels of SW-AF. The area of atrophic RPE reaches the vessel arcades. The foveal AF-attenuation due to blue-light absorption of macular pigment and RPE melanin is greatly diminished (inserts for comparison: AF images of a 44-year-old normal subject). Correspondingly, the NIR-AF image exhibits concentric contraction of the central bright area indicating loss of RPE melanin (**b**)

photoreceptors followed by changes in the RPE and glial cells, blood vessels, and neurons of the inner retina [32].

Several studies described the NIR-AF images of patients with RP [23, 27]. Early stages of RP are characterized by rings of increased SW- and NIR-AF within an area of preserved RPE at the posterior pole. In the periphery, NIR-AF is often diminished in areas of funduscopic hypopigmentation. More advanced stages show a concentric contraction of the central area of high NIR-AF, indicating the process of depigmentation progresses centrally (Fig. 7.9). Later, the SW-AF signal is also greatly diminished pointing to RPE atrophy.

7.5 Conclusion

NIR-AF imaging offers the ability to monitor ocular melanin in vivo. It provides different information when compared with that of SW-AF imaging, often reflecting different stages of progression of retinal disease. Its main disadvantage may be the lower contrast of RPE features in subjects with high ocular pigmentation. On the other hand and in contrast to SW-AF, the NIR-AF imaging modality avoids blue light exposure of the retina. This is an important advantage for patients with macular diseases.

The use of these AF imaging methods provide new tools for the detection of early degenerative changes of the RPE in patients who are at high risk for the development of age-related, hereditary, or toxic macular disorders.

Summary for the Clinician

- NIR-AF-imaging is a novel imaging modality for diagnosis of ocular disease.
- SW-AF is associated with lipofuscin in the RPE, whereas NIR-AF emanates in large part from melanin in the RPE and to a varying degree from melanin in the choroid.
- The information provided by SW-AF and NIR-AF imaging in patients with AMD and with retinal dystrophies is often complementary, and perhaps reflects different stages of progression of the retinal disease.
- Combined imaging of lipofuscin and melanin may provide a better understanding of biological changes in aging and degeneration of the retina.

References

1. von Rückmann A, Fitzke FW, Bird AC (1995) Distribution of fundus autofluorescence with a scanning laser ophthalmoscope. Br J Ophthalmol 119:543–562
2. Delori FC, Dorey CK, Staurenghi G et al (1995) In vivo fluorescence of the ocular fundus exhibits retinal pigment epithelium lipofuscin characteristics. Invest Ophthalmol Vis Sci 36:718–729
3. Piccolino FC, Borgia L, Zinicola E et al (1996) Pre-injection fluorescence in indocyanine green angiography. Ophthalmology 103(11):1837–1845

4. Keilhauer CN, Delori FC (2006) Near-infrared autofluorescence imaging of the fundus: visualization of ocular melanin. Invest Ophthalmol Vis Sci 47(8):3556–3564
5. Weinberger AWA, Lappas A, Kirschkamp T et al (2006) Fundus near infrared fluorescence is correlated to fundus near infrared reflectance. Invest Ophthalmol Vis Sci 47(7):3099–3108
6. Kellner S, Kellner U, Weber BH et al (2009) Lipofuscin- and melanin-related fundus autofluorescence in patients with ABCA4-associated retinal dystrophies. Am J Ophthalmol;147(5):895–902
7. Gibbs D, Cideciyan AV, Jacobson SG et al (2009) Retinal pigment epithelium defects in humans and mice with mutations in MYO7A: imaging melanosome-specific autofluorescence. Invest Ophthalmol Vis Sci 50(9):4386–93
8. Gabel V-P, Birngruber R, Hillenkamp F (1979) Visible and near infrared light absorption in pigment epithelium and choroid. In: Shimizu K, Oosterhuis JA (eds) XXIII Concilium ophthalmologicum: Kyoto 1978 Acta proceedings of the 23rd international congress of ophthalmology, 1978 May 14–20, Vol 14. Exerpta Medica, Amsterdam, pp 658–662
9. Docchio F, Boulton M, Cubeddu R et al (1991) Age-related changes in the fluorescence of melanin and lipofuscin granules of the retinal pigment epithelium: a time-resolved fluorescence spectroscopy study. J Photochem Photobiol 54: 247–253
10. Gallas JM, Eisner M (1987) Fluorescence of melanin dependence upon excitation wavelength and concentration. Photochem Photobiol 45(5):595–600
11. Huang Z, Zeng H, Hamzavi I et al (2006) Cutaneous melanin exhibits fluorescence emission under near-infrared light excitation. J Biomed Opt 11(3):34010
12. Kayatz P, Thumann G, Luther TT et al (2001) Oxidation causes melanin fluorescence. Invest Ophthalmol Vis Sci 42(1):241–246
13. Boulton M, Dayhaw-Barker P (2001) The role of the retinal pigment epithelium: topographical variation and ageing changes. Eye 15(Pt 3):384–389
14. Weiter JJ, Delori FC, Wing G et al (1986) Retinal pigment epithelial lipofuscin and melanin and choroidal melanin in human eyes. Invest Ophthalmol Vis Sci 27:145–152
15. Feeney-Burns L, Hilderbrand ES, Eldridge S (1984) Aging human RPE: morphometric analysis of macular, equatorial, and peripheral cells. Invest Ophthalmol Vis Sci 25: 195–200
16. Sarna T (1992) Photoperties and function of the ocular melanin: a photophysical review. J Photochem Photobiol B 12: 216–528
17. Wang Z, Dillon J, Gaillard ER (2006) Antioxidant properties of melanin in retinal pigment epithelial cells. Photochem Photobiol 82(2):474–479
18. Sarna T, Burke JM, Korytowski W et al (2003) Loss of melanin from human RPE with aging: possible role of melanin photooxidation. Exp Eye Res 76(1):89–98
19. Schraermeyer U (1993) Does melanin turnover occur in the eyes of adult vertebrates? Pigment Cell Res 6(4 Pt 1): 193–204
20. Schraermeyer U, Peters S, Thumann G et al (1999) Melanin granules of retinal pigment epithelium are connected with the lysosomal degradation pathway. Exp Eye Res 68(2): 237–245
21. Feeney-Burns L (1980) The pigments of the retinal pigment epithelium. Curr Top Eye Res 2:119–177
22. Boulton M, Docchio F, Dayhaw-Barker P, Ramponi R, Cubeddu R (1990) Age-related changes in the morphology, absorption and fluoresence of melanosomes and lipofuscin granules of the retinal pigment epithelium. Vision Res 30: 1291–1303
23. Aleman TS, Cideciyan AV, Sumaroka A et al (2007) Inner retinal abnormalities in X-linked retinitis pigmentosa with RPGR mutations. Invest Ophthalmol Vis Sci 48(10):4759–4765
24. Cideciyan AV, Swider M, Aleman TS et al (2007) Reduced-illuminance autofluorescence imaging in ABCA4-associated retinal degenerations. J Opt Soc Am A Opt Image Sci Vis 24(5):1457–1467
25. Keilhauer CN, Delori FC (2006) Infrared autofluorescence imaging in inherited macular dystrophies. Invest Ophthalmol Vis Sci ARVO E-Abstract 4045
26. Keilhauer CN, Delori FC (2008) Mapping the junctional zone of geographic atrophy with short wavelength and near-infrared autofluorescence imaging. Invest Ophthal Vis Sci 49: E-Abstract 4246
27. Kellner U, Kellner S, Weber BH et al (2008) Lipofuscin- and melanin-related fundus autofluorescence visualize different retinal pigment epithelial alterations in patients with retinitis pigmentosa. Eye 23(6):1349–59
28. Theelen T, Boon CJ, Klevering BJ et al (2008) [Fundus autofluorescence in patients with inherited retinal diseases : patterns of fluorescence at two different wavelengths] Ophthalmologe. 2008 Nov;105(11):1013–22
29. Sarks JP, Sarks SH, Killingsworth MC (1988) Evolution of geographic atrophy of the retinal pigment epithelium. Eye 2(5):552–577
30. Eagle RC, Lucier AC, Bernadino VB et al (1980) Retinal pigment epithelial abnormalities in fundus flavimaculatus: a light and electron microscopic study. Ophthalmology 87(12):1189–1200
31. O'Gorman S, Flaherty WA, Fishman GA et al (1988) Histopathologic findings in best's vitelliform dystrophy. Arch Ophthalmol 106:1261–1268
32. Milam AH, Li ZY, Fariss RN (1998) Histopathology of the human retina in retinitis pigmentosa. Prog Ret Eye Res 17(2):175–205

Chapter 8

Near-Infrared Subretinal Imaging in Choroidal Neovascularization

8

Thomas Theelen, Carel B. Hoyng, and B. Jeroen Klevering

Core Messages

- Current therapeutic strategies for treatment of choroidal neovascularization (CNV) require frequent monitoring of neovascular activity, which calls for a noninvasive, low-risk imaging technique.
- Ocular coherence tomography (OCT) focuses on static anatomical features like retinal thickening and the presence of sub- and intraretinal fluid, whereas fluorescein angiography employs a longer time frame better suited to address the dynamic aspect of active fluid leakage.
- Near-infrared imaging can be used in the general clinical setting using a commercially available confocal scanning laser device (Heidelberg Retina Angiograph 2).
- Near-infrared reflectance (NIR) imaging provides information on alterations in the retinal structure, subretinal lesions, and the accumulation of fluid within and beneath the retina and the retinal pigment epithelium (RPE). Therefore, NIR complements aspects of both fluorescein angiography and OCT in a noninvasive way.
- Increased intra- and subretinal fluid content reduces NIR and causes a characteristic dark halo around a lesion.
- A classic CNV typically shows a dark core surrounded by a bright corona on NIR imaging.
- The near-infrared image of occult neovascular membranes and detachments of the RPE are less distinctive when compared with classic neovascular membranes. An occult lesion shows an uneven signal increase; a RPE detachment typically presents with a poorly defined ring-shaped reflex.
- Following successful therapeutic intervention, certain alterations occur in the near-infrared image of the choroidal neovascular membrane. Digital subtraction analysis may be employed to enhance these alterations to accurately assess treatment efficacy.

8.1 Introduction

Choroidal neovascularization (CNV) is the hallmark feature of exudative age-related macular degeneration (AMD) and may also complicate other ocular disorders like uveitis, high myopia, and presumed ocular histoplasmosis. The visual acuity in patients with early AMD remains relatively intact until more advanced stages heralded by the arrival of geographic atrophy or CNV. Whereas there are no treatment options in geographic atrophy; most cases of wet AMD due to CNV formation are currently being treated with intravitreal injection of vascular endothelial growth factor inhibitors (anti-VEGFs). To initiate and monitor CNV treatment, careful documentation by serial imaging is necessary. This imaging technique should provide information on lesion activity and associated retinal damage with as little discomfort to the patient as possible. Currently, the most frequently employed methods are fluorescein angiography and ocular coherence tomography (OCT). The current chapter focuses on a possible alternative imaging method for choroidal neovascular membranes originating from the choroid: Near infrared reflectance (NIR).

8.1.1 Histological Characteristics of Choroidal Neovascularization

In CNV, new blood vessels grow from the choroid and invade Bruch's membrane to enter the space under the retinal pigment epithelium (RPE) and/or the subneuroretinal space [1–3]. Histological examination of excised membranes revealed the following components: vascular endothelium, blood, fibrocytes, collagen, fibrin, RPE, and retinal photoreceptors [4]. The clinical appearance of the lesion seems to depend on the localization of the CNV in relation to the other retinal layers, notably the RPE. In type 1, the CNV is located inferior to the RPE, and in type 2, the CNV penetrates the RPE layer [5]. In type 1 CNV, drusen and RPE detachment are common; however, only little RPE proliferation is found. Type 2 CNV represents a relatively sharply demarcated lesion, surrounded by a subretinal pigmentary nimbus or plaques. The histological types of CNV correlate with the angiographic subclasses of classic (type 2) and occult (type 1) CNV [6]. A distinctive characteristic of neovascular vessels in CNV is the lack of tight inter-endothelial junctions; the resulting leakage may lead to serous retinal elevation and retinal thickening owing to leakage of blood serum and small molecules [7]. The variations in anatomical structure, leakage activity, and location of the diverse CNV lesions lead to a broad variety of optical effects and resulting NIR images.

8.1.2 Current Imaging Modalities for Choroidal Neovascularization

To visualize active leakage in CNV, fluorescein angiography has firmly been established as the gold standard for diagnosing and treatment monitoring in wet AMD. Fluorescein is a relatively small chromophore, which leaks readily through neovascular endothelium and has a high quantum yield of fluorescence in the green spectrum after excitation with blue light. Therefore, even minor CNV leakage activity may be detected. However, injection of sodium fluorescein can cause significant discomfort in patients, and lead to serious adverse reactions in up to 5% of the cases [8]. The risk increases up to 49% with repeated fluorescein angiography examinations in patients who previously encountered side effects. In addition, fluorescein angiography suffers from a low inter- and intra-reader agreement [9].

To better visualize the intra-choroidal vessel structures, indocyanine green angiography (ICGA) was introduced in retinal imaging [10]. Indocyanine green is a relatively large chromophore, which does not leak through the neovascular endothelium and has a low quantum yield of fluorescence in the infrared spectrum after excitation with infrared light. Therefore, it is suitable for neovascular vessel analysis largely independent of the visible light absorbers. In contrast to fluorescein, indocyanine green has a much lower complication rate of up to 0.34% [11]. However, interpretation of ICGA images is difficult and requires significant experience.

The rapidly expanding use of anti-VEGF for the treatment of CNV has led to an exponential increase in the follow-up control visits with the need for repeated imaging of CNV activity [12]. This calls for noninvasive imaging techniques to assess CNV activity. In recent years, optical coherence tomography (OCT) has been suggested as a novel, noninvasive imaging protocol for CNV. OCT provides a pseudo-histological perspective of pathologic changes within the living retina. It has a high intra- and inter-reader agreement, and with the introduction of the spectral-domain technique, three-dimensional reconstructions of the lesions have been achievable [13, 14]. OCT and fluorescein look at different aspects of intraretinal fluid dynamics; therefore, their findings often do not concur [15]. OCT focuses on the static anatomical features like retinal thickening and the presence of sub- and intraretinal fluid, whereas fluorescein angiography employs a longer time frame better suited to address the dynamic aspect of active fluid leakage. Therefore, no clear correlations between lesion type and activity on fluorescein angiography and OCT have been established till date.

Summary for the Clinician

- Current therapeutic strategies for the treatment of CNV require frequent monitoring of neovascular activity, which calls for a noninvasive, low-risk imaging technique.
- Fluorescein angiography has a low inter- and intra-reader reliability; in addition, there is significant patient discomfort and serious adverse events occur relatively frequent.
- Indocyanine green angiography gives valuable information on intra-choroidal neovascular vessels, but the interpretation is demanding and the intra-reader agreement is low.
- Optical coherence tomography provides high intra-reader agreement and delivers a static pseudo-histological image of the retina.
- OCT and fluorescein look at different aspects of the neovascular membrane and are therefore complementary, rather than interchangeable.

8.2 The Basic Principles of Near-Infrared Reflectance Imaging of the Retina

The retina is perfectly designed to capture and process the visible spectrum of light, and therefore, main absorbance and reflectance occurs at wavelengths between 450 and 780 nm. Light of a longer wavelength such as near-infrared is invisible to the naked eye and largely avoids absorption and reflection by the layers of the neuroretina. Therefore, near infrared light penetrates relatively easily to the level of the RPE and choroid. Hence, NIR is perfectly designed for use in the imaging of subretinal structures. Probing the ocular fundus with NIR has been suggested by Dallow as early as in 1974 [16], but gained little support at that time. In 1996, Elsner and coworkers [17] demonstrated the NIR visibility of subretinal structures in macular degeneration using a confocal scanning laser ophthalmoscope (SLO). Subsequently, this technique has been extended to polarization-sensitive NIR, and only recently, NIR imaging has been used to capture the appearance of CNV in AMD patients [18–20].

8.2.1 Near-Infrared Reflectance Image Acquisition

The ocular fundus shows a high reflection of near-infrared light when compared with visible light [17]. When a normal fundus camera is employed, these reflections produce poorly contrasted images unsuitable for further analysis of subretinal pathology. Instead, imaging NIR using a confocal SLO removes the out-of-focus reflected light, which leads to a significant improvement in the image quality [21].

The Heidelberg Retina Angiograph (HRA) 2, which is currently the only available confocal SLO to achieve high-contrast NIR images, applies an 830 nm laser source to acquire reflectance images in the near-infrared. The device allows for adjustment of both laser energy and detector sensitivity to optimize the imaging process. To achieve high-quality images, an optimal balance between laser energy and detector sensitivity is necessary.

Clinical practice has shown that 25–50% of the available laser energy provides adequate illumination in the majority of cases. To properly adjust the detector sensitivity, the image needs to be adequately focused. For CNV imaging, the focal plane of the SLO should be located on the inner retinal surface. It has been shown that this provides maximum reading contrast of the images in the near-infrared [22]. To achieve this focal plane, the image focus of HRA 2 has to be positioned on the large retinal vessels. Then, the detector sensitivity can be adjusted based on the major reflecting regions, which are mainly located at the peripapillary atrophic zone. Here, colored pixels that are indicative for overexposure should be hidden. The resulting image yields a maximum contrast in the near-infrared without over- or underexposure of the structures of interest.

For fundus autofluorescence and OCT imaging, image alignment and mean image calculation have been proven to increase image detail by improving the signal-to-noise ratio [23, 24]. Even though this has not been investigated for NIR images, speckle noise does not appear to be prominent in NIR, and therefore, mean image calculation of an image series is not a promising method to further enhance image quality.

8.2.2 Near-Infrared Imaging of the Normal Retina

To correctly interpret the NIR images and to enable comparison with images in the visible spectrum, knowledge of the interactions between the light of various wavelengths and the structures of the retina is essential. In retinal photographic techniques, visible light is highly reflected by the cornea and the ever-present haze of the ocular media. In fluorescein angiography, the light used for excitation has a shorter wavelength than the light emitted by fluorescein. Therefore, reflections and absorptions of media are less important in this technique, and image quality often exceeds that of color photography. Confocal scanning laser NIR fundus imaging is also largely independent of media reflections, despite the fact that the total fundus reflectance is up to 10 times higher than that in red-free fundus photographs [17]. The fact that the healthy retina absorbs the near-infrared light to a much lower degree allows for a marked increase in contrast in the NIR images [22].

In the normal retina, NIR light is reflected by the various tissue layers as well as subretinal structures (Fig. 8.1). The inner limiting membrane demonstrates an age-dependent reflectance that relies on the curvature of the retinal surface as well as the direction of the incoming light [25, 26]. This can be illustrated at the foveal umbo, which shows an increased NIR reflectivity, especially in young individuals (Fig. 8.2). The retinal nerve fiber layer shows relatively high reflectivity in the peripapillary region (Fig. 8.2). However, it is very thin at the macula and therefore its optical impact on NIR in AMD can safely be neglected [27]. The next important reflecting layer in NIR is the retinal photoreceptor layer. Even though the reflections of an individual photoreceptor are relatively weak, the large number of retinal photoreceptors amplifies the signal to a substantial effect [28]. Within the RPE and the choroid, melanin is supposed to add to NIR fundus reflectance [29]. Finally, the sclera has to be considered as a major contributor to NIR fundus reflectivity in the healthy human eye [30].

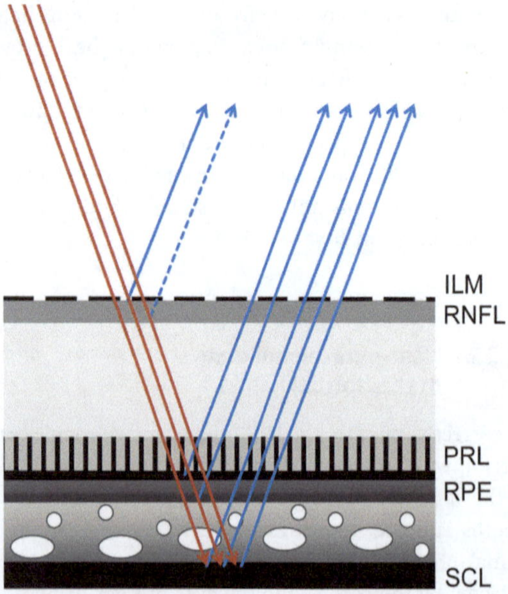

Fig. 8.1 Reflecting retinal layers in the near infrared. The illuminating beam (red arrows) is reflected by diverse intra- and subretinal layers for diverse extents. Strongest reflection is provided by the sclera (SCL), a smaller amount by the retinal photoreceptor layer (PRL) and the retinal pigment epithelium (RPE). Small amounts of reflections originate from the inner limiting membrane (ILM) while the retinal nerve fiber layer (RFNL) only gives important reflections in the near vicinity of the optic nerve. The number and length of the blue arrows indicate the degree of near infrared reflectance

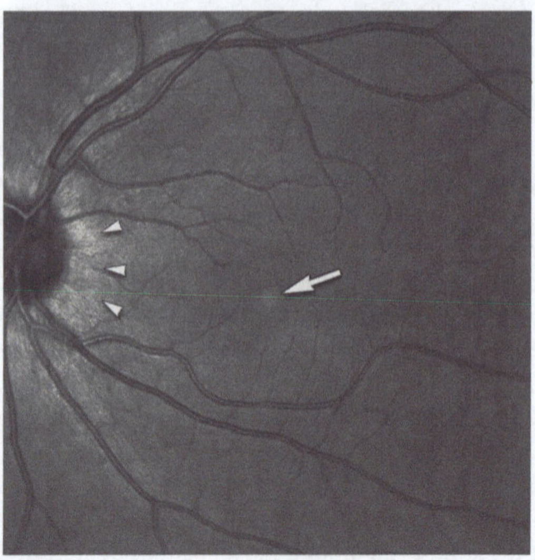

Fig. 8.2 Near infrared reflectance of the normal fundus. The NIR image of the normal fundus is predominated by a medium reflectivity originating from deep layers, like sclera, photoreceptors and retinal pigment epithelium. Even though, these are the strongest reflectors in the near infrared, the reflected light is diffused by intra-retinal, blood-related absorbance and scattering. Therefore, the superficial peripapillary and perivascular retinal nerve fibers (arrowheads) and the prefoveal inner limiting membrane (arrow) as superficial reflectors in the near infrared, outshine the image

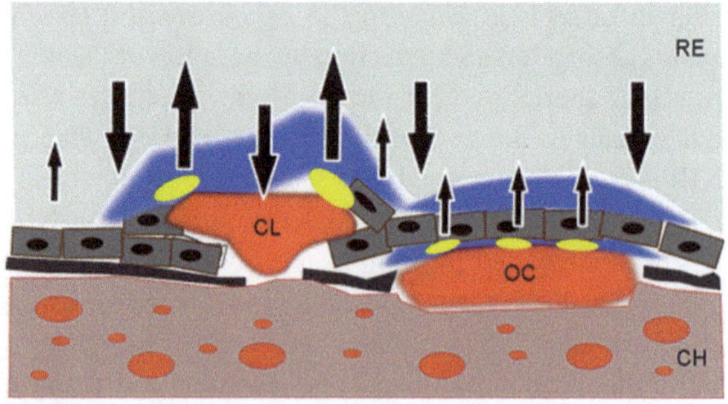

Fig. 8.3 Near-infrared reflectors and absorbers in choroidal neovascularization. A multitude of reflecting (arrows point up) and absorbing (arrows point down) elements add to the near-infrared reflectance image of a choroidal neaovascularization (CNV). The length of the arrows indicated the strength of the optical effects. Unmasked fibrin (yellow dots) is a strong reflector while fluid appears main the absorber. CL=classic CNV; CH= choroidea; OC= occult CNV; RE= retina

Blood and fluid are the main absorbers in the near-infrared spectrum and will therefore look dark on NIR imaging. Other CNV components, such as melanin, fibrin, and collagen, are strong NIR reflectors and will therefore appear bright on the NIR image (Fig. 8.3). Similar to fluorescein angiography, the anatomical setting of the neovascular membrane, i.e., above or below the RPE, is of influence on the NIR image.

Summary for the Clinician

- In NIR imaging with the Heidelberg Retina Angiograph, the confocal laser should be focused on the inner surface of the retina, i.e., the large retinal vessels.
- The NIR image of the normal ocular fundus is defined by a variety of optical tissue interfaces and natural reflectors, such as the inner limiting membrane, the photoreceptors layer, melanin in the RPE and choroid, and finally, the sclera.
- The various components of a CNV membrane may absorb (blood and other fluids) or reflect the infrared light (melanin, fibrin, and collagen).

8.3 Clinical Practice of Near-Infrared Subretinal Imaging

NIR imaging in exudative AMD yields very diverse pictures. This section illustrates the near-infrared properties of all types of CNVs in exudative AMD. The NIR features of neovascular macular degeneration (including idiopathic polypoidal choroidal vasculopathy (IPCV)) are summarized in Table 8.1.

Table 8.1. Key features of near-infrared reflectance in exudative macular degeneration

	NIR appearance				
Lesion type	Dark halo	Bright corona with dark core	Speckled hyper-reflectivity	Diffuse signal increase	Large area of strong signal
Classic CNV	+	+	–	–	–
Occult CNV	+	–	+	–	–
Predominant/minimal classic CNV	+	+	+[2]	–	–
RPE detachment	+	–	+[2]	+[3]	–
RAP	+	–	+	–	–
IPCV	+	–	–	+[4]	–
Fibrovascular scar	±[1]	–	–	–	+

CNV choroidal neovascularization; *IPCV* idiopathic polypoidal choroidal vasculopathy; *RPE* retinal pigment epithelium; *RAP* retinal angiomatous proliferation

[1]Dependent on residual leakage activity

[2]Only occult lesion parts

[3]Poor-defined, ring-like appearance

[4]Vascular, elongated structures

8.3.1 Exudative Age-Related Macular Degeneration

In general, active leakage from a CNV will result in fluid accumulation beneath and within the neuroretina [31]. Visual function in macular edema, however, depends on the integrity of the retinal photoreceptor layer [32]. In NIR imaging, the increased fluid content at the posterior pole amplifies the near-infrared light absorption and scattering [17]. As a result, less light will reach the camera detector, causing regions with increased fluid exudation to appear darker on the NIR image [33]. This reduced photoreceptor reflectivity in NIR in patients with macular edema is directly related to the severity of edema [34]. The area of leakage and edema on the fluorescein angiogram corresponds to a dark, poorly defined halo around the CNV lesion on NIR imaging (Fig. 8.4). We will now discuss the appearance of various types of CNV in AMD on the NIR image. The entity of IPCV will be discussed separately in the following section.

8.3.1.1 Classic Choroidal Neovascularization

Before the introduction of anti-VEGF treatment of neovascular AMD, only classic CNV cases with well-defined borders were applicable for treatment by either focal laser coagulation or photodynamic therapy [35, 36]. Classic cases show high blood flow within the lesion and are surrounded by a characteristic pigmented halo [4, 37]. These features account for the characteristic findings on NIR imaging of classic CNVs [19, 38].

Classic CNVs are typically located anterior to the RPE [4] and therefore only little NIR light reflection and absorbance occurs, which accounts for a good visibility of the classic CNV lesion in the near-infrared. A main attribute of classic CNV lesions in NIR appearance is the combination of a central dark core surrounded by a bright corona (Fig. 8.5). The ring-shaped bright corona may be incomplete in up to one-third of the cases [19]. The active neovascular process is depicted as a dark core due to the blood- and fluid-related light absorption in this area.

It has been shown that neovascular changes due to AMD may not only lead to hypertrophic RPE reactions, but also to exudation of fibrin in the area adjacent to the CNV [6, 39]. More so than melanin, fibrin is a relatively strong reflector in the near-infrared [29]. The bright nimbus surrounding the classic membranes is only partially co-located with the funduscopically visible pigmented halo. Hence, the bright corona on NIR imaging of classic CNV lesions may probably reflect not only the hypertrophic RPE reaction, but also the fibrin exudation.

8.3.1.2 Occult Choroidal Neovascularization

The occult form of CNV is the most frequent neovascular lesion type in AMD [40]. On fluorescein angiogram, occult CNVs are typically characterized by the phrase "late leakage of undetermined source"; however, they may appear as shallow fibrovascular detachments when examined by OCT. Based on the exact anatomical position of the membrane, light reflection, scattering, and absorption all add to the near-infrared image [27]. Contrary to classic lesions, occult neovascular membranes are poorly demarked and show overlying scattered NIR increase (Fig. 8.6). With regard to histology, occult

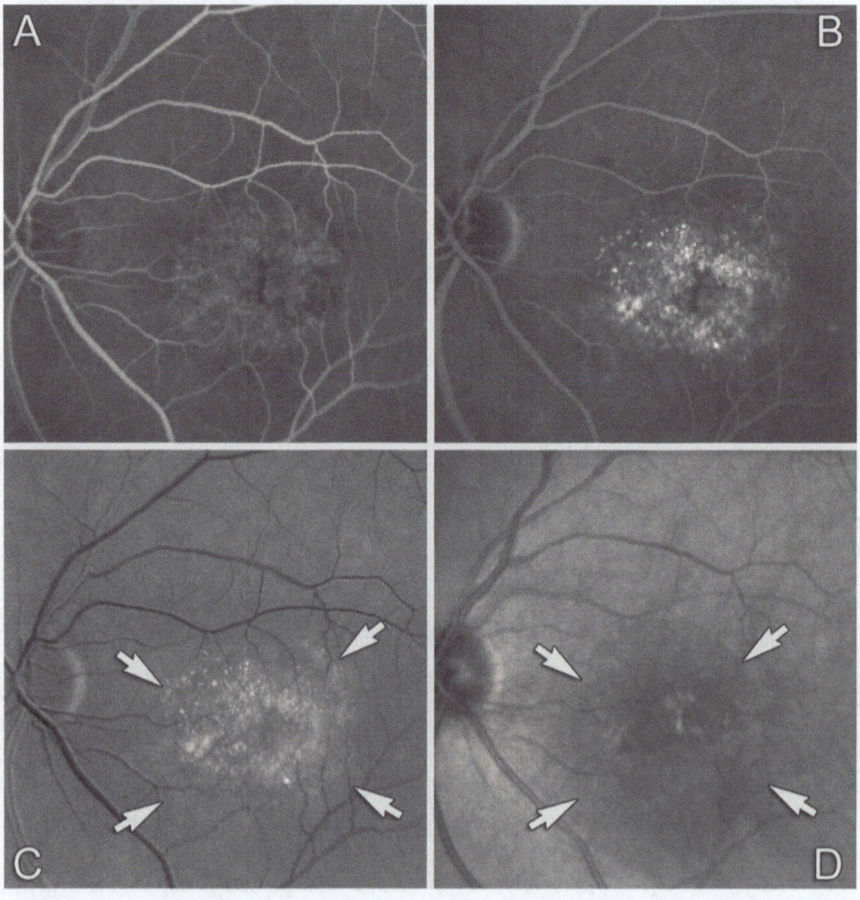

Fig. 8.4 Effect of fluid leakage on the NIR image of a CNV. A case of active leaking CNV documented by fluorescein angiography (A, B). The poorly demarked CNV (A) is surrounded by diffuse staining in the late phase angiography (B). The digital subtraction analysis clearly demarcates this fluorescein leakage area (C, arrows), which correlates with the reduced near-infrared reflectance around the lesion (D, arrows). Note that the central part of stronger leakage is associated with a darker innermost NIR area

CNV membranes are largely located posterior to the RPE [1, 2]. On the surface of the occult CNV, disseminated fibrin coagulates have been found [6], which may be related to the spotted NIR increase. Frequently observed alterations of the RPE and small drusen in occult CNV cases may also add to their NIR appearance. RPE loss, for instance, will cause increased choroidal reflectivity and drusen may decrease NIR focally.

8.3.1.3 Vascularized Detachment of the Retinal Pigment Epithelium

If fluid is trapped beneath the RPE, an occult CNV may cause a dome-shaped RPE detachment, despite slow vessel proliferation and only mild leakage. Typically, a peripheral hyperfluorescent notch on fluorescein angiography suggests the presence of a CNV associated with such an RPE detachment [37]. The optical appearance of an RPE detachment on NIR is determined by its anatomical contour, melanin content, and turbidity of the sub-RPE fluid. In addition, the appearance of the lesion is largely determined by the focus of the SLO [41]. If the focal plane of the image is near the apex of the RPE elevation, then the lesion appears bright due to the light scattered by the pigment epithelium. However, if the image is focused deep to Bruch's membrane, a dark core caused by light absorption within the turbid sub-RPE fluid will dominate the lesion center. The edges of the RPE elevation will appear bright due to the oblique position and associated scattering of the incoming light. This summation of melanin reflectance and light scattering results in a strong NIR signal. Usually, a thin dark halo caused by a discrete serous retinal elevation surrounds the RPE detachment (Fig. 8.7). In general, an RPE detachment will appear as round lesion with a centrally decreased reflectivity by turbid sub-RPE fluid, delimited by a thin, brighter nimbus and bordered by a dark, irregular halo [42]. As in occult lesions without RPE detachment, the CNV membrane is poorly defined.

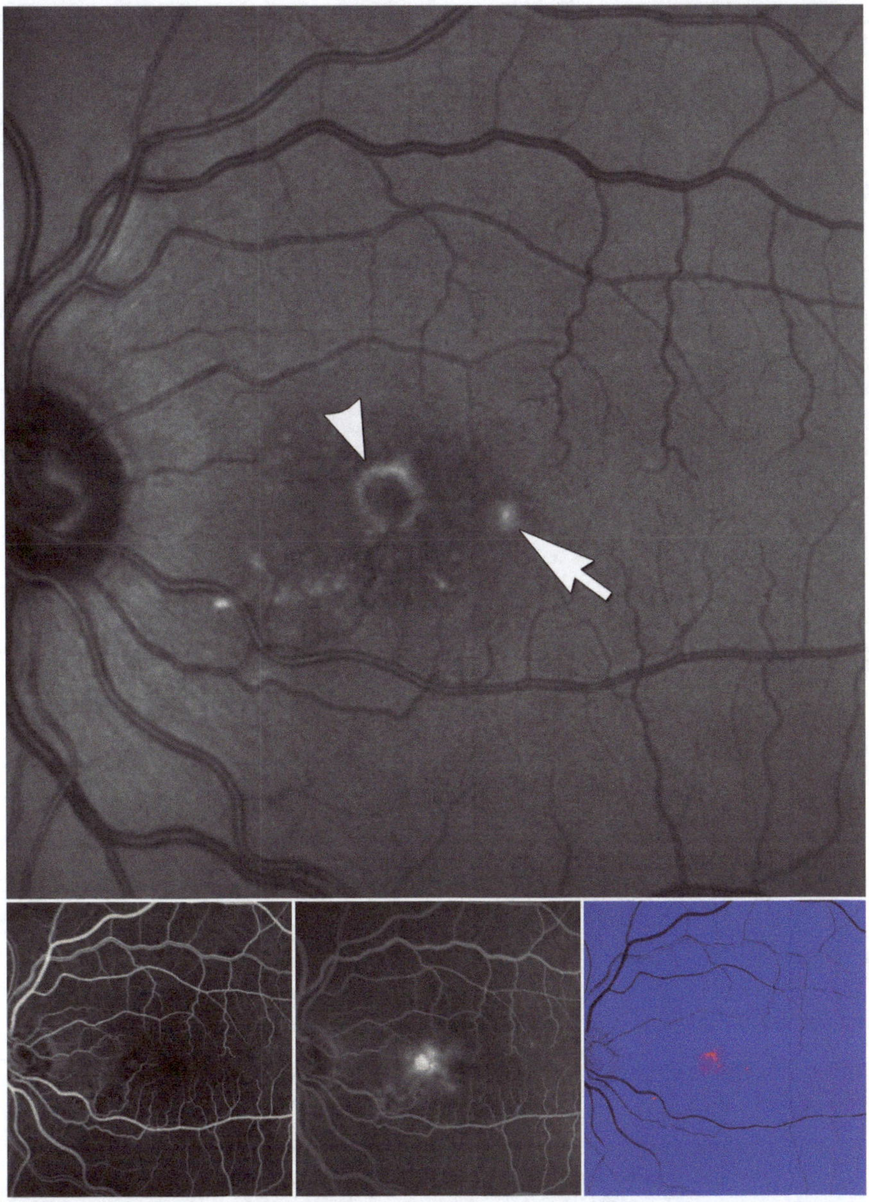

Fig. 8.5 NIR appearance of classic CNV as compared to fluorescein angiography. This case of classic, parafoveal CNV shows a ring of increased NIR (upper panel, arrowhead) that is co-located with early staining on FA (lower panel, left). The leakage zone on FA (lower panel, middle) and the dark halo on NIR (upper panel) match properly. The increased NIR at the fovea (arrow) points to a virtual anatomical integrity of this area (visual acuity 20/25). As indicated by the red color on the difference map between FA leakage and NIR (lower panel, right), fluid accumulation is only underestimated on NIR at hyper-reflective areas, however, comparable information on leakage is provided at the remaining fundus (blue hues)

8.3.1.4 Mixed-Type Choroidal Neovascularization

In a minority of cases, a nonuniform type of CNV will occur [43]. In fluorescein angiography, these membranes are classified into minimal classic and predominantly classic CNV lesions. In NIR, these mixed types show characteristics of both classic and occult CNVs (Fig. 8.8). As in fluorescein angiography, the lesion type may be estimated by the area covered by the classic and occult portion, respectively.

8.3.1.5 Retinal Angiomatous Proliferation

Unlike regular exudative AMD, the neovascular membrane in retinal angiomatous proliferation (RAP) originates from the neuroretina [44]. The formation of a CNV

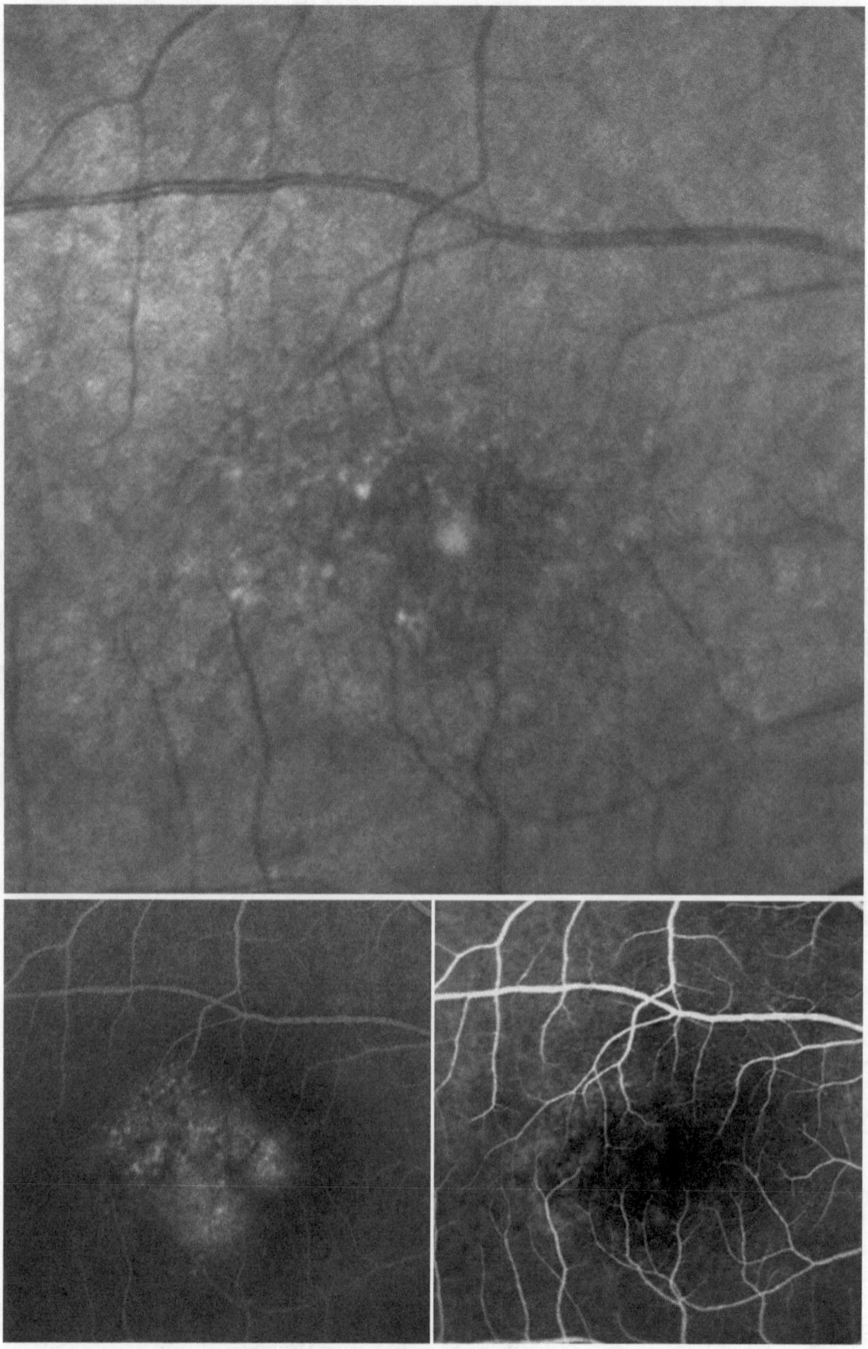

Fig. 8.6 NIR appearance of occult CNV. An eye with occult CNV on FA (lower panels) shows characteristic jagged NIR elevations within an area of decreased NIR signal (upper panel). Note that the lesion is poorly demarcated on NIR as well as on FA. In contrast to the majority of classic lesions, the dark halo on NIR in most occult CNV is less prominent due to only mild leakage activity

in RAP is therefore an inherently secondary process. Once the CNV has formed, the differentiation between non-RAP and RAP lesions on NIR may become impossible. The neovascular membrane in the early pre-CNV stages of RAP, on the other hand, may show unique optical properties. In these early RAP cases, focally increased NIR signals within a darkened, ill-defined area can be observed (Fig. 8.9). This hyperreflection is most likely associated with the fibrinous material located within the edematous swollen retina surrounding the lesion, as demonstrated in the histological preparations of RAP patients [39]. Interestingly, some RAP cases show a much

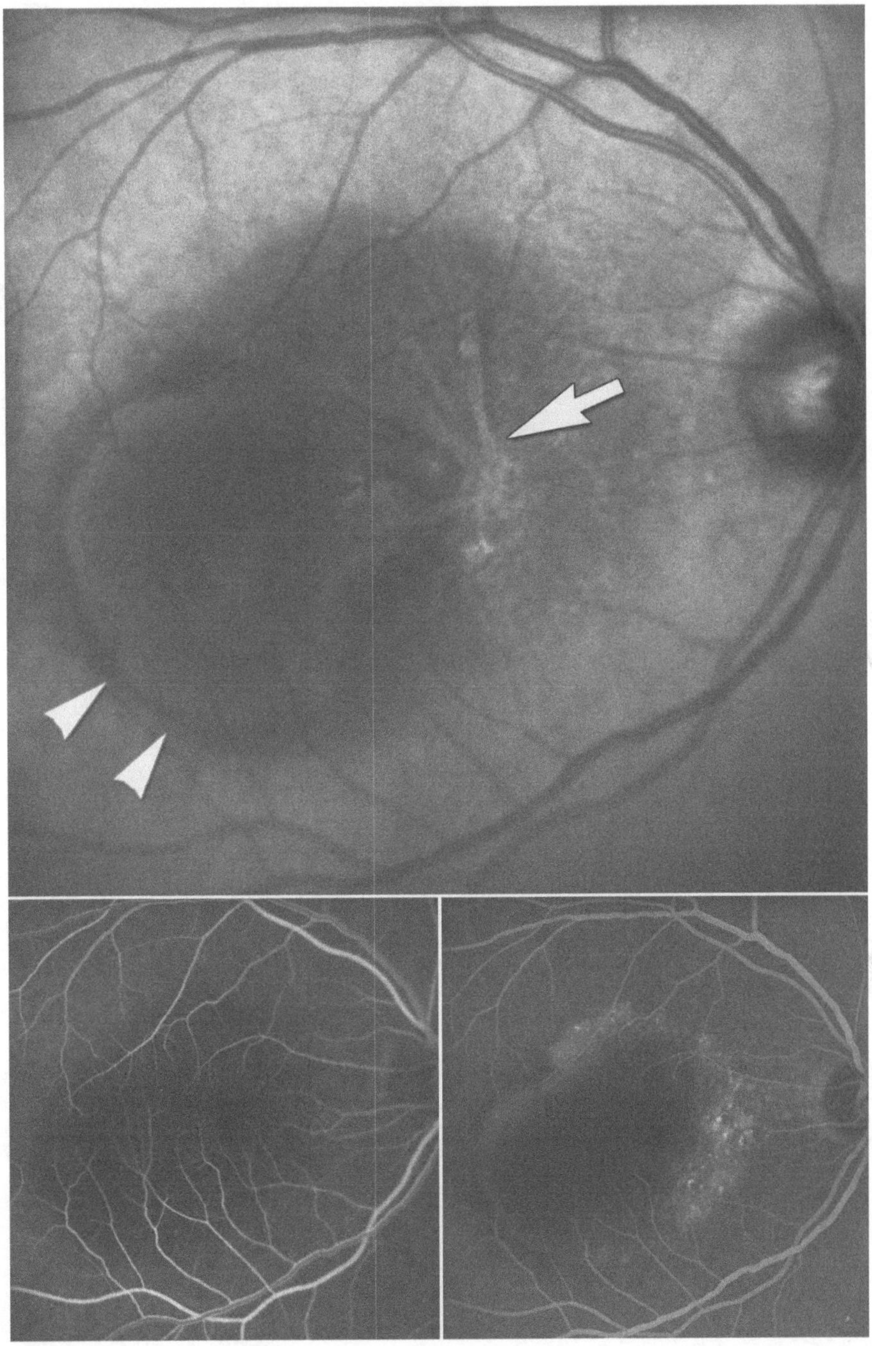

Fig. 8.7 Vascularized RPE detachment. A case of occult CNV with associated serous RPE detachment (NIR, upper panel; FA, lower panels). The occult lesion has called up a fibrotic reaction with secondary retinal folds (arrow), leading to increased scattering and reflectivity in the near-infrared. The edges of the RPE detachment (arrowheads) appear brighter than the surrounding dark halo caused by sub-retinal fluid. The focal plane of the cSLO is located deep in the retina. Therefore, the turbid sub-RPE fluid causes the center of the RPE detachment to appear dark

larger zone of decreased NIR than is to be expected from the corresponding fluorescein angiogram. This may be caused by abnormalities in the Müller cell population, resulting in an increase in the NIR light absorption prior to macroscopic thickening of the neuroretina or leakage on the fluorescein angiogram [45, 46].

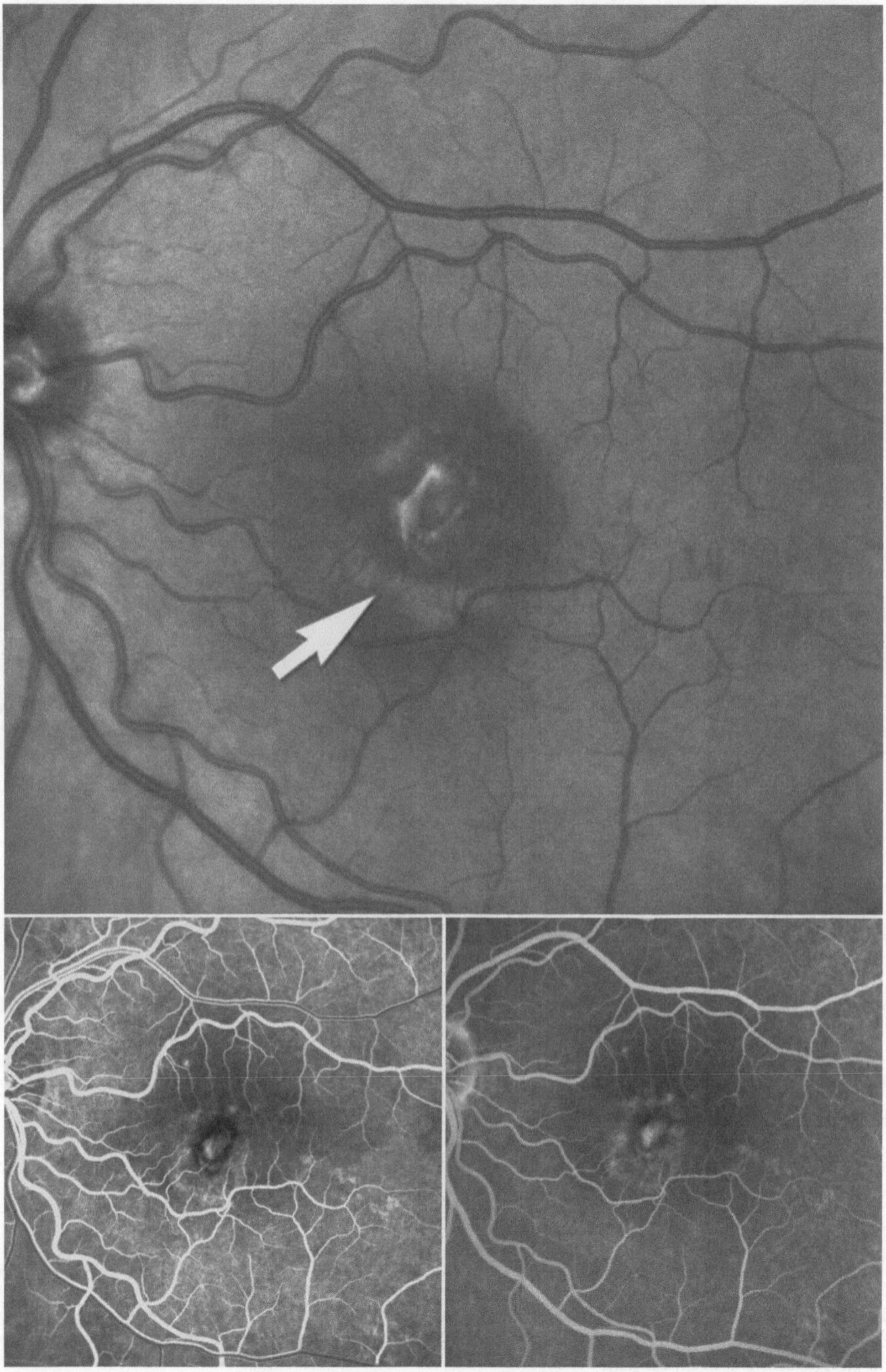

Fig. 8.8 Minimal classic CNV lesion. In partial classic CNV cases, NIR (upper panel) shows properties of classic and occult membranes. Note that the area corresponding to the classic component on FA (lower panels) appears as incomplete bright ring with a dark halo on NIR, while the occult parts cause poorly demarcated, incomplete NIR elevation within the darkened area of sub-retinal fluid (arrow)

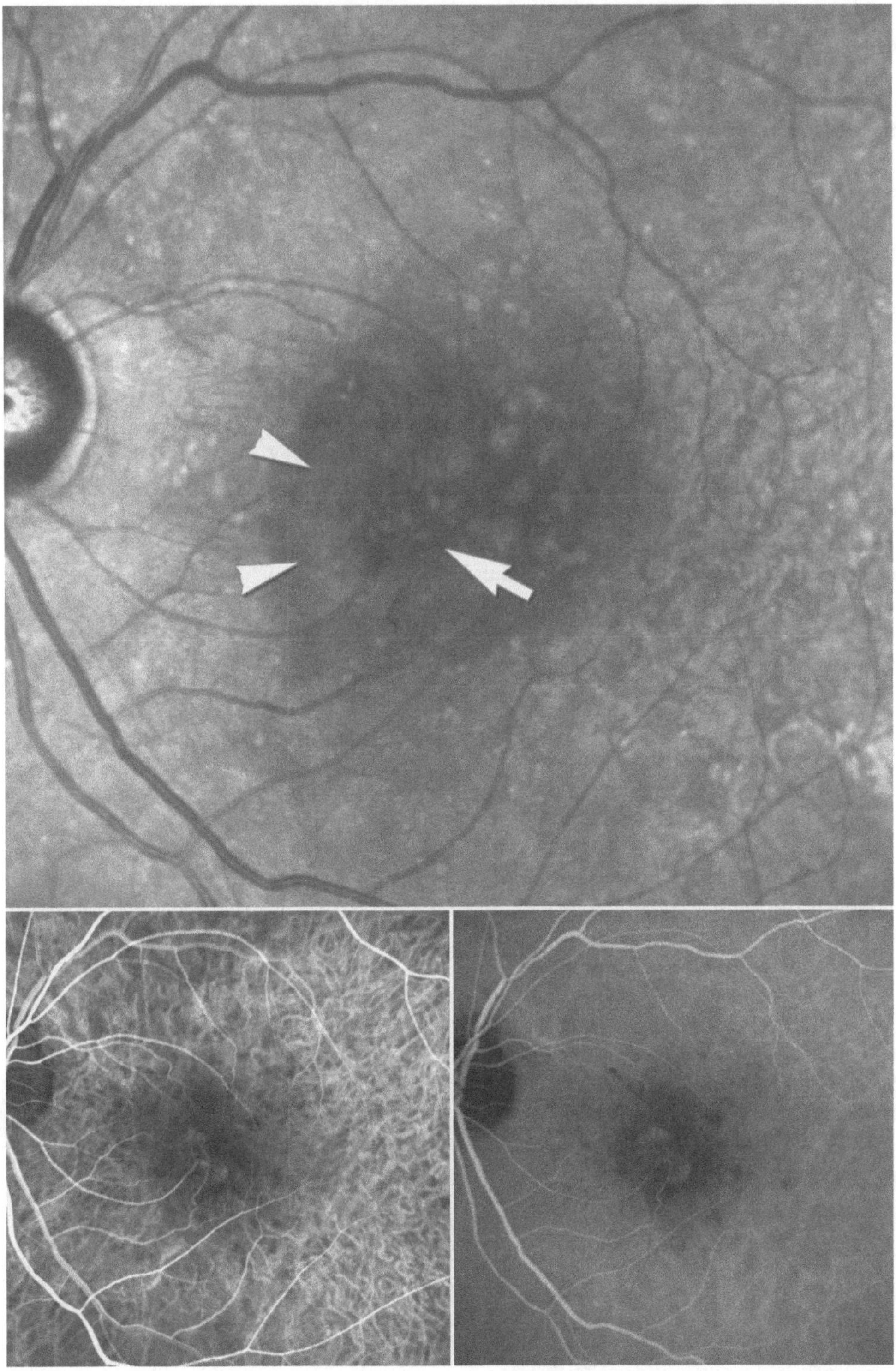

Fig. 8.9 Retinal angiomatous proliferation. RAP lesions are typically best visualized on indocyanine green angiography (ICGA, lower panels). The new vessels initiate within the neuroretina and grow to the RPE and choroid, eventually leading to secondary CNV formation. The intra-retinal vascular complex causes jagged NIR elevation within the halo of fluid exudation (upper panel, arrow). The additional RPE detachment without signs of CNV on ICGA is visible on NIR (upper panel, arrowheads)

8.3.2 Idiopathic Polypoidal Choroidal Vasculopathy

The term IPCV stands for a separate clinical entity that differs clinically and demographically from AMD [47]. ICG and OCT studies revealed that polypoidal vascular lesions of the choroid are associated with serous and hemorrhagic RPE detachments [48, 49]

The variable presentation of IPCV gives rise to equally variable NIR images. RPE detachments and serous retinal elevations have a similar aspect as vascularized RPE detachments in AMD (Sect. 8.3.1.3). However, the localization and the source of the underlying subretinal structures separate IPCV from a regular AMD-associated RPE detachment on NIR imaging (Fig. 8.10). The polypoidal structures can be identified by their increased signal on NIR that collocates with their position on ICGA. The bright reflex represents the typically elongated, large vessel-like structures, as opposed to the adjacent small-sized signals of RPE alterations and the large, round reflexes of RPE detachments.

8.3.3 Fibrovascular Scar

Following treatment or in the later stages of a wet AMD, a degenerative process will lead to vessel occlusion and the development of scar tissue within the neovascular lesion. This scar consists of dense fibrous tissue, possibly surrounded by fibrinous exudations [50]. Higher levels of collagen fibers will lead to increased scattering and reflectance within the tissue, consequently enlarging the NIR signal [51]. Therefore, fibrovascular scars can be identified by their exceedingly bright appearance on NIR imaging (Fig. 8.11). Depending on a residual elevation of the overlying retina, a dark halo may be observed in the vicinity of the scar. In addition, there may be co-existing active parts of a CNV with the typical NIR manifestations as described in Sect. 8.3.1.1 through 8.3.4.

Summary for the Clinician

- The location of the neovascular membrane in relation to the RPE has its effects on the resultant NIR image.
- A dark, often poorly defined halo around the lesion is a frequent finding in the NIR of exudative macular degeneration and correlates with active CNV leakage on fluorescein angiography.
- On the NIR image, a bright corona surrounding a dark core is the characteristic sign of a well-defined, classic CNV.
- Occult CNV lesions show poorly demarked areas of scattered NIR increase with an underlying dark halo.
- In RPE detachments, a thin, lighter corona encircles an area of normal to low reflectivity, including scattered NIR increase at the area of the CNV.
- The darkened halo in RAP often exceeds the leakage zone on fluorescein angiography, possibly as a result of pre-edematous Müller cell disease. The RAP lesion itself appears as an irregular, increased NIR signal.
- Abnormal vessels in IPCV are mirrored by relatively high-reflective, elongated structures on NIR imaging.
- In the end stage of CNV membranes, the dense-packed collagen fibers in fibrovascular scars produce a very strong NIR signal.

8.3.4 Choroidal Neovascularization Not Associated with AMD

A variety of other disorders like high myopia, retinal dystrophies, uveitis, or idiopathic genesis may account for the development of CNV [52–54]. The majority of these neovascularization appear to be of the well-defined classic type. Coexisting retinal changes associated with underlying disorder, however, may confuse the interpretation of the NIR image. For instance, non-neovascular fundus lesions like inflammatory spots may also have increased fluid content and cause a locally elevated retina, giving rise to NIR abnormalities not unlike CNVs.

8.4 Evaluating Therapeutic Effects with Near-Infrared Reflectance Imaging

The evolving new therapeutic strategies in CNV treatment require repeated imaging of the fundus to monitor the treatment effects and to aid in the appropriate timing for re-treatment [55]. Besides fluorescein angiography as the gold-standard for the assessment of CNV activity, OCT has become a widely accepted noninvasive tool in the evaluation of AMD therapy [56]. However, OCT data are not directly comparable with fluorescein angiography results due to their essential differences. Besides the static character of the anatomical OCT image, the huge memory capacity needed for modern three-dimensional OCT may be a drawback. Fluorescein angiography evaluates the functional aspects of the CNV by dynamic imaging

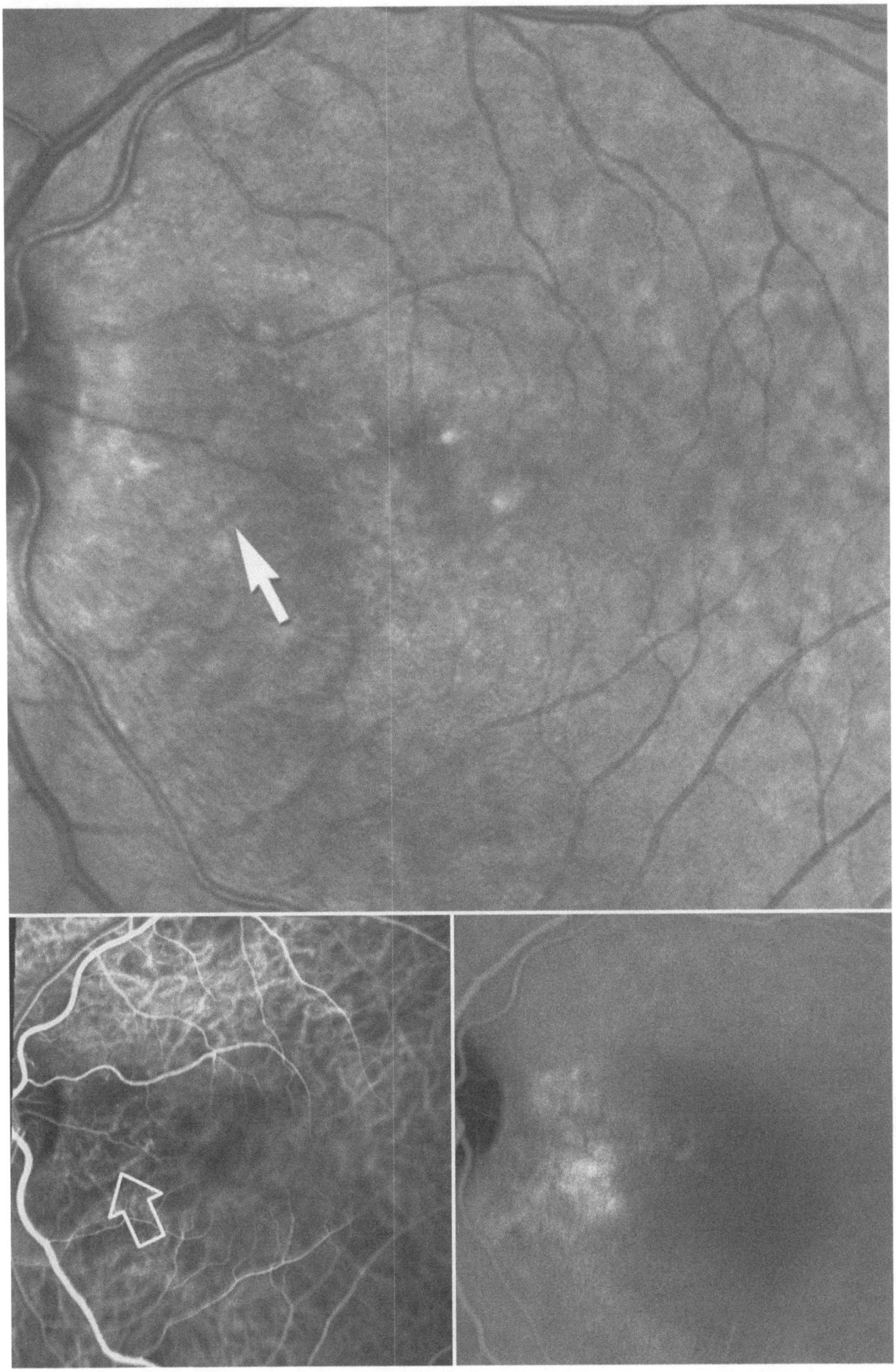

Fig. 8.10 Idiopathic polypoidal choroidal vasculopathy. In idiopathic polypoidal choroidal vasculopathy vascular structures may be detected in NIR (upper panel, arrow), typically located nasally from the macular area. These structures correlate with the polypoidal vessel abnormalities identified on ICGA in the early phase (lower panel, open arrow). A corresponding RPE detachment causes characteristic NIR affections comparable to those in Fig. 8.8

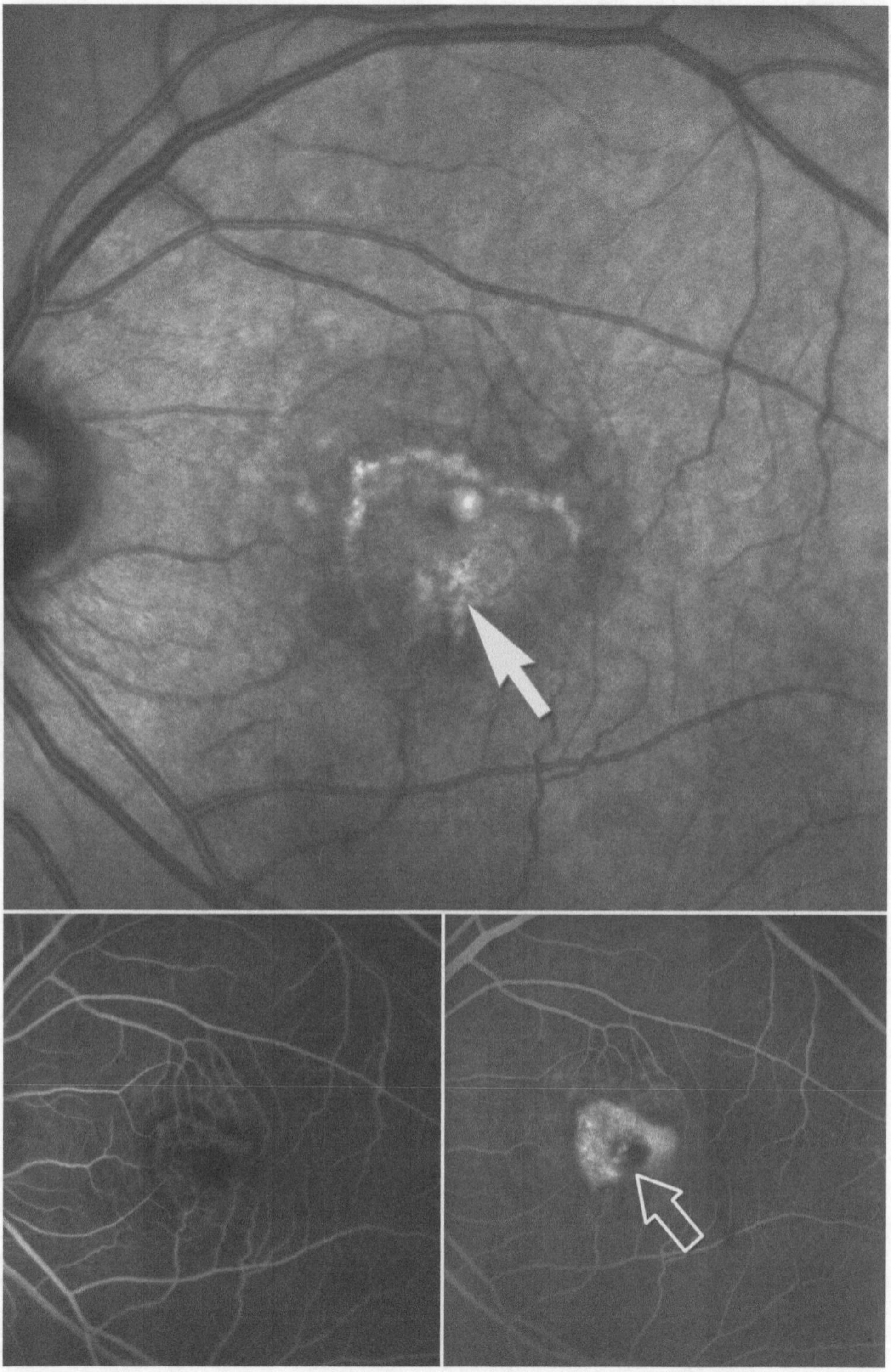

Fig. 8.11 Fibrovascular scar. After treatment a fibrovascular scar remains as leftover of the CNV. This formerly classic lesion has partially kept the appearance of a bright ring on NIR (upper panel). Some parts of the membrane still show some perfusion on FA (lower panel), however others do not (open arrow). These avascular components appear highly reflective on NIR due to their increased content of collage fibers (arrow)

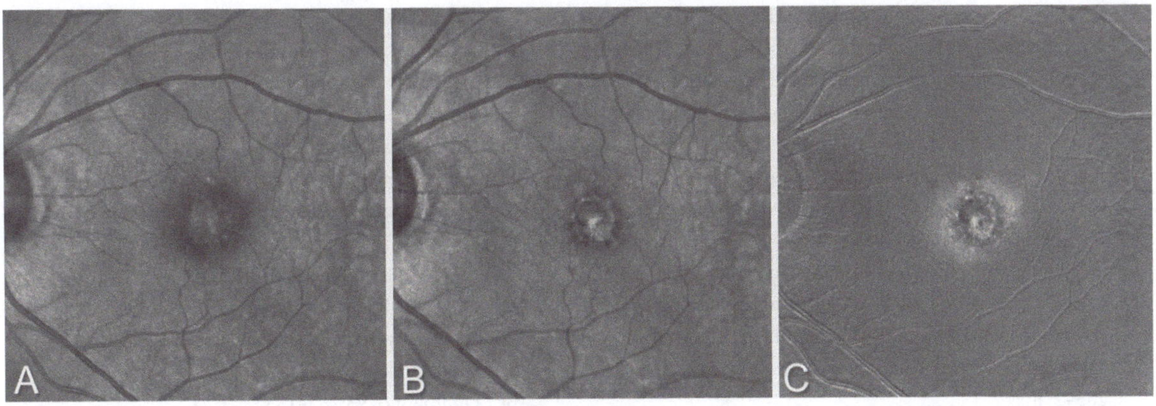

Fig. 8.12 Follow-up of bevacizumab therapy with NIR. During successful treatment of active CNV leakage of fluid will regress and scarring may come up. This example illustrates the accompanying NIR changes in a patient with a small, occult lesion. Pre treatment (**A**) a considerable dark halo is present around the CNV. After three sessions of intravitreal bevacizumab, the dark halo has largely disappeared (**B**). In addition, the center of the lesion shows increased NIR due to scarring. The difference in NIR can be illustrated by a subtraction map, which shows increased NIR, thus reduced fluid leakage, as white pixels (**C**)

of the amount of exudation, but does not provide anatomic information on retinal thickening [15].

NIR imaging, on the other hand, will cover both functional (leakage) and anatomical (thickening) aspects of CNV membranes by noninvasive means. The amount of storage capacity needed is minimal when compared with 3D OCT (usually between 20 and 800 kilobytes as JPEG and TIFF files, respectively). Changes in leakage as well as decrease in the retinal thickening both will influence the NIR signal. These changes can be assessed by digital subtraction analysis and may be used for monitoring the CNV treatment (Fig. 8.12). Just as in fluorescein angiography, an *en face* image is provided and allows mapping of sub- and intraretinal fluid and thickening. Other than OCT volume scan, the rapid image acquisition minimizes artifacts due to eye movements. Still, the specificity and sensitivity of NIR in CNV treatment monitoring has to be verified by prospective studies.

Summary for the Clinician

- NIR imaging is capable of detecting both the changes in the amount of leakage as well as the amount of fluid accumulation in the retina or under the RPE. In this, it combines the aspects of both fluorescein angiography and OCT.
- Regressive changes within a neovascular membrane lead to increased near-infrared reflectivity, which can be measured by subtraction analysis.
- The sensitivity and specificity of NIR imaging still has to be verified by prospective studies, and until that time, fluorescein angiography and OCT should complementarily be used.

8.5 Conclusions

NIR imaging by confocal scanning laser opthalmoscopy offers a rapid and noninvasive way to depict subretinal changes of the ocular fundus in exudative macular degeneration. As in fluorescein angiography, NIR provides information on the area of leakage, which appears as a dark halo around a lesion. In addition, data on the nature of the CNV (well-defined or occult) could be derived by NIR in a noninvasive way. Retinal thickening, inherently invisible on fluorescein angiography, also leads to changes in the NIR images and could be correlated to OCT findings. Following successful CNV treatment, the NIR image changes occur due to reduction of leakage and the formation of the fibrinous scar. Even though NIR study results seem promising, the clinical significance of NIR imaging in CNV evaluation and treatment remains to be proven in large patient samples in a masked, prospective way. The sensitivity and specificity of this promising new technique still needs to be compared with established methods of investigation, such as fluorescein angiography and OCT.

References

1. Grossniklaus HE, Miskala PH, Green WR, Bressler SB, Hawkins BS, Toth C, Wilson DJ, Bressler NM (2005) Histopathologic and ultrastructural features of surgically excised subfoveal choroidal neovascular lesions: submacular surgery trials report no. 7. Arch Ophthalmol 123:914–921
2. Grossniklaus HE, Wilson DJ, Bressler SB, Bressler NM, Toth CA, Green WR, Miskala P (2006) Clinicopathologic studies of eyes that were obtained postmortem from four patients who were enrolled in the submacular surgery trials: SST Report No. 16. Am J Ophthalmol 141:93–104

3. Spraul CW, Lang GE, Grossniklaus HE, Lang GK (1999) Histologic and morphometric analysis of the choroid, Bruch's membrane, and retinal pigment epithelium in postmortem eyes with age-related macular degeneration and histologic examination of surgically excised choroidal neovascular membranes. Surv Ophthalmol 44(Suppl 1):S10–S32
4. Grossniklaus HE, Gass JD (1998) Clinicopathologic correlations of surgically excised type 1 and type 2 submacular choroidal neovascular membranes. Am J Ophthalmol 126:59–69
5. Gass JD (1994) Biomicroscopic and histopathologic considerations regarding the feasibility of surgical excision of subfoveal neovascular membranes. Am J Ophthalmol 118: 285–298
6. Lafaut BA, Bartz-Schmidt KU, Vanden BC, Aisenbrey S, De Laey JJ, Heimann K (2000) Clinicopathological correlation in exudative age related macular degeneration: histological differentiation between classic and occult choroidal neovascularisation. Br J Ophthalmol 84:239–243
7. Campochiaro PA (2000) Retinal and choroidal neovascularization. J Cell Physiol 184:301–310
8. Kwiterovich KA, Maguire MG, Murphy RP, Schachat AP, Bressler NM, Bressler SB, Fine SL (1991) Frequency of adverse systemic reactions after fluorescein angiography. Results of a prospective study. Ophthalmology 98:1139–1142
9. Holz FG, Jorzik J, Schutt F, Flach U, Unnebrink K (2003) Agreement among ophthalmologists in evaluating fluorescein angiograms in patients with neovascular age-related macular degeneration for photodynamic therapy eligibility (FLAP-study). Ophthalmology 110:400–405
10. Slakter JS, Yannuzzi LA, Guyer DR, Sorenson JA, Orlock DA (1995) Indocyanine-green angiography. Curr Opin Ophthalmol 6:25–32
11. Obana A, Miki T, Hayashi K, Takeda M, Kawamura A, Mutoh T, Harino S, Fukushima I, Komatsu H, Takaku Y (1994) Survey of complications of indocyanine green angiography in Japan. Am J Ophthalmol 118:749–753
12. Andreoli CM, Miller JW (2007) Anti-vascular endothelial growth factor therapy for ocular neovascular disease. Curr Opin Ophthalmol 18:502–508
13. Wojtkowski M, Srinivasan V, Fujimoto JG, Ko T, Schuman JS, Kowalczyk A, Duker JS (2005) Three-dimensional retinal imaging with high-speed ultrahigh-resolution optical coherence tomography. Ophthalmology 112:1734–1746
14. Zhang N, Hoffmeyer GC, Young ES, Burns RE, Winter KP, Stinnett SS, Toth CA, Jaffe GJ (2007) Optical coherence tomography reader agreement in neovascular age-related macular degeneration. Am J Ophthalmol 144:37–44
15. van Velthoven ME, de Smet MD, Schlingemann RO, Magnani M, Verbraak FD (2006) Added value of OCT in evaluating the presence of leakage in patients with age-related macular degeneration treated with PDT. Graefes Arch Clin Exp Ophthalmol 244:1119–1123
16. Dallow RL (1974) Color infrared photography of the ocular fundus. Arch Ophthalmol 92:254–258
17. Elsner AE, Burns SA, Weiter JJ, Delori FC (1996) Infrared imaging of sub-retinal structures in the human ocular fundus. Vision Res 36:191–205
18. Elsner AE, Weber A, Cheney MC, Vannasdale DA, Miura M (2007) Imaging polarimetry in patients with neovascular age-related macular degeneration. J Opt Soc Am A Opt Image Sci Vis 24:1468–1480
19. Semoun O, Guigui B, Tick S, Coscas G, Soubrane G, Souied EH (2009) Infrared features of classic choroidal neovascularisation in exudative age-related macular degeneration. Br J Ophthalmol 93:182–185
20. Theelen T, Berendschot TT, Hoyng CB, Boon CJ, Klevering BJ (2009) Near-infrared reflectance imaging of neovascular age-related macular degeneration. Graefes Arch Clin Exp Ophthalmol. 2009 (in press)
21. Webb RH, Hughes GW, Delori FC (1987) Confocal scanning laser ophthalmoscope. Appl Opt 26:1492–1499
22. Miura M, Elsner AE, Beausencourt E, Kunze C, Hartnett ME, Lashkari K, Trempe CL (2002) Grading of infrared confocal scanning laser tomography and video displays of digitized color slides in exudative age-related macular degeneration. Retina 22:300–308
23. Hangai M, Yamamoto M, Sakamoto A, Yoshimura N (2009) Ultrahigh-resolution versus speckle noise-reduction in spectral-domain optical coherence tomography. Opt Express 17:4221–4235
24. Jorzik JJ, Bindewald A, Dithmar S, Holz FG (2005) Digital simultaneous fluorescein and indocyanine green angiography, autofluorescence, and red-free imaging with a solid-state laser-based confocal scanning laser ophthalmoscope. Retina 25:405–416
25. Gorrand JM, Alfieri R, Boire JY (1984) Diffusion of the retinal layers of the living human eye. Vision Res 24:1097–1106
26. Gorrand JM, Delori FC (1999) Reflectance and curvature of the inner limiting membrane at the foveola. J Opt Soc Am A Opt Image Sci Vis 16:1229–1237
27. Berendschot TT, De Lint PJ, van Norren D (2003) Fundus reflectance – historical and present ideas. Prog Retin Eye Res 22:171–200
28. van de Kraats J, Berendschot TT, van Norren D (1996) The pathways of light measured in fundus reflectometry. Vision Res 36:2229–2247
29. Weinberger AW, Lappas A, Kirschkamp T, Mazinani BA, Huth JK, Mohammadi B, Walter P (2006) Fundus near infrared fluorescence correlates with fundus near infrared reflectance. Invest Ophthalmol Vis Sci 47:3098–3108
30. Delori FC, Pflibsen KP (1989) Spectral reflectance of the human ocular fundus. Appl Opt 28:1061–1077
31. Eter N, Spaide RF (2005) Comparison of fluorescein angiography and optical coherence tomography for

patients with choroidal neovascularization after photodynamic therapy. Retina 25:691–696

32. Murakami T, Tsujikawa A, Ohta M, Miyamoto K, Kita M, Watanabe D, Takagi H, Yoshimura N (2007) Photoreceptor status after resolved macular edema in branch retinal vein occlusion treated with tissue plasminogen activator. Am J Ophthalmol 143:171–173
33. Elsner AE, Zhou Q, Beck F, Tornambe PE, Burns SA, Weiter JJ, Dreher AW (2001) Detecting AMD with multiply scattered light tomography. Int Ophthalmol 23:245–250
34. Lardenoye CW, Probst K, DeLint PJ, Rothova A (2000) Photoreceptor function in eyes with macular edema. Invest Ophthalmol Vis Sci 41:4048–4053
35. The Macular Photocoagulation Study Group (1994) Laser photocoagulation for juxtafoveal choroidal neovascularization. Five-year results from randomized clinical trials. Arch Ophthalmol 112:500–509
36. Bressler NM (2001) Photodynamic therapy of subfoveal choroidal neovascularization in age-related macular degeneration with verteporfin: two-year results of 2 randomized clinical trials-tap report 2. Arch Ophthalmol 119:198–207
37. Gass JD (1997) Stereoscopic atlas of macular diseases, 4th edn. Mosby, St Louis
38. Hartnett ME, Elsner AE (1996) Characteristics of exudative age-related macular degeneration determined in vivo with confocal and indirect infrared imaging. Ophthalmology 103:58–71
39. Lafaut BA, Aisenbrey S, Vanden BC, Bartz-Schmidt KU (2000) Clinicopathological correlation of deep retinal vascular anomalous complex in age related macular degeneration. Br J Ophthalmol 84:1269–1274
40. Olsen TW, Feng X, Kasper TJ, Rath PP, Steuer ER (2004) Fluorescein angiographic lesion type frequency in neovascular age-related macular degeneration. Ophthalmology 111:250–255
41. Kunze C, Elsner AE, Beausencourt E, Moraes L, Hartnett ME, Trempe CL (1999) Spatial extent of pigment epithelial detachments in age-related macular degeneration. Ophthalmology 106:1830–1840
42. Miura M, Yamanari M, Iwasaki T, Elsner AE, Makita S, Yatagai T, Yasuno Y (2008) Imaging polarimetry in age-related macular degeneration. Invest Ophthalmol Vis Sci 49:2661–2667
43. Olsen TW, Feng X, Kasper TJ, Rath PP, Steuer ER (2004) Fluorescein angiographic lesion type frequency in neovascular age-related macular degeneration. Ophthalmology 111:250–255
44. Yannuzzi LA, Negrao S, Iida T, Carvalho C, Rodriguez-Coleman H, Slakter J, Freund KB, Sorenson J, Orlock D, Borodoker N (2001) Retinal angiomatous proliferation in age-related macular degeneration. Retina 21:416–434
45. Bringmann A, Pannicke T, Grosche J, Francke M, Wiedemann P, Skatchkov SN, Osborne NN, Reichenbach A (2006) Muller cells in the healthy and diseased retina. Prog Retin Eye Res 25:397–424
46. Reichenbach A, Wurm A, Pannicke T, Iandiev I, Wiedemann P, Bringmann A (2007) Muller cells as players in retinal degeneration and edema. Graefes Arch Clin Exp Ophthalmol 245:627–636
47. Yannuzzi LA, Ciardella A, Spaide RF, Rabb M, Freund KB, Orlock DA (1997) The expanding clinical spectrum of idiopathic polypoidal choroidal vasculopathy. Arch Ophthalmol 115:478–485
48. Iijima H, Iida T, Imai M, Gohdo T, Tsukahara S (2000) Optical coherence tomography of orange–red subretinal lesions in eyes with idiopathic polypoidal choroidal vasculopathy. Am J Ophthalmol 129:21–26
49. Yannuzzi LA, Sorenson J, Spaide RF, Lipson B (1990) Idiopathic polypoidal choroidal vasculopathy (IPCV). Retina 10:1–8
50. Lafaut BA, Aisenbrey S, Vanden BC, Di TF, Bartz-Schmidt KU (2001) Clinicopathological correlation in exudative age-related macular degeneration: recurrent choroidal neovascularization. Graefes Arch Clin Exp Ophthalmol 239:5–11
51. Weingarten MS, Papazoglou ES, Zubkov L, Zhu L, Neidrauer M, Savir G, Peace K, Newby JG, Pourrezaei K (2008) Correlation of near infrared absorption and diffuse reflectance spectroscopy scattering with tissue neovascularization and collagen concentration in a diabetic rat wound healing model. Wound Repair Regen 16:234–242
52. Marano F, Deutman AF, Leys A, Aandekerk AL (2000) Hereditary retinal dystrophies and choroidal neovascularization. Graefes Arch Clin Exp Ophthalmol 238:760–764
53. O'Toole L, Tufail A, Pavesio C (2005) Management of choroidal neovascularization in uveitis. Int Ophthalmol Clin 45:157–177
54. Soubrane G (2008) Choroidal neovascularization in pathologic myopia: recent developments in diagnosis and treatment. Surv Ophthalmol 53:121–138
55. Jager RD, Mieler WF, Miller JW (2008) Age-related macular degeneration. N Engl J Med 358:2606–2617
56. Meyer CH, Helb HM, Eter N (2008) [Monitoring of AMD patients on anti-vascular endothelial growth factor (VEGF) treatment. Practical notes on functional and anatomical examination parameters from drug approval studies, specialist information and case series]. Ophthalmologe 105: 125–38

Chapter 9

RetCam™ Imaging of Pediatric Intraocular Tumors[1]

Carol L. Shields, Aparna Ramasubramanian, Sarah Harmon, and Sara Lally

Core Messages

- Photographic imaging of the pediatric fundus can be performed with one of several cameras, including noncontact imaging devices such as standard 30, 45, 50, and 60 cameras or Optos™, or they can be imaged with contact systems using RetCam™ or Panoret™.
- RetCam™ imaging depends on a light source that emanates from the lens handpiece.
- RetCam™ can provide a 30°, 80°, 120°, or 130° image of the retina or even a full face portrait depending on the lens employed.
- RetCam™ can provide high-resolution wide-angle fluorescein angiography images using an appropriate filter.
- RetCam™ can provide gonioscopic images using the standard lens, contact gel, and defocusing to the front of the eye.
- RetCam™ can provide anterior segment images of the conjunctiva, cornea, or iris with removal of the lens.
- RetCam™ is usually performed with the child under anesthesia, but can be performed in the office with secure child restraint, topical anesthesia, and eyelid speculum.
- Ideal fundus images with RetCam™ are obtained in young children with wide dilation and without crystalline lens or media opacity.
- Poor fundus images with RetCam™ are the result of inadequate dilation leading to poor transmission of light and a central dark spot on imaging. Media opacity in the cornea, lens, or vitreous precludes sufficient light transmission for fundus illumination and results in poor image. Reflections off intraocular lens cause substantial glare and poor image.

9.1 Fundus Cameras

Imaging of the ocular fundus is important for documentation of numerous retinal and choroidal conditions. Fundus photography is especially important for documentation of intraocular tumors in children and adults. Photograph can be used to judge tumor size and extent, related features, and quantify response following therapy. However, fundus photography can be especially challenging in children because of the lack of cooperation for a still photograph of the interior of the eye. Most fundus photography on young children, under the age of 5 years, is performed in the operating suite with the child under general anesthesia.

One important limiting factor of fundus imaging is adequate fundus illumination. The small pupillary aperture, even when fully dilated, can inhibit adequate illumination of the interior of the eye for image capture. In most photographic systems, transpupillary light transmission is employed, where the light is aimed through the pupil, whereas in other systems, transcleral light transmission is used, where a brilliant light source is directed through the sclera. There are currently several fundus imaging systems available for children, most of which use transpupillary illumination techniques, and include standard fundus photography, RetCam™, and Optos™ imaging. Those that use the transcleral technique include Pomerantzeff and Panoret™ systems. Other considerations for fundus imaging

[1]Support provided by the Retina Research Foundation of the Retina Society in Cape Town, South Africa, a donation from Michael, Bruce, and Ellen Ratner, New York, NY, Mellon Charitable Giving from the Martha W. Rogers Charitable Trust, Philadelphia, PA, the LuEsther Mertz Retina Research Foundation, New York, NY, and the Eye Tumor Research Foundation, Philadelphia, PA.

is the image landscape extent whether it be small-angle or wide-angle as well as the patient contact issue whether it be lens contact to the cornea or noncontact lens. Most standard cameras provide small-angle viewing, whereas a few specialized systems that provide wide-angle viewing include Pomerantzeff equator plus camera, RetCam™, Panoret™, Optos™, and manual montage or auto-montage on standard cameras. Most standard cameras and the Optos™ systems are noncontact, whereas Pomerantzeff camera, RetCam™, and Panoret™require contact with the eye using either a panoramic contact lens, camera lens, or transillumination probe.

9.1.1 Standard Images

Several standard slit lamp camera systems provide small-angle, high-resolution photography of the posterior pole, measuring approximately 30°, 45°, 65°, and 80° of the posterior segment (measured from the center of the vitreous cavity). Photography of the fundus anterior to the equator of the eye is particularly difficult with standard slit lamp photography systems. Additionally, imaging of large fundus abnormalities is sometimes inadequate with these systems as the abnormality is documented in a piecemeal fashion without the desired broad perspective of the entire lesion. To document larger fundus abnormalities, manual or automatic montage capabilities have been designed.

9.1.2 Wide-Angle Images

There are three wide-angle color digital imaging systems currently available, including RetCam™, Panoret™, and Optos™. The Pomerantzeff camera and the Panoret™ system are still used at some institutions but no longer manufactured.

9.1.2.1 Pomerantzeff Equator Plus

The Pomerantzeff camera, or technique, was the first true wide-angle imaging system for the ocular fundus. Pomerantzeff and associates designed this new concept wide-angle imaging system in the early 1970s, in which they separated the illumination source from the camera observation aperture [1–4]. Using a panoramic contact lens on the eye, their "Equator Plus" camera was capable of photographing a field of approximately 148° from equator to equator. With experience, imaging of the retina near the ora serrata and occasionally into the ciliary body was achieved. In this method, the intraocular lighting was provided with an external fiber-optic source placed on the sclera to transilluminate the globe. Next, a standard camera with images through a panoramic lens allowed for wide-angle images. The transillumination technique was key to this technique, as it provided illumination without glare or reflection from the lens. Satisfactory photographs with adequate resolution were obtained in 87% of the 700 eyes imaged in this fashion and there were no local ocular complications [1]. In retrospect, this breakthrough in fundus wide-angle photography provided remarkably broad, film photographs of large portions of the fundus. However, details were often limited, because the necessary brilliant transillumination bleached out adjacent details; therefore, strategic placement of the light source distant from relevant details was important. This nondigital technique continues to be used at a few centers in the United States and is applicable only in the clinic setting as a slit lamp camera is required. Cooperative children can occasionally be imaged in this way.

9.1.2.2 RetCam™

RetCam™ is a novel, wide-angle fundus imaging system designed mainly for retinal imaging in children. There have been many reports on its use for retinopathy of prematurity screening, retinoblastoma evaluation, shaken baby syndrome, and many other pediatric conditions [5–12]. This system is regarded as simple, easy to manipulate, and with high-quality digital imaging. We have used this system for approximately 6,000 sessions, mostly in children with retinoblastoma, Coats disease, and other pediatric retinal congenital and vascular abnormalities. The system is manageable by the surgeon without the need for a dedicated photographer. We have used RetCam™ in young adults and older adults, but the older the patient and greater the lens opacity, the poorer the image.

RetCam™ Camera Description

RetCam™ is a mobile camera on wheels that can be transported to an operating room. The imaging is most often performed on children under anesthesia, but occasionally it can be used in the office with proper restraint of the child. The unit involves a console with dual DVD-RAM for backup, camera light box, fluorescein angiography light box, storage drawer for lens, color printer, tri-function foot-control for adjusting light intensity, focus, and video or image capture, and a standard hand-control panel for image adjustment and capture (Fig. 9.1). Atop the console is an LCD display with real-time video. The image is taken with a hand-held video camera that is lightweight, with a long fiber-optic cable, and five changeable lens. The lens include the standard baby lens for pediatric and young

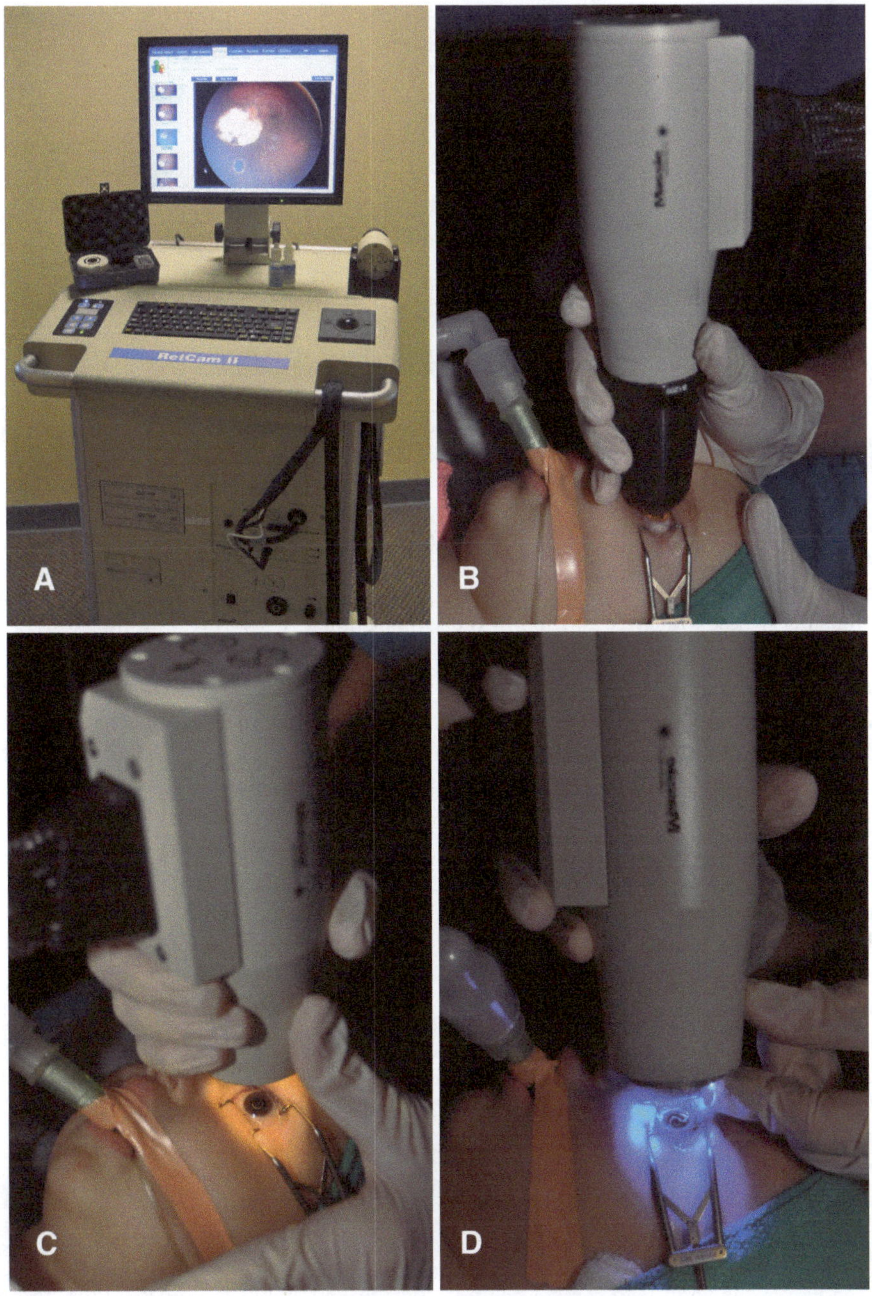

Fig. 9.1 Techniques of RetCam™ photography. (**a**) RetCam™ with keyboard, control panel, LCD display, hand-held camera, fiber-optic cord, and lens. (**b**) Hand-held camera in place for fundus photography with lubricating gel on the cornea. (**c**) Camera with conical lens removed to image the anterior segment. (**d**) Camera with conical lens removed and blue filter light for anterior segment fluorescein angiography

adult patients providing 120° images, the premature infant lens with smaller lens contact area and 130° field of view, the high magnification lens to evaluate fine detail of 30° field of view, the 80° lens for higher contrast, and the flat portrait lens for external full face or cutaneous imaging. All lens are simply clicked into place for rapid usage.

RetCam™ Technique of Image Capture

The hand-held camera is placed gently and directly on the corneal surface atop ophthalmic lubricant or gel (Fig. 9.1). The fundus view will be immediately visualized on the display and should be adjusted so that the image is upright and properly oriented. Focus and lighting can be

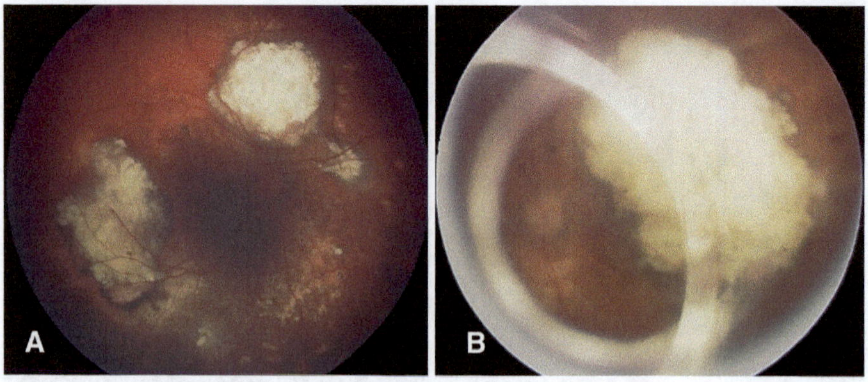

Fig. 9.2 Artifacts of RetCam™ photography. (**a**) Small, poorly dilated pupil can lead to a dark central spot in the image. (**b**) Intraocular lens causes reflections in the fundus image

adjusted with the foot-controls or hand-controls. An image is taken with the image capture button. Another alternative is to capture video and later select the appropriate images. Imaging is best with wide dilation of the pupil, clear crystalline lens, and minimal media opacity. Imaging through corneal opacity, lens opacity, pseudophakic lens, or other media opacities yield suboptimal images due to inability to adequately illuminate the interior of the globe or difficulties with light reflection off irregular or artificial surfaces.

Special imaging with the RetCam™ unit includes gonioscopy, anterior segment and iris imaging, and fluorescein angiography imaging. Gonioscopy imaging is usually performed with the standard lens and a moderate amount of lubricant gel. For best images, the lens is placed atop the gel without pressure, pointing toward the angle, and the camera is defocused to the anterior segment. Iris images can be obtained in the same fashion but are somewhat distorted, so we prefer to remove the conical lens and take the iris photos with reduced lighting (Fig. 9.1). Focus can be obtained for iris images by the control panel or by simply moving the camera slightly toward or away from the globe.

Fluorescein angiography is performed with a filter disc that is placed within the hand-held camera behind the removable lens. The fluorescein angiography light source is connected by a fiber-optic cord and the fluorescein program is selected from the display screen. For fundus fluorescein angiography, a blue light is transmitted through the hand-held piece and detected by the video camera. For iris fluorescein angiography, the snap-on lens is removed and the filter disc held in place with a finger so that a nondistorted image of the anterior segment is obtained (Fig. 9.1). This is especially important while imaging neovascularization of the iris.

RetCam™ Problems

There are problems that should be recognized with the RetCam™ system. First, any media opacity will reduce image quality as this minimizes light transmission. Patients with corneal or lens opacity, vitreous hemorrhage, or vitreous opacity will have reduced image quality with dark images and patchy details. Second, poor pupillary dilation reduces light transmission and leads to a central dark spot in the middle of the imaging field (Fig. 9.2). Third, pseudophakic intraocular lens cause prominent light reflections and lead to suboptimal images with glare and bleached images (Fig. 9.2). Fourth, the DVD storage system is generally adequate if the anticipated databank will be small, but for a busy practice that might take numerous images on several patients daily, the DVD will most likely not be capable of keeping up with the enormous storage needs. In our busy practice, we have found that RetCam™ software slows with increasing data banking.

9.1.2.3 Panoret™

Panoret™ is a wide-angle fundus imaging system based on the Pomerantzeff "Equator Plus" technique of transcleral illumination. Panoret™ is so-named as it can capture panoramic retinal images [13, 14]. Panoret™ differs from the "Equator Plus" camera with adaptations of a comfortable contact camera using digital capture, providing acclaimed image resolution of 20 μm on the retina with little glare or scleral brightness at the illumination site. Panoret™ can capture approximately 130° of the fundus using digital imaging, with a potential capability for wide-angle fluorescein angiography and indocyanine green angiography. This somewhat portable camera is useful for both adults in the office setting and children at examination under anesthesia. Because of the transcleral illumination method, the quality of images can be maintained in those patients with cataract, pseudophakia, some corneal opacities, and even those with small pupil, as the light is delivered posterior to these abnormalities, avoiding reflection and diminution of light. Imaging of extensive diabetic retinopathy, retinal detachment, peripheral retinal abnormalities, and intraocular tumors is excellent with this system. Clear panoramic images from the optic disc to the ora serrata can be obtained in each quadrant.

For Panoret™ imaging, the patient is reclined to a supine position and topical anesthesia followed by an eyelid speculum is applied by the gloved photographer. The cylindrical camera, attached to a retractable arm is brought in proximity with the patient's cornea, while at the same time a thin, transillumination probe is applied to the conjunctival fornix to illuminate the interior of the globe 180° opposite the lesion to be imaged. Using a foot pedal, rapid sequence, automatic-focus, video imaging of the patient's fundus is viewed on a monitor by the photographer. When the image is of good alignment, a second press on the foot pedal freezes and captures the image.

We have performed over 5,000 studies with this camera on 3,000 patients with various intraocular conditions [13, 14]. The patients ranged in age from 3 months to 92 years of age. Patients under age 5 years were generally imaged while under anesthetic examination. The youngest patient imaged in the office with Panoret™ was a cooperative 4-year-old. The technique of camera application was favorable with regard to patient comfort, minimal time commitment, and rapid image capture. The camera technique was somewhat cumbersome with regard to learning to the "three-hand" method of image capture using one hand for light source, one hand for camera placement, and one foot for image capture. After using the system for 40 or 50 studies, excellent, aligned image capture could be achieved within 3 min of reclining a cooperative patient.

The quality of Panoret™ images can be outstanding with regard to wide-angle viewing, fine resolution, and realistic color match. The camera can view the macula to the ora serrata in one image, achieving an angle of at least 130° of the fundus. Fundus features such as subretinal fluid, exudation, retinoschisis, and retinal pigment epithelial changes can be clearly depicted in a single image remote from the main condition of focus and with little distortion. There is often some brilliance of the transillumination probe at the site of its application through the wall of the eye, but this does not usually affect resolution of details. We have had no complications with this contact imaging system. Despite the contact camera, there have been no patients with symptomatic corneal abrasion, corneal or conjunctival infection, or pain. One notable drawback, however, was that imaging through a darkly pigmented uvea such as in Asian or African–American patients lead to poorer, darker images due to reduced light transmission.

9.1.2.4 Optos™

Optos™ is a noncontact wide-angle imaging system that relies on the patient alignment of their head on a chinrest, then viewing a target, then pressing a button to self-take their fundus image. This camera provides a global view of the fundus for approximately 200°. This versatile system can perform wide-angle color images as well as wide-angle fluorescein angiography [15–17]. This device incorporates low-powered laser wavelengths of red 633 nm and green 532 nm to provide high-resolution images. The blue laser wavelength (488 nm) allows for the addition of fluorescein angiography. Optos™ has been found to be helpful in the identification of fundus abnormalities for screening of patients or for those who prefer no dilation. This approach is ideal for cooperative adults but less useful for children, as it requires a level of cooperation and understanding. Additionally, interference by imaging of eyelashes can cause disturbance in the far peripheral fundus region and slightly skewed fundus images have been a challenge with this system. There is occasionally a red/green laser mismatch that leads to unnatural coloration of the fundus image.

Summary for the Clinician

- Imaging of intraocular tumors in children requires a high-resolution wide-angle system with rapid image capture that is portable and can be used in infants and children. There are several available systems and RetCam™ offers the ideal one as it is portable, easy to use by the surgeon or technician, and with rapid image capture.
- For best RetCam™ images, the pupil should be widely dilated.
- RetCam™ can provide several views of the fundus depending on the lens and the patient age from 60 to 130°.

9.2 RetCam™ Imaging for Specific Pediatric Intraocular Tumors

9.2.1 Retinal Tumors

There are several retinal tumors that can occur in children including retinoblastoma, astrocytic hamartoma, acquired astrocytoma, and the vascular tumors such as retinal hemangioblastoma, cavernous hemangioma, racemose hemangioma, and vasoproliferative tumor [18, 19].

9.2.1.1 Retinoblastoma

Retinoblastoma is the most common intraocular malignancy of childhood. It affects approximately 300 children in the USA each year and about 5,000 children worldwide. If detected while the tumor is contained within the eye, survival is excellent (Fig. 9.3). Risks for metastases include optic nerve invasion, choroidal invasion, scleral invasion, anterior chamber invasion, and orbital invasion. Treatment of retinoblastoma included enucleation,

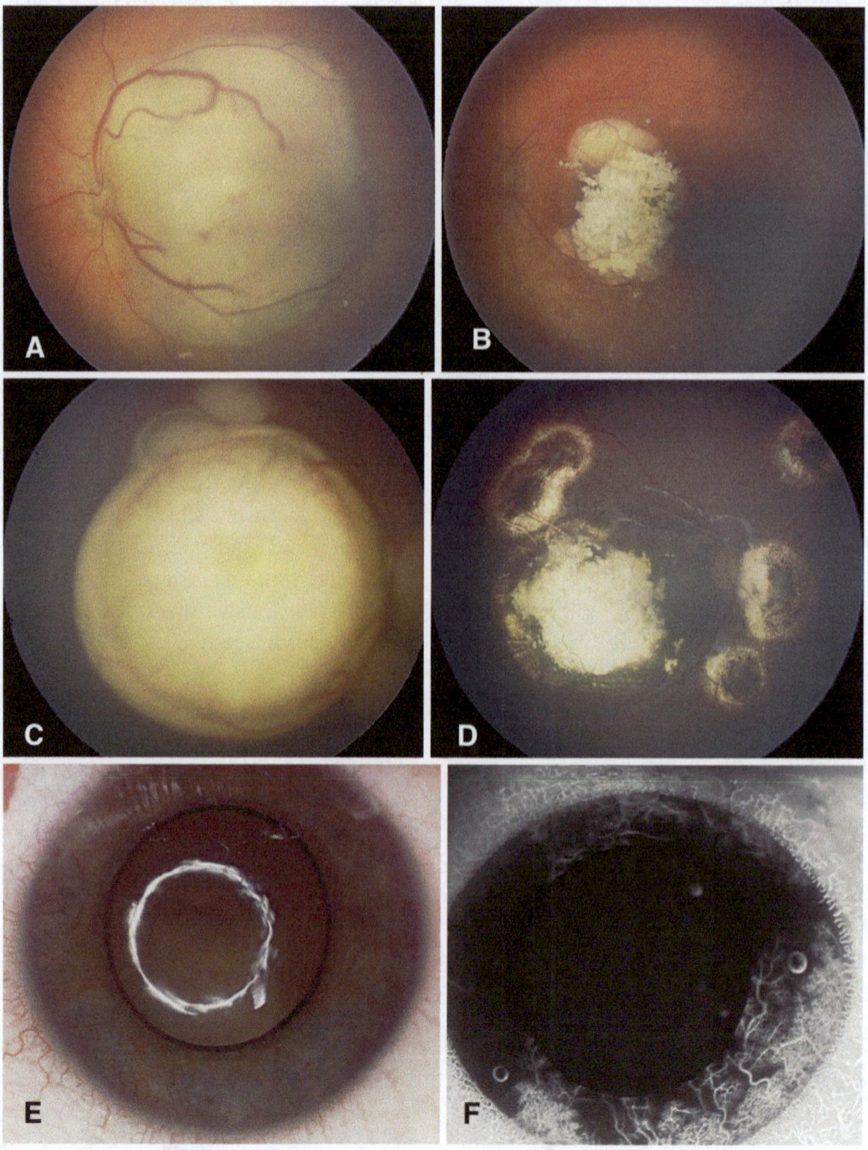

Fig. 9.3 Retinoblastoma imaged with RetCam™. Macular retinoblastoma before (**a**) and after chemoreduction (**b**). Multifocal retinoblastoma before (**c**) and after chemoreduction (**d**). Iris neovascularization in an eye with retinoblastoma imaged on RetCam™ with anterior segment photography (**e**) and fluorescein angiography (**f**)

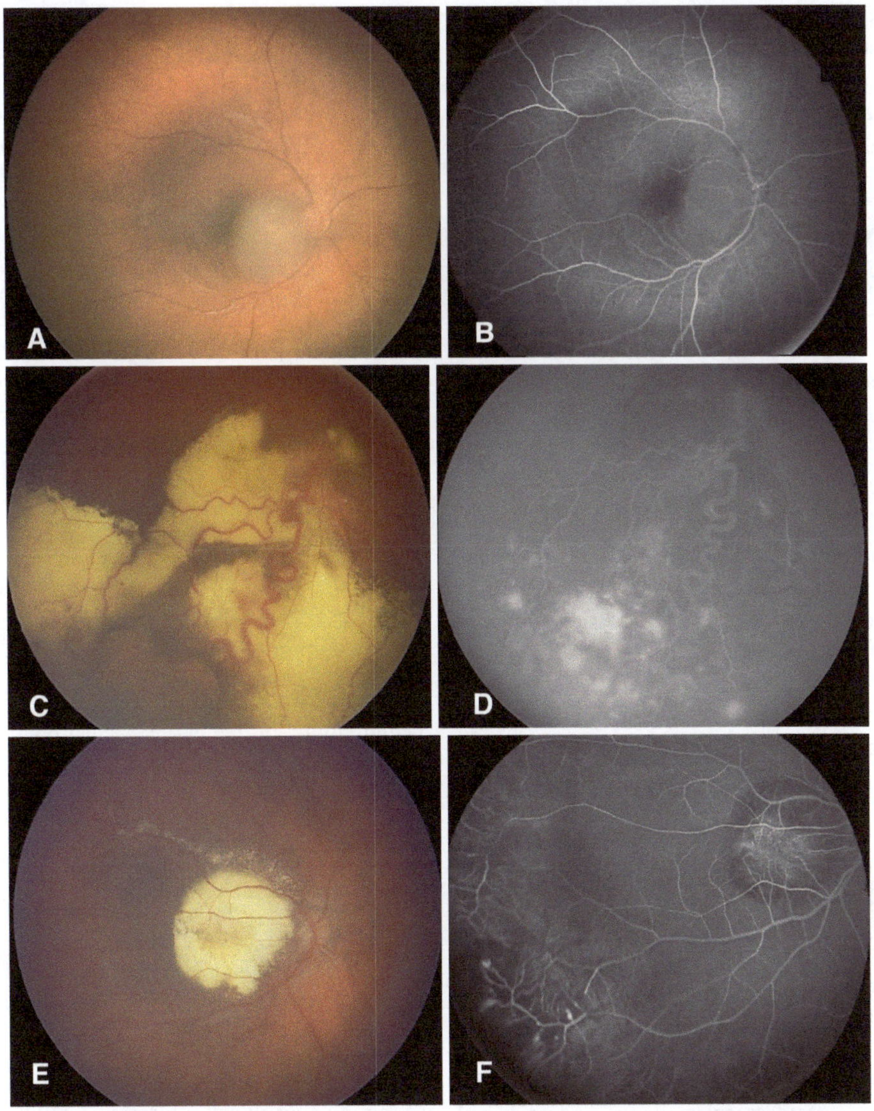

Fig. 9.4 Simulators of retinoblastoma imaged with RetCam™. Macular astrocytic hamartoma (**a**) showing minimal angiographic fluorescence (**b**). Retinal hemangioblastoma (**c**) with marked exudative retinopathy showing multifocal leakage on fluorescein angiography (**d**). Coats disease with macular exudation (**e**) showing peripheral light bulb telangiectasia, retinal edema, and nonperfusion (**f**)

chemoreduction plus thermotherapy or cryotherapy, intraarterial chemotherapy, external beam radiotherapy, plaque radiotherapy, laser photocoagulation, and cryotherapy [20]. Enucleation is often necessary for unilateral retinoblastoma, whereas chemoreduction is used for most bilateral cases.

9.2.1.2 *Astrocytic Hamartoma*

Retinal astrocytic hamartoma is a tumor of glial origin and can be found in patients with tuberous sclerosis or neurofibromatosis. In some instances, it is sporadic. Astrocytic hamartoma tends to develop in the nerve fiber layer and can cause slight traction with minimal if any dilation of the retinal vessels (Fig. 9.4).

9.2.1.3 *Retinal Capillary Hemangioma (hemangioblastoma)*

Retinal capillary hemangioma (hemangioblastoma) is a reddish orange, vascular tumor that can produce retinal and vitreous exudation, subretinal fluid, and macular edema, often leading to poor visual acuity [21] (Fig. 9.4). New genetic information has found that this tumor is stimulated by vascular endothelial growth factor (VEGF) that is secreted by the stromal tumor cells. This tumor generally presents in children and young adults. Retinal hemangioblastoma can occur as a sporadic tumor or as part of von Hippel–Lindau disease, especially if there are two or more retinal tumors. Such patients should have lifelong screening for related brain and visceral tumors.

9.2.1.4 Retinal Cavernous Hemangioma

The retinal cavernous hemangioma is a dark red–blue, low flow vascular tumor. Occasionally, it can rupture and produce vitreous hemorrhage. Some cases are associated with the phakomatosis in which there are cavernous hemangiomas of the retina, brain, and skin.

9.2.1.5 Retinal Racemose Hemangioma

Retinal racemose hemangioma is a congenital vascular malformation in which some or all of the retinal vessels are dilated, often to the point that the arterial system cannot be distinguished from the venous system. Visual acuity can be normal for extrafoveal tumors and poor for those with foveal involvement. This tumor can be associated with the Wyburn–Mason syndrome in which similar racemose hemangiomas are found in the midbrain, leading to stroke, and in the mandible, leading to bleeding at dental work.

9.2.1.6 Vasoproliferative Tumor

The retinal vasoproliferative tumor is a vascular mass typically located in the inferotemporal periphery of the fundus near the ora serrata in middle-aged and older patients [22]. Occasionally, it is found in children. This benign tumor can produce intraretinal and subretinal exudation, subretinal fluid, cystoid macular edema, and epiretinal membrane, leading to poor visual acuity. This tumor is not associated with von Hippel–Lindau disease. This tumor can be idiopathic or related to pars planitis, retinitis pigmentosa, and inflammatory or traumatic conditions.

Summary for the Clinician

- Retinoblastoma is a serious intraocular malignancy in children that can lead to death if there is optic nerve or choroidal invasion.
- Retinal astrocytic hamartoma can appear like retinoblastoma, but the vessels are not dilated and show traction and the calcification is glistening and not chalky.
- Retinal vascular tumors have different clinical features and can be associated with severe systemic consequences.

9.2.2 Retinal Pigment Epithelium Tumors

There are few retinal pigment epithelium (RPE) tumors that can occur in children including congenital hypertrophy of the RPE, congenital simple hamartoma of the RPE, and combined hamartoma of the retina and RPE [18, 19].

9.2.2.1 Congenital Hypertrophy of the Retinal Pigment Epithelium

Congenital hypertrophy of the RPE (CHRPE) is a flat pigmented lesion arising deep in the retina, typically in the peripheral fundus [23]. It is often discovered coincidentally on ocular examination. CHRPE can display clinical features that resemble choroidal nevus or choroidal melanoma. CHRPE is generally a stable lesion, but can slowly grow over many years.

9.2.2.2 Congenital Simple Hamartoma of the Retinal Pigment Epithelium

Congenital simple hamartoma of the RPE is a dark black benign tumor located in the macular region, often immediately adjacent to the foveola [24]. It appears like a black ink spot involving full thickness retina. Fine retinal traction can be noted surrounding the mass. Often, there are slightly dilated feeding and draining retinal vessels. This tumor usually remains stable.

9.2.2.3 Combined Hamartoma of the Retinal Pigment Epithelium

Combined hamartoma of the retinal and RPE is a tractional mass located in the juxtapapillary region more so than the periphery, often associated with poor visual acuity [25, 26]. This gray–green ill-defined mass displays corkscrew, twisted vessels and retinal traction. Optical coherence tomography reveals peaked and folded retina from traction. Rarely, retinal exudation or hemorrh age is found. This lesion can be associated with neurofibromatosis type 2.

Summary for the Clinician

- CHRPE appears as a flat mass often in the periphery and can show slow enlargement over decades.
- Congenital simple hamartoma of the RPE is found in the macula.
- Combine hamartoma of the RPE and retina can produce poor visual acuity if there is macular involvement.

9.2.3 Choroidal Tumors

The two most important choroidal tumors in children include nevus and melanoma [18, 19].

9.2.3.1 *Choroidal Nevus*

Choroidal nevus is found in children and adults. It appears as a brown, tan, or yellow mass in the choroid, with an oval or round shape, less than 2 mm thickness [27] (Fig. 9.5). Features of overlying RPE atrophy, hyperplasia, fibrous metaplasia, osseous metaplasia, and drusen imply a chronic nevus. Features such as subretinal fluid or overlying orange pigment imply an active mass and could represent a small choroidal melanoma. Growth of choroidal nevus into melanoma is estimated to occur at a rate of 1/5,000.

9.2.3.2 *Choroidal Melanoma*

Choroidal melanoma are generally found in adults, but <1% are discovered in children [28]. Choroidal melanoma is classified into small (≤3 mm thickness), medium (3.1–8 mm thickness), and large (>8 mm thickness) and the mortality depends on tumor thickness. Melanoma appears as a pigmented or nonpigmented mass, often with overlying subretinal fluid (Fig. 9.5). The tumor can assume a dome,

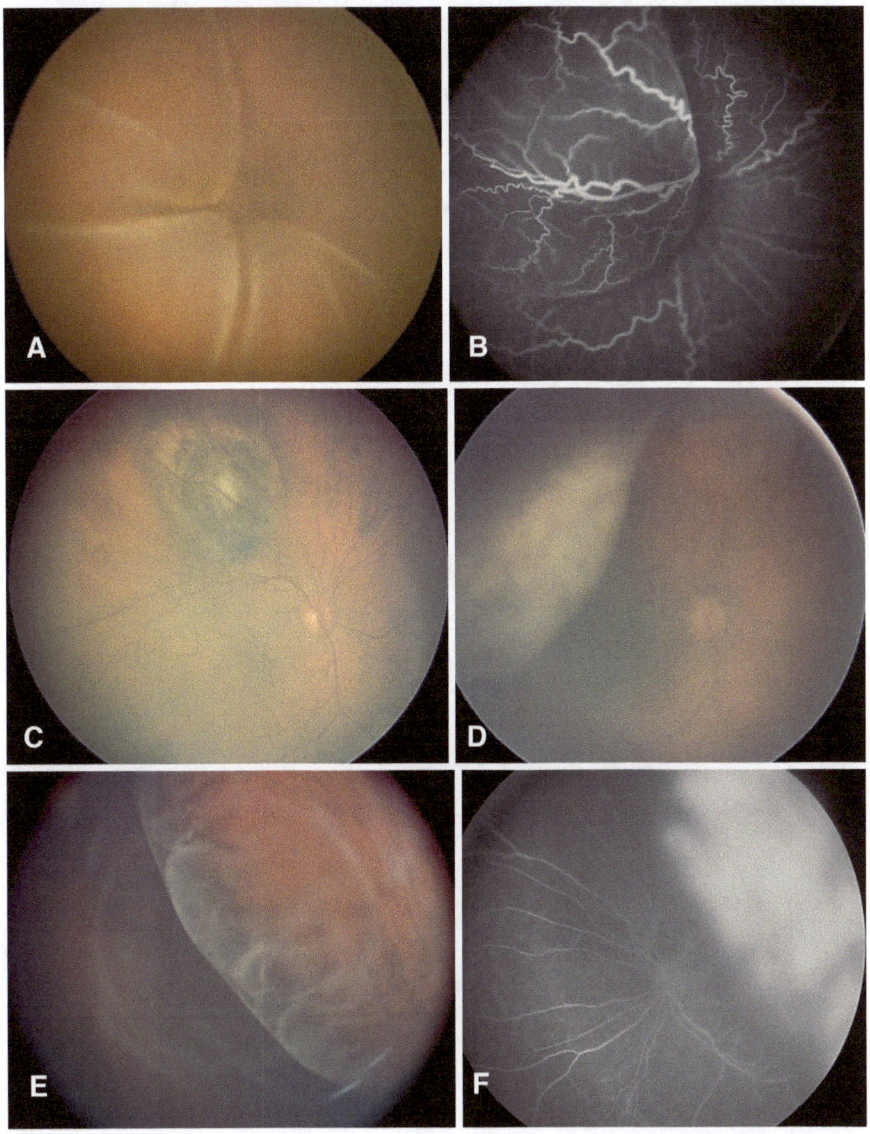

Fig. 9.5 Choroidal tumors imaged with RetCam™. Diffuse choroidal hemangioma (**a**) with total serous retinal detachment confirmed on fluorescein angiography (**b**). (**c**) Choroidal nevus with overlying fibrous metaplasia of the retinal pigment epithelium. (**d**) Choroidal melanoma with mushroom shape in an 8-year-old girl. Large choroidal melanoma (**e**) with serous retinal detachment and hyperfluorescence (**f**) in a 6-year-old boy

mushroom, or diffuse (flat) growth pattern. Metastasis to the liver, lung, and skin should be screened.

9

> **Summary for the Clinician**
>
> - Choroidal nevus in children typically appears as a pigmented mass under 2 mm thickness.
> - Choroidal melanoma in children is rare, measuring over 2 mm thickness and often producing subretinal fluid.

9.2.4 Anterior Segment Lesions

9.2.4.1 Iris Lesions

There are several iris lesions that can be found in children including nevus, melanoma, iris pigment epithelial cyst, iris stromal cyst, juvenile xanthogranuloma, and other rarer conditions such as choristomas [18, 19] (Fig. 9.6). Ciliary body medulloepithelioma can involve the anterior segment or manifest as a fleshy vascularized mass behind the clear lens (Fig. 9.6). Occasionally, congenital malformations such

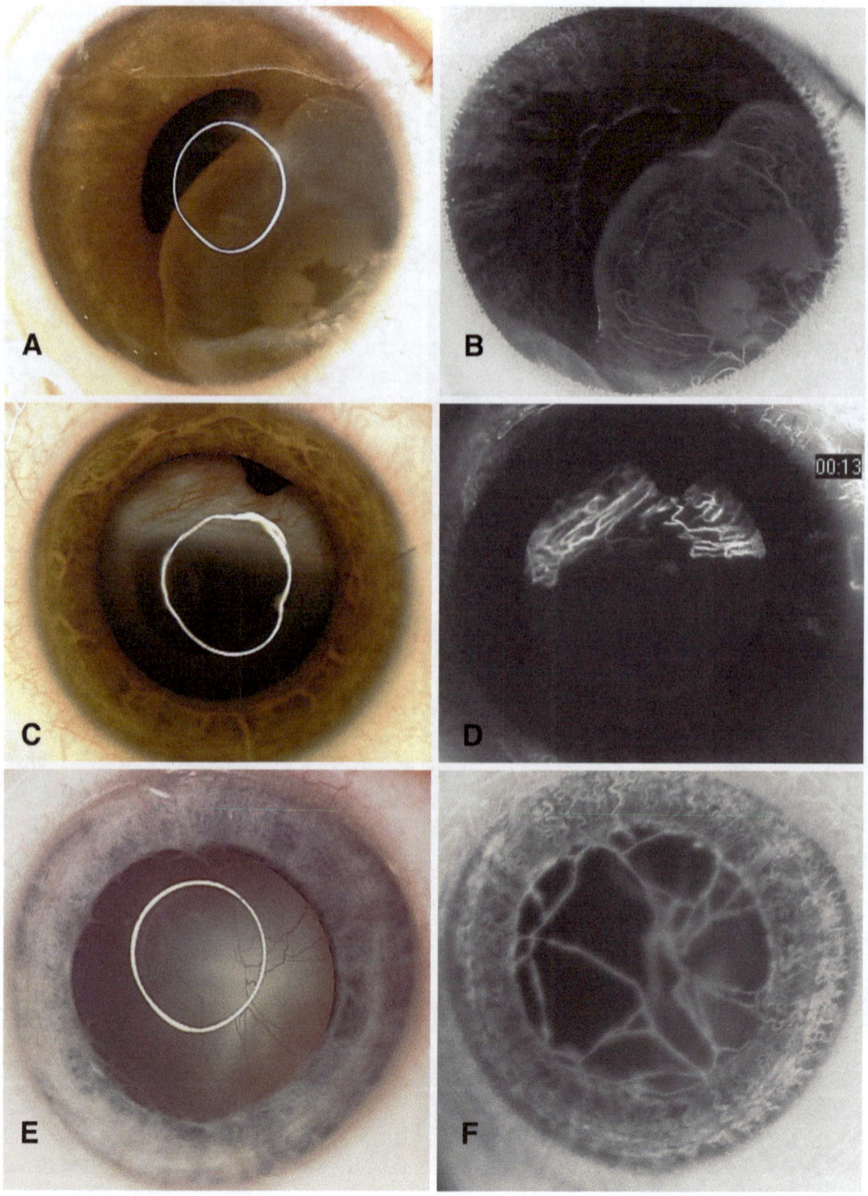

Fig. 9.6 Anterior segment imaging with RetCam™. Iris stromal cyst (**a**) with band keratopathy showing fluorescence of the cyst wall (**b**). Medulloepithelioma (**c**) of the nonpigmented ciliary epithelium with prominent vascularity (**d**). Persistent hyperplastic primary vitreous (PHPV; persistent fetal vasculature, PFV) displaying remnants of the tunica vasculosa lentis (**e**) with fluorescein-confirmed perfusion (**f**)

as persistent hyperplastic primary vitreous (PHPV; persistent fetal vasculature, PFV), iris coloboma, Peters anomaly, and others can simulate an iris tumor (Fig. 9.6).

References

1. Ducrey N, Pomerantzeff O, Schepens Cl, Delori FC, Schneider J (1977) Clinical trials with the equator-plus camera. Am J Ophthalmol 84:840–846
2. Pomerantzeff O (1975) Equator-plus camera. Invest Ophthalmol 4:401–406
3. Pomerantzeff O (1980) Wide-angle noncontact and small-angle contact cameras. Invest Ophthalmol Vis Sci 19:973–979
4. Pomerantzeff O, Webb RH, Delori FC (1979) Image formation in fundus cameras. Invest Ophthalmol Vis Sci 18: 630–637
5. Azad R, Chandra P, Khan MA, Darswal A (2008) Role of intravenous fluorescein angiography in early detection and regression of retinopathy of prematurity. J Pediatr Ophthalmol Strabismus 45:36–39
6. Dhaliwal C, Wright E, Graham C, McIntosh N, Fleck BW (2009) Wide-field digital retinal imaging versus binocular indirect ophthalmoscopy of rretinopathy of prematureity screening: a two-observer prospective, randomized comparison. Br J Ophthalmol 93:355–359
7. Hussein MAW, Coats DK, Paysse EA (2004) Use of the RetCam 120 for fundus evaluation in uncooperative children. Am J Ophthalmol 137:354–355
8. Kemper AR, Wallace DK, Quinn GE (2008) Systematic review of digital imaging screening strategies for retinopathy of prematurity. Pediatrics 122:825–830
9. Murakami Y, Jain A, Silva RA, Lad EM, Gandhi J, Moshfeghi DM (2008) Stanford University network for diagnosis of retinopathy of prematurity (SUNDROP): 12 month experience with telemedicine screening. Br J Ophthalmol 92:1456–1460
10. Nakagawa TA, Skrinska R (2001) Improved documentation of retinal hemorrhages using a wide-field digital ophthalmic camera in patients who experienced abusive head trauma. Arch Pediatr Adolesc Med 155:1149–1152
11. Roth DB, Morales D, Feuer WJ, Hess D, Johnson RA, Flynn JT (2001) Screening for retinopathy of prematurity employeing the RetCam 120. Sensitivity and specificity. Arch Ophthalmol 119:268–272
12. Saleh M, Schoenlaub S, Desprez P, Bourcier T, Gaucher D, Astruc D, Speeg-Schatz C (2009) Use of digital camera imaging of eye fundus for telemedicine in children suspected of abusive head injury. Br J Ophthalmol 93:424–428
13. Shields CL, Materin M, Epstein J, Shields JA (2003) Wide-angle imaging of the ocular fundus. Rev Ophthalmol 2:66–70
14. Shields CL, Materin M, Shields JA (2003) Panoramic imaging of the ocular fundus. Arch Ophthalmol 121:1603–1607
15. Jain A, Shah SP, Tsui I, McCannel TA (2009) The value of optos panoramic 200MA imaging for the monitoring of large suspicious choroidal lesions. Semin Ophthalmol 24:43–44
16. Mackenzie PJ, Russell M, Ma PE, Isbister CM, Maberley DA (2007) Sensitivity and specificity of the optos optomap for detecting peripheral retinal lesions. Retina 27:1119–1124
17. Manivannan A, Plskova J, Farrow A, Mckay S, Sharp PF, Forrester JV (2005) Ultra-wide-field fluorescein angiography of the ocular fundus. Am J Ophthalmol 140:525–527
18. Shields JA, Shields CL (2008) Intraocular tumors. An atlas and textbook, 2nd edition. Lippincott Williams & Wilkins, Philadelphia, pp 13–502
19. Shields JA, Shields CL (1992) Intraocular tumors: a text and atlas. WB Saunders, Philadelphia, pp 45–488
20. Shields CL, Shields JA (2006) Basic understanding of current classification and management of retinoblastoma. Curr Opin Ophthalmol 17:228–234
21. Singh AD, Shields CL, Shields JA (2001) Major review: Von Hippel–Lindau disease. Surv Ophthalmol 46:117–142
22. Shields CL, Shields JA, Barrett J, De Potter P (1995) Vasoproliferative tumors of the ocular fundus. Classification and clinical manifestations in 103 patients. Arch Ophthalmol 113: 615–623
23. Shields CL, Mashayekhi A, Ho T, Cater J, Shields JA (2003) Solitary congenital hypertrophy of the retinal pigment epithelium: clinical features and frequency of enlargement in 330 patients. Ophthalmology 110:1968–1976
24. Shields CL, Shields JA, Marr BP, Sperber DE, Gass JDM (2003) Congenital simple hamartoma of the retinal pigment epithelium. A study of five cases. Ophthalmology 110:1005–1011
25. Schachat AP, Shields JA, Fine SL, Sanborn GE, Weingeist TA, Valenzuela RE, Brucker AJ (1984) Combined hamartomas of the retina and retinal pigment epithelium. Ophthalmology 91:1609–1615
26. Shields CL, Thangappan A, Hartzell K, Valente P, Pirondini C, Shields JA Shields JA (2008) Combined hamartoma of the retina and retinal pigment epithelium in 77 consecutive patients. Visual outcome based on macular versus extramacular tumor location. Ophthalmology 115: 2246–2252
27. Shields CL, Furuta M, Mashayekhi A, Berman EL, Zahler JD, Hoberman DM, Dinh DH, Shields JA (2008) Clinical spectrum of choroidal nevi based on age at presentation in 3422 consecutive eyes. Ophthalmology 115:(3) 546–552
28. Shields CL, Shields JA, Milite J, Depotter P, Sabbagh R, Menduke H (1991) Uveal melanoma in teenagers and children. A report of 40 cases. Ophthalmology 98:1662–1666

10 Metabolic Mapping

Dietrich Schweitzer

Core Messages

- Studies of metabolism can be performed with regard to the external or the internal aspect at the fundus.
- The external aspect of metabolism is characterised by parameters of microcirculation (blood flow, oxygen saturation).
- The internal aspect describes the cellular metabolism.
- The cellular metabolic state can be determined by the fluorescence of endogenous fluorophores.
- The fluorescence of redox pairs NAD^+ / NADH and FAD/FADH depends on the availability of the dissolved oxygen.
- Several other substances fluoresce in ocular tissue.
- Fluorophores can be discriminated by excitation and emission spectra as well as by decay of fluorescence intensity (lifetime).
- The transmission of ocular media hinders the excitation of fluorophores in their maxima below 400 nm.
- Several fluorophores emit a weak fluorescence below 560 nm.
- The fundus fluorescence above 560 nm is dominated by lipofuscin.
- Lifetime measurements are independent of fluorophore concentration and absorption into the surrounding tissue.
- Lifetime measurements permit the discrimination of a weakly emitting fluorophore whose emission spectrum is covered by a strongly emitting fluorophore.
- A fluorescence lifetime mapping ophthalmoscope permits excitation at different wavelengths and time-resolved fluorescence measurements of two spectral ranges (490–560 nm, 560–700 nm).
- The results of up to three exponential approximations of fluorescence decay can be presented in images, histograms and cluster diagrams of lifetimes or of amplitudes.
- Early phases of age-related macular degeneration (AMD) can be discriminated from healthy subjects by lifetimes $\tau 1$ and $\tau 2$ in the short-wavelength channel and by $\tau 2$ in the long-wavelength channel.
- Reduced metabolic activity can be demonstrated in arterial branch occlusion.
- Regions of reduced metabolism can be found in mild non-exudative diabetic retinopathy.

10.1 Aspects of Metabolism

The first pathological signs occur in metabolism. Thus, an important goal in ophthalmic research is to find the methods of objective evaluation of retinal metabolism. The metabolism in the retina can be considered with regard to the external and the internal aspects. The external aspect is characterised by blood flow in arterioles and in venules. The blood flow as blood volume/time can be calculated from measurements of the physical parameters, such as blood velocity and vessel diameter. In addition to blood flow, the concentration of metabolites is important in the blood, e.g. oxygen saturation. In this way, the supply and the consumption of oxygen can be determined in retinal tissue according to (10.1) [1]:

$$Q \cdot \mathrm{OS} \cdot c_{\mathrm{total}} \cdot \eta_0 = \frac{V}{t} \cdot \frac{c_{\mathrm{HbO_2}}}{c_{\mathrm{HbO_2}} + c_{\mathrm{Hb}}} \cdot c_{\mathrm{total}} \cdot \eta_o. \qquad (10.1)$$

Assuming a blood flow $Q = 21$ µL/s, an arterial oxygen saturation $\mathrm{OS}_a = 95\%$, a total haemoglobin concentration/4 $c_{\mathrm{total}} = 8.9$ mmol/L and a transport effectiveness η_0, which means that 1 mol O_2 (32 g) is transported by 1 mol haemoglobin (≈16,100 g), and the tissue is supplied with 0.358 ng/s of oxygen. If the arterio-venous difference

OSa–v = 35%, then the consumption of oxygen is about 0.132 ng/s in the supplied retinal tissue.

Different methods for the measurement of the blood flow have been published, determined as volume/time. Most accurate in clinical application is the measurement of blood velocity by bi-directional laser Doppler anemometry and the simultaneous determination of vessel diameter [2]. New developments in optical coherence tomography are promising for the determination of blood flow simultaneously in multiple vessels of a 3D retina volume [3].

The measurement of oxygen saturation in the retinal vessels has been a subject of research for several years. The simplest methods are based on reflection measurements at two wavelengths. One measurement is performed at an isosbestic point, where the extinction coefficients of reduced and oxygenated haemoglobin are identical. The other is done at a wavelength with the largest difference between the two components of haemoglobin. Despite this latter method being a raw approximation of the interaction between light and blood, several studies use the algorithm, which is described in Beach et al. [4]. In the most accurate method for the measurement of oxygen saturation, a complete reflection spectrum is detected [1, 5]. The oxygen saturation is then calculated by an approximation of this spectrum by the complete extinction spectrum of haemoglobin and oxyhaemoglobin. In addition to the absorption, the scattering of light is also included in the model function. The oxygen saturation can be determined in an artery, a vein and also in the retinal tissue, simultaneously.

On studying the oxygen saturation in the retinal vessels in early diabetes, no change in arterial oxygen saturation was found in relation to age-matched controls, but venous oxygen saturation was increased [6]. In other words, the consumption of oxygen was reduced, indicating a virtual over-supplying of the retinal tissue. These measurements demonstrate the limitation of measurements of oxygen saturation, because in diabetic tissue, there is a lack of oxygen.

There has been no technical solution for the simultaneous measurement of blood flow and oxygen saturation until now. Such a solution would be helpful for the interpretation of the complicated control mechanism of blood flow and oxygen saturation.

Measurements of the external aspect of metabolism are necessary, but they are not sufficient.

The internal aspect of metabolism describes the basic mechanisms, e.g. of energy production. These processes are glycolysis, the citrate acid cycle, the respiratory chain and oxidative phosphorylation, and act inside the cells in cytosol (glycolysis) and mitochondria (citrate acid cycle) [7]. They require metabolites, e.g. glucose and dissolved oxygen, which have to diffuse through the vessel wall and cell membranes. Here, an increased resistance of diffusion might explain the discrepancy between increased venous oxygen saturation and lack of oxygen in the cells in diabetes.

Besides the mechanisms of energy production, the internal aspect of metabolism also includes processes like accumulation of pigments, e.g. the macular pigment xanthophyll, as protection against energy-rich radiation, metabolic end products like lipofuscin, or advanced glycation end products (AGEs). The formation of scars can also be considered a result of changed internal metabolism.

The internal aspect of metabolism can be studied by the fluorescence of endogenous fluorophores. Of special interest are changes in the fluorescence of the redox pairs NAD^+/NADH (oxidised and reduced nicotinamide adenine dinucleotide) and FAD/$FADH_2$ (flavin adenine dinucleotide). These redox pairs act as electron transporters in the basic mechanisms of energy production. The change in fluorescence of both the redox pairs allows an estimation of the availability of oxygen inside the cells. The reduced form, NADH, emits fluorescence if there is a relative lack of oxygen, whereas the oxidised NAD is non-fluorescent. In contrast, the oxidised FAD fluoresces if there is sufficient oxygen and the reduced $FADH_2$ exhibits no fluorescence. Unfortunately, the fluorescence of these redox pairs is covered by the fluorescence of several other fluorophores in the ocular tissue. Most prominent is the fluorescence of lipofuscin, which accumulates in the cells of the retinal pigment epithelium, especially in age-related macular degeneration (AMD). Glycolised proteins (AGEs) are found in the lens and fundus tissue in diabetic patients. All connective tissues contain the fluorophores collagens and elastin. The fluorophores pyridoxal and protoporphyrin IX act in haem synthesis. The amino acids such as tryptophan, tyrosine, and kynurenine also emit strong fluorescence.

However, the problem is how these fluorophores, can be discriminated from each other. There are three properties that are characteristic of each fluorophore. The excitation spectrum describes the wavelength range in which the energy of light is high enough to move the electrons from the singlet ground state, S0, to an excited singlet state, S1 or higher. The excitation spectrum characterises the structure of the excited state. Through a radiation-less internal conversation, the electrons move from the higher excited states in the first excited state, S1. It is also possible for the electrons to move from higher excited singlet states into excited triplet states via intersystem crossing.

The electrons go back from the S1 state to the singlet ground state S0 in the time scale of ps- to ns-emitting fluorescence light. This fluorescence spectrum is the second characteristic parameter of each fluorophore. It characterises the structure of the ground state. The wavelength of the fluorescence light is longer than the excitation light. Besides the emission of fluorescence light, there is also a radiation-less relaxation. Both processes depopulate the excited singlet state S1. The inverse sum of the emission rate Γ and the non-radiative decay rate k_{nr} is the mean lifetime τ of electrons in the excited state (10.2):

$$\tau = \frac{1}{\Gamma + k_{nr}}. \qquad (10.2)$$

The lifetime τ is the third parameter for characterising each fluorophore.

The lifetime τ is detectable as the decay rate of normalised fluorescence intensity. On the other hand, the spin orientation of electrons is anti-parallel in S1 and S0, and the spins are parallel in the excited triplet state T1 and the singlet state S0. Hence, relaxation from T1 to S0 is forbidden and occurs much longer than fluorescence as phosphorescence in the millisecond time scale.

The shape of both the excitation and the emission spectrum are influenced by the absorption spectrum of the neighbouring substances. Furthermore, a strongly emitted fluorescence spectrum covers the fluorescence spectra of weakly emitting fluorophores. Thus, the discrimination of a single fluorophore is difficult in a mixture of absorbing and fluorescing substances. In contrast, the fluorescence lifetime is independent of the absorption in the neighbourhood. Strongly and weakly emitting fluorophores can be separated from each other, if the lifetimes are sufficiently different. The lifetime is independent of the fluorophore concentration. As the lifetime depends on viscosity, pH and temperature, information can be attained about the embedding matrix of the cells.

10.2 Limiting Conditions for the Discrimination of Fluorophores at the Ocular Fundus

The discrimination of fluorophores according to the excitation and emission spectra, and according to fluorescence lifetime, is limited under the conditions of the measurements at the ocular fundus. There are four specific limitations. First, the transmission of the ocular media permits spectral measurements at the fundus only between 400 and 900 nm [8]. The absorption edge of the crystalline lens is at 400 nm and the cornea absorbs the light for wavelengths shorter than 350 nm. Above 900 nm, the light is absorbed by water. Second, the eye is a moving object. That is, measurements of long duration, which are required for a good signal-to-noise ratio (SNR), are impossible at the same position of the fundus. Thus, eye trackers or methods of image registration are required. The next limitation is related to the anatomy of the eye. The eye consists of several layers, e.g. cornea, lens, vitreous, nerve fibre layer, receptor layer, retinal pigment epithelium and choroid. Nearly the same fluorophores act in all these layers. Thus, in the fluorescence detected, all the emission spectra are superimposed, independent of the point of origin. The influence of lens fluorescence during fundus measurements can be suppressed to a certain degree by confocal laser scanning or by the principle of aperture division. By applying two-photon excitation, the fluorescence is observed to originate only at the focus of the imaging system. Thus, a discrimination of emitting layers is possible in principle. As the threshold between obtaining fluorescence and damaging the fundus tissue is low, the two- or multi-photon technique is a subject of research for fundus imaging [9]. The most important limitation is the maximal permissible exposure for fluorescence measurements in the eye [10]. To obtain an SNR that is high enough, a number of fluorescence images taken under weak excitation should be averaged. The eye movement during the measurement must be compensated for by image registration.

10.3 Excitation and Emission Spectra and Fluorescence Lifetimes of Expected Endogenous Fluorophores and Ocular Tissue

Optimal discrimination of fluorophores should include specific excitation and emission as well as measurement of fluorescence lifetime. To find the required spectral ranges and lifetime scale, the excitation and emission spectra and the lifetimes of the isolated substances were determined by Schweitzer et al. [11].

Table 10.1 shows these data. The excitation and emission maxima for collagen and elastin are given by Sionkowska et al. [12]. The absorbance spectra of both components of connective tissue are partly detectable in the visible spectrum. The corresponding emission spectra are detectable up to 650 nm. The lifetime of FAD and NADH changes between the free and the protein-bound state. Besides own measurements [11], the lifetime of free FAD is given as 2.05 ns [13] and 2.3 ns [14]. According to Nakashima et al. [15], the lifetime of the FAD monomer is 140 ps and that of the FAD dimer 40 ps. The quantum yield of the FAD monomer is higher than that of the FAD dimer. Skala et al. [13] determined the lifetime of protein-bound FAD to be about 100 ps.

Reversed behaviour is valid for NADH. The fluorescence lifetime of free NADH was determined to be 300 ps [16] and 400–500 ps [17]. The fluorescence lifetime of protein-bound NADH increases to 1 ns [18], 2 ns [16] and 2–2.5 ns [17].

Table 10.1. Excitation and emission as well as fluorescence decay times of expected fundus substances and ocular tissue

Substance	Maximum excitation (nm)	Maximum emission in nm	Amplitude α1 (%)	Lifetime τ1 (ps)	Amplitude α 2 (%)	Lifetime τ2 (ps)
Free NADH	350	450	73	387	27	3,650
Free FAD	370, 446	525	18	330	82	2,810
AGE	360	505	62	865	28	4,170
A2E	437	600	98	170	2	1,120
Lipofuscin			48	390	52	2,240
Melanin	360	436	70	280	30	2,400
Elastin	275	304	72	380	28	3,590
Collagen 1	275	304	68	670	32	4,040
Collagen 2			64	470	36	3,150
Collagen 3			69	345	31	2,800
Collagen 4			70	740	30	3,670
Ocular tissue						
Retina			90	260	10	2,790
RPE			96	210	4	1,800
Choroid			70	500	30	3,400
Sclera			65	450	35	3,110
Cornea			70	570	30	3,760
Lens			69	490	31	3,600

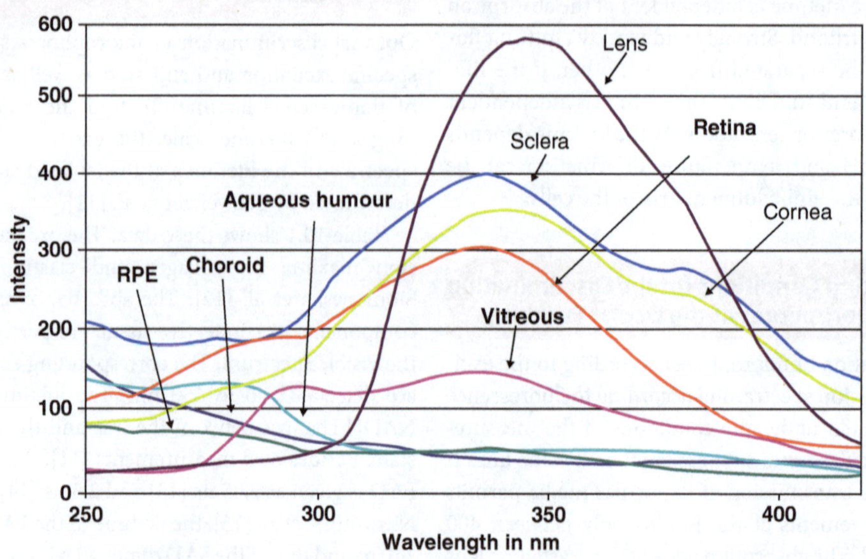

Fig. 10.1 Excitation spectra of the structures in porcine eyes

The ratio of amplitudes of free and protein-bound NADH is an indicator of cellular metabolism [18]. It gets reduced if the energy is increasingly delivered under anaerobic conditions.

To investigate whether discrimination of ocular structures might be possible according to the excitation and emission spectra as well as the fluorescence lifetime, these parameters were measured in isolated structures of porcine eyes [19]. Figure 10.1 shows the excitation spectra, detected by the changes in the fluorescence intensity at 460 nm. This wavelength was chosen because it corresponds to the emission maximum of NADH.

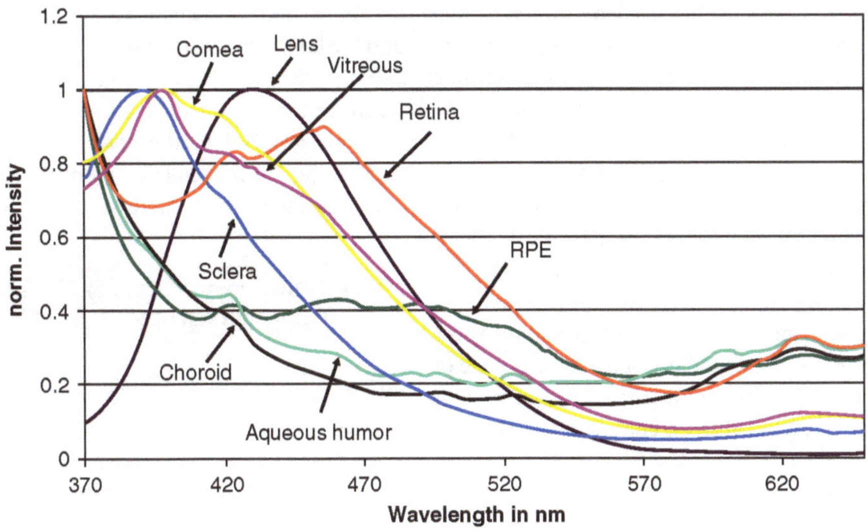

Fig. 10.2 Emission spectra of the structures in porcine eyes

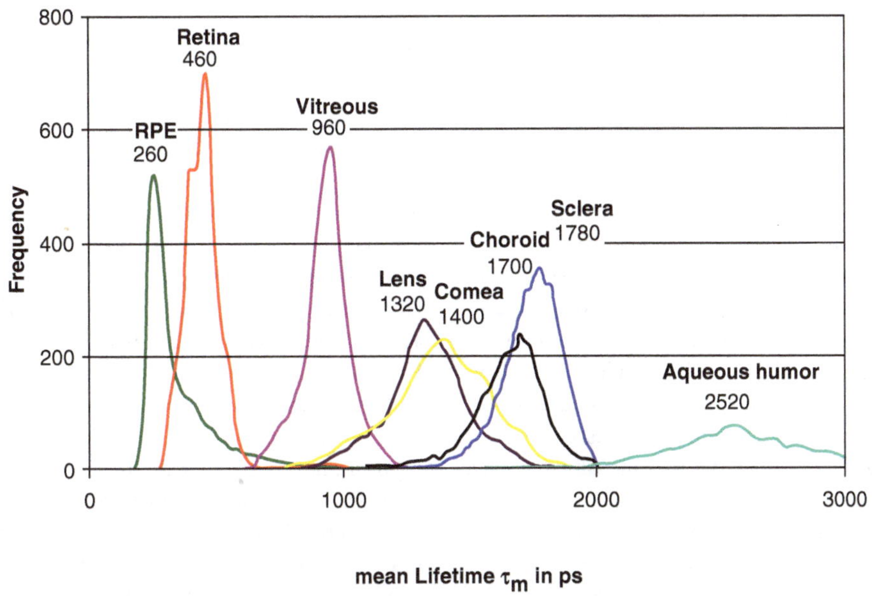

Fig. 10.3 Mean fluorescence lifetime of the structures in porcine eyes

The fluorescence spectra of these tissues are presented in Fig. 10.2. The excitation was at 350 nm. As demonstrated in these diagrams, spectral discrimination of the ocular structures is quite difficult. No accumulation of ageing pigment lipofuscin was detectable in the retinal pigment epithelium of these young animals. The strong fluorescence of the crystalline lens is remarkable up to 520 nm.

Better discrimination of ocular structures was reached by fluorescence lifetime measurements, as demonstrated in Fig. 10.3. The fluorescence was excited by laser pulses of 100 ps full width at half maximum at 446 nm. The dynamic emission was detected in the spectrum from 490 to 700 nm.

The decay of fluorescence intensity was bi-exponentially approximated. The shortest lifetimes were detected in the RPE (maximal τ_m = 260 ps) and the neuronal retina (maximal τ_m = 460 ps). The lifetime histograms of lens (maximal τ_m = 1,320 ps) and cornea (maximal τ_m = 1,420) are quite similar just as of choroid (maximal τ_m = 1,700 ps) and sclera (maximal τ_m = 1,780 ps).

From studies on expected fundus fluorophores as well as those on ocular structures, the technical parameters can be derived for excitation, emission and for the time range of decay times. Taking into account the transmission of the ocular media, the optimal excitation of fundus fluorophores is around 440 nm up to 490 nm. A certain discrimination of fluorophores is possible if the emission is detected within a short wavelength range of 490–560 nm and within a long wavelength range of 560–700 nm. The fluorescence of NADH, AGE, FAD and connective tissue (collagen, elastin) contributes to the emission in the short wavelength interval. The possibility of the fluorescence of the lens covering the fundus fluorescence to a certain degree cannot be excluded. As a consequence, different results can be expected from eyes with crystalline lens and those with implanted intra-ocular lens. The fluorescence in the long wavelength range is dominated by lipofuscin. The influence of all other fluorophores is considerably reduced. As the longest detected lifetime was about 4 ns, 12.5 ns was sufficient time between the two excitation pulses according to a repetition rate of 80 MHz.

The autofluorescence signal is very weak. The number of fluorescence photons as a result of excitation has been calculated by Schweitzer et al. [20]. Less than one fluorescence photon can be expected when the fundus is excited by a series of ten pulses near the maximal permissible exposure [21]. This result leads to two conclusions. First, the signal is too weak to measure the fluorescence decay in the frequency domain [22]. In the frequency domain, the fluorescence lifetime is calculated from the phase shift or demodulation between the modulated excitation laser radiation and the modulated fluorescence light. This principle would require at least three fluorescence photons for construction of a half wave. The very weak detectable fundus fluorescence signal is optimally suited for the application of the time-correlated single photon counting technique (TCSPC) [22, 23]. In the TCSPC, the time is measured between the excitation pulse and the first and only fluorescence photon detected. According to this time, the content of the added photons in the corresponding time channel is increased by number 1 for each detected photon. After a certain measuring time, the content in all the time channels represents the probability density function of the fluorescence decay from the excited singlet state S1 to the ground state S0. According to this principle, the original decay process is transformed from the sub-nanosecond decay in the well-detectable time scale of seconds or minutes. The goal is now to detect such decay signals in the fundus fluorescence images for each pixel in, for example, a 150 × 150 pixel matrix. It can be estimated that the measuring time would have to last for several minutes to get a good SNR. As this detection of single photons is a Poisson process, the SNR is equal to the square root of the signal. That is, 10, 000 photons are required for SNR = 100.

The second consequence of the weak detectable signal and the long measuring time that is necessary is the application of the methods of image registration. That is, each fluorescence photon detected must be collected in the right image pixel in the corresponding time channel, despite the eye movements. From these basic investigations, the fluorescence lifetime mapper was developed.

10.4 Fluorescence Lifetime Mapping Ophthalmoscopy

10.4.1 Technical Solution

A fluorescence lifetime laser scanner ophthalmoscope was developed at the Department of Experimental Ophthalmology at the University Eye Clinic, Jena, Germany. It works in the time domain. According to previous investigations, all parameters required for the discrimination of fluorophores are combined. Thus, two wavelengths can be used for excitation, and the time-resolved autofluorescence is measured within two spectral ranges in the TCSPC technique. Furthermore, an online image registration is realised, allowing measurements over a period of minutes despite eye movements and blinking. A short technical description follows.

The opto-mechanical basis is a laser scanner ophthalmoscope (HRA II; Heidelberg Engineering, Heidelberg, Germany). This device was added by a unit for the fibre adoption of pulse laser diodes (HLD 440 or HLD 470; Lasos, Jena, Germany; Becker & Hickl, Berlin, Germany). These diodes emit pulses at 448 or 468 nm (75 ps FWHM, 80 MHz). The fibre end (3 μm) is imaged at the fundus during the scanning process. The average radiation power is about 120 μW in the corneal plane. Thus, the applied exposure is about 1% of the maximal permissible exposure. The fluorescence light is confocally detected via a 100 μm fibre. In addition, the fundus is irradiated by an IR Laser (820 nm) permitting contrast-rich fundus images, also in cases of cataracts. As the acquisition time is short for single images, it is unlikely that eye movements will interfere with the measurement. Subsequent images are registered in relation to the IR reference image. The calculated image transformation is also used for the registration of weak images of the dynamic fluorescence. As shown in Fig. 10.4, the IR light is separated from fluorescence light by a dichroic mirror, DM1. The excitation light is blocked by a razor filter (Laser 2000, Wesseling, Germany) at 488 nm from the fluorescence light. The fluorescence light is separated by a second dichroic mirror, DM2, in two spectral ranges, K1 = 490–560 nm and K2 = 560–700 nm. In both channels, the time-resolved fluorescence is detected by a multi-channel photomultiplier (MCP-PMT, HAM-R 3809U-50; Hamamatsu, Herrsching, Germany).

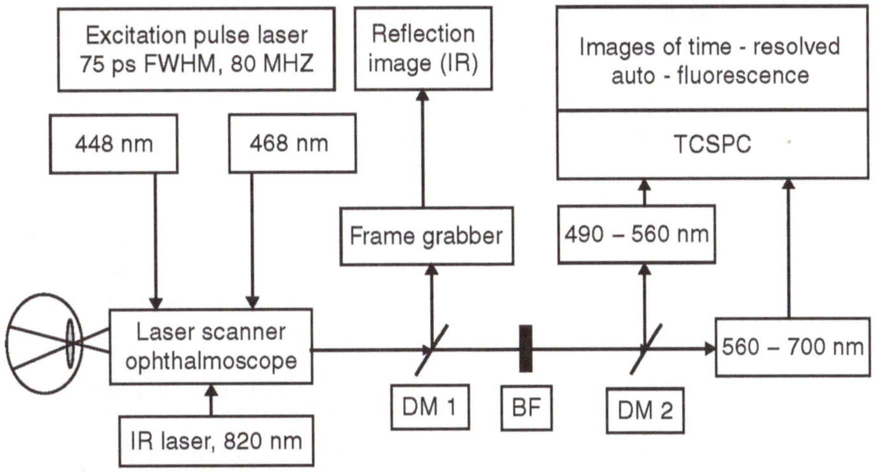

Fig. 10.4 Schema of the fluorescence lifetime mapping ophthalmoscope

A TCSPC board SPC 150 (Becker & Hickl, Berlin, Germany) detects the fluorescence decay. This board works in first-in first-out mode and has direct memory access. Thus, continuous measurements are possible and no interruption is required for data-saving. During the measuring process, online image registration is performed in both channels. The measuring time is determined by the number of collected photons required for the evaluation of the decay process. The number of collected photons in each time channel depends on the time resolution and spatial resolution selected. In the case of a constant width of the time channels, the smallest expected fluorescence lifetime determines the number of time channels. As the time between the two excitation pulses is divided into 1,024 time channels, the time resolution is 12.5 ps in the device described.

The better the image resolution, the longer the measuring time. A good compromise is a 40 µm × 40 µm resolution in 30 fundus images. This spatial resolution corresponds to one-fourth of a vessel diameter. Regions of changed metabolism are much more extensive. On the other hand, a thrombus or deposits in the retinal vessels are smaller than a vessel diameter. If a large number of photons is required for the calculation of lifetime parameters, several small pixels can be added to one extended pixel.

10.4.2 Calculation of the Parameters of Time-Resolved Fluorescence

As result of measurements of dynamic fluorescence, histograms of fluorescence decay are detected at each pixel in the fundus image. These histograms represent the decay of fluorescence intensity as the function of time.

The process is mostly assumed to be exponential decay, which can be approximated by a sum of e-functions (10.3):

$$\frac{I(t)}{I_0} = \sum_{i=1}^{p} \alpha_i \cdot e^{-\frac{t}{\tau_i}} + b, \qquad (10.3)$$

where:

α_i is the pre-exponential factor of exponent i or amplitude

τ_i is the lifetime of exponent i

b is the background

p is the degree of exponential function

As the excitation is not a Dirac pulse, the measured decay of fluorescence is the convolution of the excitation pulse with the decay process. Hence, the criterion for the fitting process is the minimisation of χ_r^2 (10.4):

$$\chi_r^2 = \frac{1}{n-q} \cdot \sum_{j=1}^{n} \frac{\left[N(t_j) - N_c(t_j)\right]^2}{N(t_j)}. \qquad (10.4)$$

In this equation, $N(t_j)$ is the number of photons measured in the time channel j. $N_c(t_j)$ is the number of expected photons, which is calculated by the convolution of the instrumental response function and the model function. n is the number of time channels and q is the number of free parameters (α_i, τ_i, b).

If the detection of the photons is a Poisson process, the mean square root error between the detected photons and the calculated photons is equal to the square root of the detected events:

$$\text{Noise} = \sqrt{[N(t_j) - N_c(t_j)]^2} = \sqrt{N(t_j)}. \qquad (10.5)$$

Thus, the ratio in the sum of (10.4) is 1 for each time channel and the sum is n, that is, the limiting value of χ_r^2 is 1.

The algorithm is independent of the degree of exponential function, but the calculation time increases with the number of exponents.

For the evaluation of lifetime measurements, in addition to the single amplitudes and lifetimes, parameters such as mean lifetime τ_{mean} and relative contribution Q_i are helpful. Here, the mean lifetime is defined as

$$\tau_{mean} = \frac{\sum_{i=1}^{p} \alpha_i \cdot \tau_i}{\sum_{i=1}^{p} \alpha_i}. \quad (10.6)$$

The relative contribution Qi of the component i corresponds to the area under the decay curve, as determined by the component i. This value is calculated according to (10.7):

$$Q_i = \frac{\alpha_i \cdot \tau_i}{\sum_{i=1}^{p} \alpha_i \cdot \tau_i}. \quad (10.7)$$

After the fitting calculation is completed, a two-dimensional (2D) data matrix is determined for each basic parameter τ_i and α_i, as well as for the derived parameter τ_{mean} and Q_i. 2D or quasi-three-dimensional (3D) images can be presented from these data for visual inspection. In particular, for images of amplitudes, there are two different possibilities for presentations. In images of absolute values of amplitudes, regions are visible that exhibit high or low fluorescence intensity. Unfortunately, these images also represent non-homogeneous illumination. Images of relative amplitudes are independent of the illumination. These images demonstrate the position at which a certain amplitude is dominating and whether another amplitude is missing. By comparing such a relation with the anatomical structure of the fundus, the original layer of the specific amplitude can be determined. For more quantitative evaluation, histograms of lifetimes, amplitudes or relative contribution can be calculated. Such a histogram shows how often, for example, a certain lifetime was determined in the fundus image. Despite the lack of relation to the location at the fundus, such histograms can be used for statistical comparison between healthy subjects and patients. If the degree of the e-function is higher than 1, then pairs of lifetimes or amplitudes are calculated for the same pixel in the fundus image. These pairs can be presented as cluster diagrams with, for example, $\tau 1$ as the abscissa and $\tau 2$, $\tau 3$ as the ordinate. Isolated fluorophores and ocular structures form specific lifetime and amplitude clusters. In clusters $\alpha 2$ vs $\alpha 1$, gradients can be calculated specifically for each ocular structure [19]. The lifetime clusters of a young and a middle-aged subject have been compared with the lifetime cluster of an AMD patient and the lifetime cluster of lipofuscin by Schweitzer et al. [24].

10.5 Clinical Results

In comparing measurements, the crystalline lens was found to have an influence on lifetimes in the short-wavelength detection channel related to eyes with implanted intra-ocular lenses. The lifetimes are longer in cases of natural lens and increase with age as a result of metabolic changes during cataract formation. Hence, healthy subjects and patients can be compared if they have the same kind of lenses and are of comparable age.

10.5.1 Age-Related Macular Degeneration

10.5.1.1 Detection of Alterations in Early AMD

The importance of the lifetimes and amplitudes in both detection channels was investigated in a comparison study of healthy subjects and patients suffering from the early phases of AMD [25]. Nine healthy subjects at the mean age of 63.2 years (41–85 years) were considered as controls.

Fifteen patients in the early phases of AMD [26] had a mean age of 74.7 years (65–87 years). All the eyes had crystalline lenses. The mean lifetimes in K1 and K2 are given for healthy subjects in Table 10.2 and for patients with the early phases of AMD in Table 10.3.

Table 10.2. Mean and standard deviation of the summarised lifetime histograms of healthy subjects

Lifetime	Spectral channel	Mean (ps)	Standard deviation (ps)
τ1	K1	118	23
τ1	K2	104	31
τ2	K1	584	184
τ2	K2	477	82
τ3	K1	2,826	583
τ3	K2	1,623	242

Table 10.3. Mean and standard deviation of the summarised lifetime histograms in patients with early age-related macular degeneration (AMD)

Lifetime	Spectral channel	Mean (ps)	Standard deviation (ps)
τ1	K1	166	51
τ1	K2	137	55
τ2	K1	986	408
τ2	K2	583	218
τ3	K1	3,309	989
τ3	K2	1,924	540

Table 10.4. Significance of lifetimes for the detection of early AMD

Lifetime	Spectral channel	Significance
τ1	K1	$p < 0.01$
τ1	K2	Not significant
τ2	K1	$p < 0.01$
τ2	K2	$p < 0.05$
τ3	K1	Not significant
τ3	K2	$p < 0.05$

A statistical comparison was based on lifetime histograms in K1 and K2 of both the groups.

As shown in Table 10.4, τ1 and τ2 in the short-wavelength channel K1 are best suited to discovering early pathological alterations in AMD. No discrimination is possible based on τ3 in the short-wavelength channel K1 and on τ1 in the long-wavelength channel. If the amplitudes were additionally included, the discrimination of both the groups would further improve.

The best separation of healthy subjects and patients with early AMD in the short-wavelength channel confirms the studies on isolated fluorophores, taking into account the spectral transmission of the ocular media. According to these studies, most weakly emitting endogenous fundus fluorophores can be excited by wavelengths around 450 nm. The time-resolved fluorescence detection in the short-wavelength spectral channel permits the detection of weakly emitting fluorophores simultaneously with lipofuscin, which mostly emits strongly in the long-wavelength channel. The lifetime τ1 = 118 ps in healthy subjects is determined by protein-bound FAD in the short-wavelength channel. In AMD, this lifetime is increased to τ1 = 166 ps by the influence of A2E, the component VIII of lipofuscin [27], which is τ1 = 170 ps in Table 10.1.

The increases in lifetime τ2 = 584 ps in the short-wavelength emission range in healthy subjects up to τ2 = 982 ps in early AMD is interpretable as an increase in the protein-bound NADH. The contribution of protein-bound NADH increases in the case of a lack of oxygen, when more energy is produced by glycolysis.

As the measurements were performed in 30° fundus images and were not limited to the macula, it can be concluded that early alterations in AMD occur in the whole fundus. These alterations are prominent in the macula for both the patient and the investigator in the late phases of AMD.

10.5.1.2 Lifetime Images in Late AMD

Non-Exudative AMD and Geographic Atrophy

Measurements of fluorescence lifetime in different spectral channels lead to new information that might be helpful in discovering the patho-mechanism in AMD. For example, images of lifetime τ3 are demonstrated, which were measured from a 77-year-old woman [28]. The patient was suffering from non-exudative AMD. The decimal visual acuity was 0.8 in the IOL-wearing eye. As demonstrated in Fig. 10.5, reverse distribution of lifetime in the macula was determined in the short-wavelength and long-wavelength spectral channels. In the short-wavelength channel, the lifetime τ3 was prolonged in the papillo-macular bundle and around the macula, but was normal in a central circular field. In contrast, the lifetime τ3 was prolonged in the central macular field and was normal in the papillo-macular region in the long-wavelength channel. The prolonged lifetime τ3 in the short-wavelength channel is interpretable as an accumulation of connective tissue. The prolonged lifetime τ3 in the long-wavelength channel is caused by a fluorophore that emits in the long-wavelength spectral range. This might be a component of lipofuscin, but not A2E. The lifetime of A2E is 170 ps and the lifetime of this unknown fluorophore is up to 4 ns. The difference in the lifetime in both the spectral channels is also denoted in the comparison of a colour fundus image and an infrared fundus image, to a certain degree. In the colour image, a dark central macular range is surrounded by bright reflecting spots of drusen. In contrast, there are bright spots in the central macular area in the infrared image (Fig. 10.5).

Local alterations of autofluorescence in the geographic atrophy are detectable by time-resolved measurements as demonstrated in a 61-year-old patient with natural crystalline lens (Fig. 10.6). His decimal visual acuity was 0.3, despite the massive macular alteration. The strongest alterations were detectable in the images of lifetime τ2 in the short-wavelength channel. While only reduced amplitudes of α1 were detectable in the atrophic range (Fig. 10.6a), detailed local differences were visible in the images of lifetime τ2 (Fig. 10.6b). The prolonged lifetime τ2 in the macula was reduced to normal values in the fovea, which might be the reason for the relatively good vision. This foveal range was omitted from atrophy visible in the corresponding fluorescence angiogram (Fig. 10.6c). Early atrophic alterations were already verifiable in the lifetime image of the inferior fovea, but not visible in the fluorescence angiogram. The lifetime image of τ2 in the short-wavelength channel of a 38-year-old healthy subject is given for comparison (Fig. 10.6d). Here, besides the optic disc, τ2 is around 400 ps and is reduced in the macula to a certain degree.

Exudative AMD

Local macular alterations are detectable in exudative AMD by time-resolved fluorescence measurement as demonstrated in Fig. 10.7. In this example, a 78-year-old

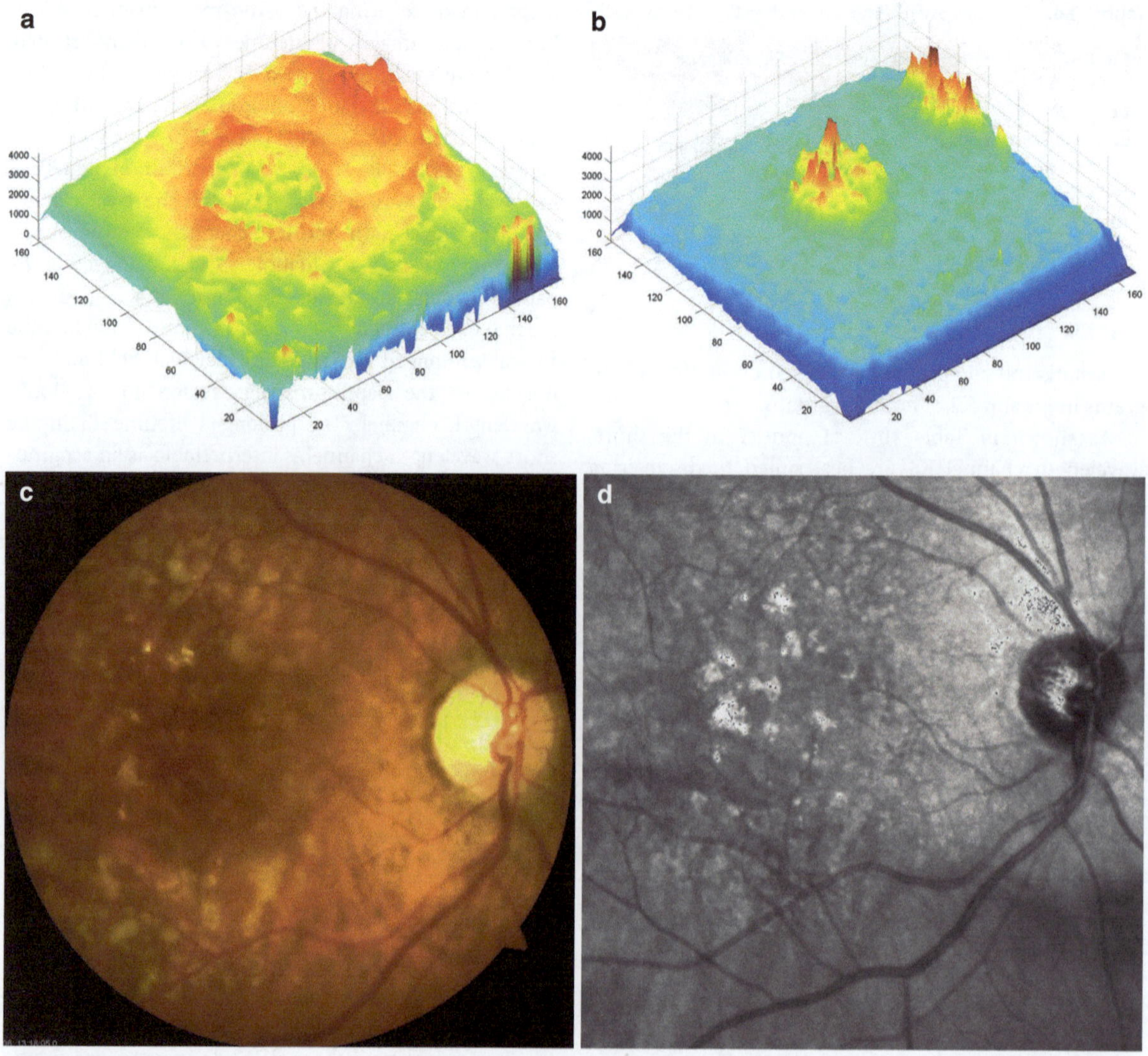

Fig. 10.5 Fluorescence lifetime $\tau 3$ in non-exudative < (AMD). **a** $\tau 3$ in K1 (490–560 nm), **b** $\tau 3$ in K2 (560–700 nm), **c** colour fundus image, **d** infrared fundus image

woman suffering from exudative AMD was considered. The decimal visual acuity was 0.2 in this eye with crystalline lens. This time, changes in the long-wavelength channel K2 (560–700 nm) were considered. The amplitude $\alpha 1 = 90\%$ dominates the fluorescence decay. Images of amplitude $\alpha 1$ are comparable with the images of static fluorescence, as evaluated by Bindewald et al. [29]. In Fig. 10.7a, the values of $\alpha 1$ are continuously reduced in the macula to the minimum in the fovea. In contrast, the values of lifetime $\tau 2$ in Fig. 10.7b were widely normal at the whole fundus. Only a peak of $\tau 2$ appeared in the central macular range. A membrane is visible at this position in the fluorescence angiogram (Fig. 10.7c). Thus, the increased lifetime $\tau 2$ probably originates from this membrane. As demonstrated for comparison, the lifetime $\tau 2$ of a 60-year-old man is reduced in the macula (Fig. 10.7d).

10.5.2 Metabolic Changes in Retinal Vessel Occlusion

10.5.2.1 Arterial Branch Occlusion

The supply of oxygen is reduced or interrupted in arterial occlusion. This state can be considered a provocation of metabolism. Of special interest are metabolic changes in the arterial branch occlusion. As each quadrant of the fundus is supplied in principle by a pair of an artery and a vein, a comparison of the metabolic state is possible

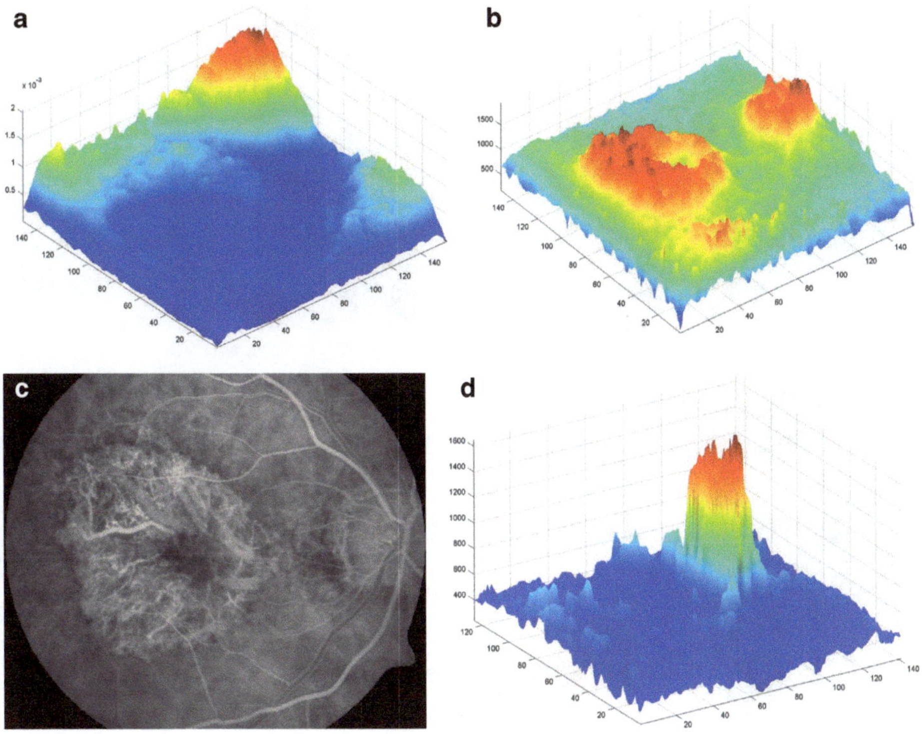

Fig. 10.6 Time-resolved autofluorescence in geographic atrophy. **a** Amplitude α1 and **b** lifetime τ2 in K1 (490–560 nm), **c** fluorescence angiogram, **d** lifetime τ2 of a healthy subject in K1 (490–560 nm)

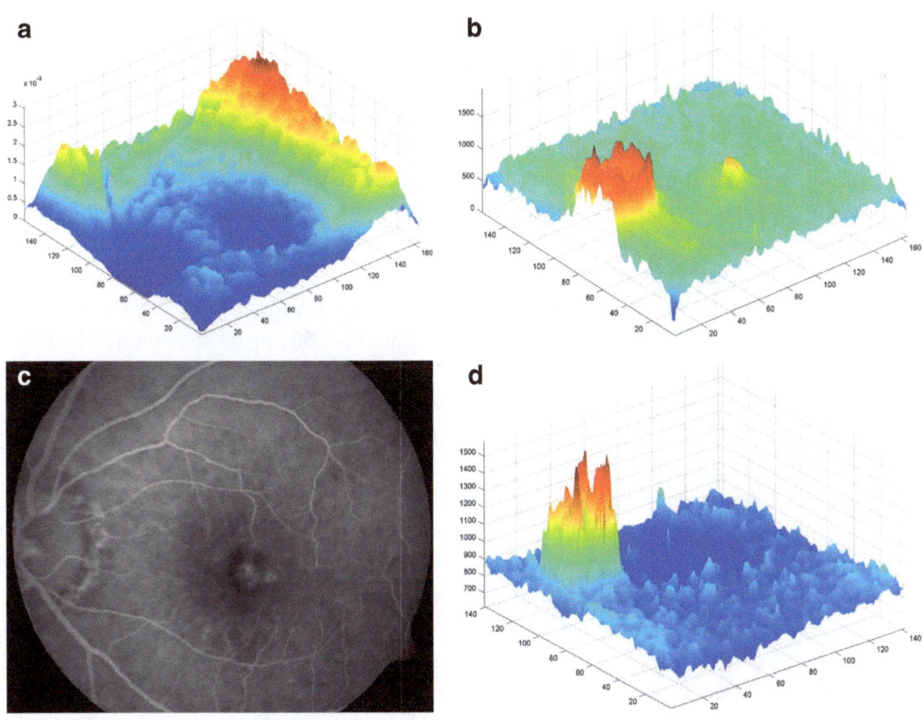

Fig. 10.7 Time-resolved autofluorescence in exudative AMD. **a** Amplitude α1, **b** lifetime τ2 in K2 (560–700 nm), **c** fluorescence angiogram, **d** lifetime τ2 in K2 of a healthy subject

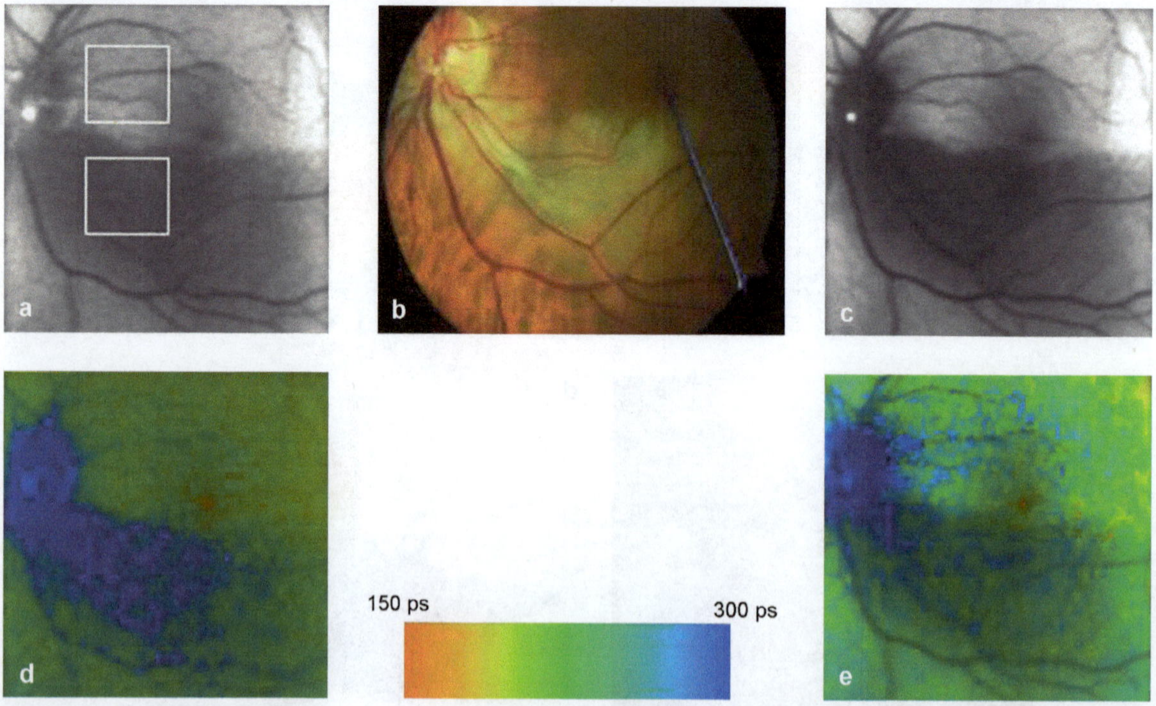

Fig. 10.8 Time-resolved autofluorescence in arterial branch occlusion. **a** Fluorescence intensity in K1 (490–560 nm), **b** colour fundus image, **c** fluorescence intensity in K2 (560–700 nm), **d, e** images of mean lifetime τ_m in K1 and K2

between a supplied and a non-supplied region. For example, Fig. 10.8 demonstrates an arterial branch occlusion in the temporal inferior quadrant. The decimal visual acuity of a 69-year-old woman was 1.0. The natural crystalline lens was in the eye. Figure 10.8a and c are the images of fluorescence intensity in K1 and K2 in which the thrombus appears as a bright spot. The non-supplied range is dark in both the images. whereas, structures are visible in the optic disc in the fluorescence intensity image of K1, the fluorescence intensity is very weak in the optic disc in K2. In the colour fundus image (Fig. 10.8b), the non-supplied quadrant appears bright. The non-supplied region exhibits a long lifetime in the image of the mean lifetime τ_m in K1 (Fig. 10.8d). The borderlines of the non-supplied range are much better visible in the lifetime image of K1 than in the mean lifetime τ_m of K2 (Fig. 10.8e). The longest lifetime was detected in the optic disc and the shortest one in the macula in both the spectral channels.

The fluorescence decay was approximated three-exponentially. Histograms of lifetimes were considered for the quantitative evaluation of metabolic changes. These histograms were determined in areas of the same size, both in the supplied superior and in the non-supplied inferior quadrants (Fig. 10.8a). Clear differences between the histograms of lifetimes in the supplied and non-supplied areas were detectable only in the short-wavelength channel, especially for the lifetime $\tau 2$.

As demonstrated in Fig. 10.9, the most frequent lifetime was $\tau 2$ = 508 ps in the supplied area. The distribution of $\tau 2$ was extended in the non-supplied field with a maximum at $\tau 2$ = 1,233 ps. Based on the comparison of anatomical fundus structure and lifetimes, it follows that $\tau 2$ originates to a certain degree in the neuronal retina. Furthermore, NADH and FAD emit in the short-wavelength spectral range. Thus, the alterations of lifetime $\tau 2$ in K1 are caused by these co-enzymes. The lifetime $\tau 2$ = 508 ps of the supplied field is in the order of the mean lifetime τ_m = 460 ps, determined for porcine neuronal retina (Fig. 10.3). This lifetime is probably determined by free NADH [17]. The longer lifetime $\tau 2$ = 1,233 ps in K1 of the non-supplied field is interpretable as an increase in the protein-bound NADH, as observed in the glycolysis. The lifetime of protein-bound NADH was determined to be between 1 and 2.5 ns in the literature [16–18]. It is also remarkable that the pH value decreases in the non-supplied ocular tissue in arterial occlusion [30]. As the fluorescence lifetime depends on pH, its decrease leads to longer lifetimes [31]. In an animal model, apoptosis was demonstrated in the inner retinal layers caused by under-supplying as a result of occlusion in the central retinal artery [21].

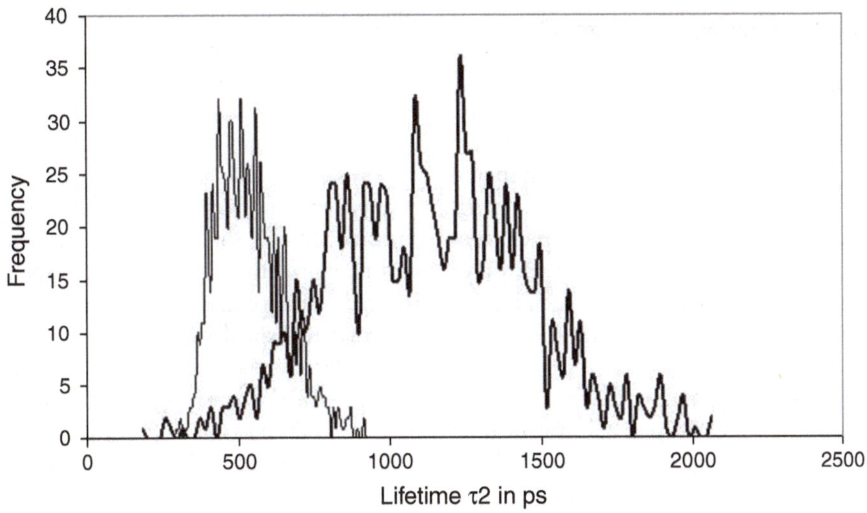

Fig. 10.9 Histogram of lifetime τ2 in K1 (490–560 nm) of the supplied (maximum 508 ps) and non-supplied range (maximum 1,233 ps)

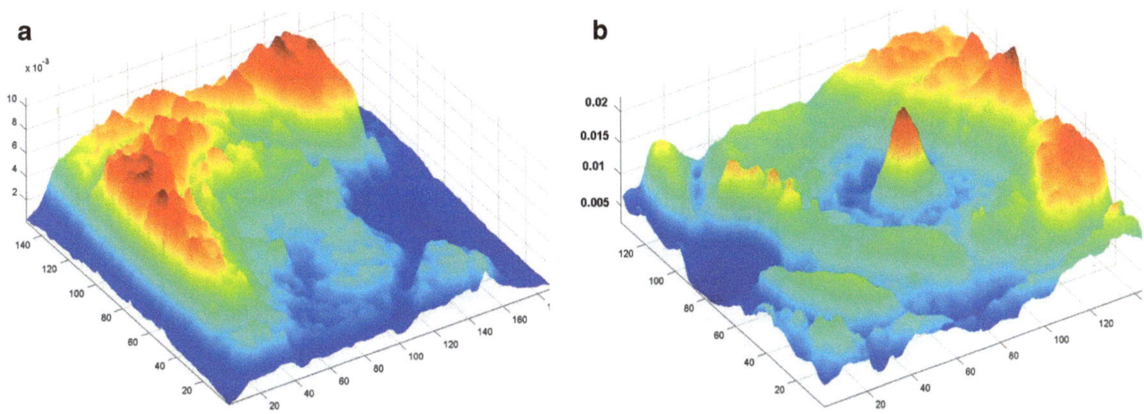

Fig. 10.10 Images of amplitude α1 in K1 (490–560 nm). **a** Healthy subject, **b** central arterial occlusion

This result supports the assumption that τ2 is related to the neuronal retina. On the other hand, although the lifetime is prolonged in apoptosis, it stays constant in necrosis [32]. Considering the lifetimes, a differentiation of damaging mechanisms might be possible, leading to therapy optimisation.

10.5.2.2 Images of Lifetime Amplitudes in Central Arterial Occlusion

Besides lifetime images and corresponding histograms, the amplitudes also deliver helpful information. For example, images of the amplitude α1 in the short-wavelength channel in a healthy subject (aged 82 years, Fig. 10.10a) and a patient suffering from central retinal artery occlusion (aged 79 years, Fig. 10.10b) are compared. An intra-ocular lens was in the patient's eye, but the visual acuity was only finger counting.

The fluorescence intensity in the optic disc is generally weak in all cases. The fluorescence τ1 and the corresponding amplitude α1 originate predominantly in the retinal pigment epithelium. Hence, the amplitude α1 is blocked by retinal vessels. In the macula of this old healthy eye, the amplitude α1 is at the same level as in the surrounding tissue. It decreases somewhat in the inferior part. In contrast, the absolute amplitude α1 peaks in the macula in central retinal artery occlusion.

10.5.3 Metabolic Alteration in Diabetes Mellitus

10.5.3.1 Detection of Fields of Reduced Metabolism

Pathological alterations of the cellular metabolism are expected in diabetes. The lack of dissolved oxygen should lead to comparable lifetimes, as demonstrated in arterial branch occlusion. Thus, early detection of such changes should be possible by fluorescence lifetime measurements. It is conceivable to be able to detect such unsupplied fields. In individually adapted therapy, these fields might be coagulated first.

To find such alterations, time-resolved fluorescence measurements were performed on a 77-year-old male diabetic type II patient. There were few signs of early non-exudative diabetic retinopathy in the eye with crystalline lens. Fluorescence lifetime measurements were considered for comparison of an 82-year-old healthy subject. As in arterial branch occlusion, a definite difference was detectable in lifetime $\tau 2$ in the short-wavelength channel. Figure 10.11 shows the histograms of $\tau 2$ in K1 of both subjects.

The distribution of the lifetime $\tau 2$ in K1 of the older healthy subject exhibits a single maximum at 497 ps. In diabetic patients, the maximum of $\tau 2$ in K1 is shifted to 662 ps and an additional shoulder appears around 1,200 ps. This lifetime range around 1,200 ps was expected as a sign of reduced oxidative metabolism. It corresponds to the lifetime $\tau 2$ in K1, which was detected in the non-supplied area in the arterial branch occlusion. This prolonged lifetime $\tau 2$ is the result of an increasing contribution of protein-bound NADH, produced as an augmented effect of glycolysis.

The fields of reduced metabolic activity can be selected at the fundus. Figure 10.12 shows an image of lifetime $\tau 2$ in K1. In this image, regions with lifetimes shorter than

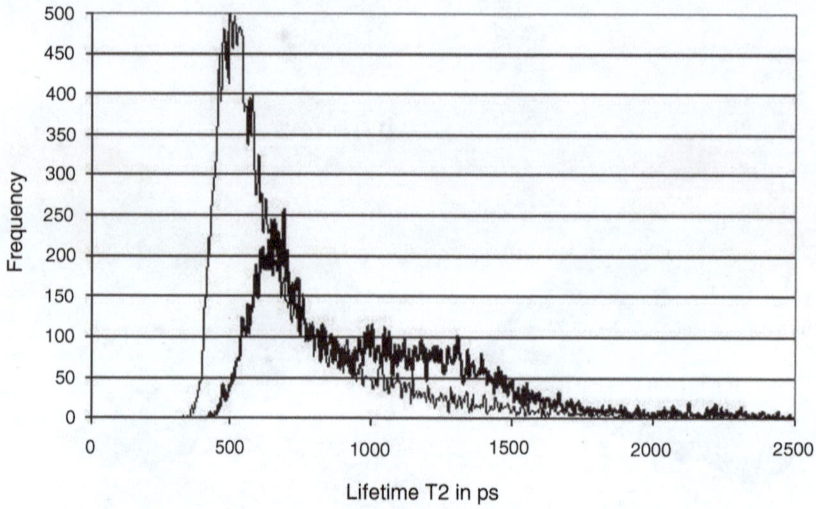

Fig. 10.11 Histogram of lifetime $\tau 2$ in K1 (490–560 nm). Healthy subject maximum of $\tau 2$ at 497 ps, diabetic maximum at 662 ps with shoulder at1,200 ps

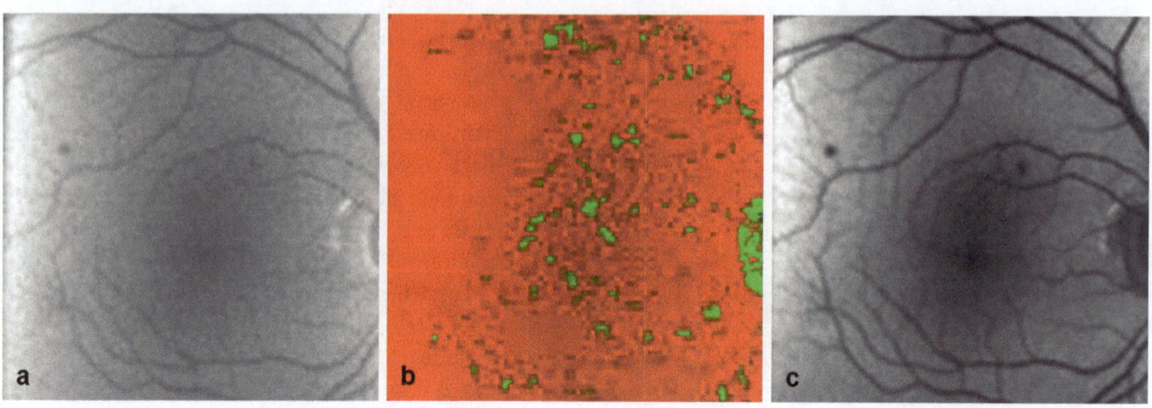

Fig. 10.12 Detection of ranges with reduced metabolism. **a** Fluorescence intensity in K1 (490–560 nm), **b** fluorescence lifetime $\tau 2$ in K1, **c** fluorescence intensity in K2 (560–700 nm)

1,000 ps are red and fields of reduced metabolism with lifetimes longer than 1,000 ps are marked in green. For better orientation, the images of fluorescence intensity are also given. The contrast is weak in the image of fluorescence intensity in K1 (490–560 nm) because of the fluorescence of the lens. The contrast is much better in the long-wavelength channel, where no fluorescence of the crystalline lens is detectable. The coagulations of the fields of reduced metabolism might be a subject of further research into individually adapted therapy.

The histograms of lifetime τ2 in K2 are identical to maxima at 467 ps. Further typical changes in lifetime in diabetic and healthy subjects were detected for τ1 also. In channel 1 (490–560 nm), the frequency of τ1 was maximal at 92 ps in the healthy subjects. For the diabetic subjects, this histogram was double humped at 97 and 132 ps. In K2 (560–700 nm), the most frequent lifetime τ1 = 92 ps in diabetics was shorter than τ1 = 102 ps in the healthy subject.

Large differences between the diabetic and healthy subjects were detectable for lifetime τ3 in K1. The most frequent lifetime τ3 = 5,530 ps in diabetic subjects was considerably longer than τ3 = 4,000 ps in the healthy subjects. In K2 (560–700 nm), the difference was much smaller in the diabetic subjects (τ3 = 2,980 ps) than in healthy subject (τ3 = 2,590 ps). As the lifetime τ3 in eyes with crystalline lens is predominantly determined by the fluorescence lifetime of the lens, the prolonged lifetime in diabetic subjects is caused by metabolic changes in the lens. The main reason is the forming of glycolysed proteins (AGE), exhibiting long lifetime. An early sign of diabetic metabolic alteration is observable in the lens. Owing to excitation by blue light at 448 nm, diabetic lenses emit a strong green fluorescence.

10.5.3.2 Lifetime Images in Diabetes After Laser Coagulation

Laser coagulation is the most frequent therapy in severe diabetic retinopathy. Changes in time-resolved autofluorescence after laser coagulation have been demonstrated in a 77-year-old diabetic patient in Fig. 10.13. An intra-

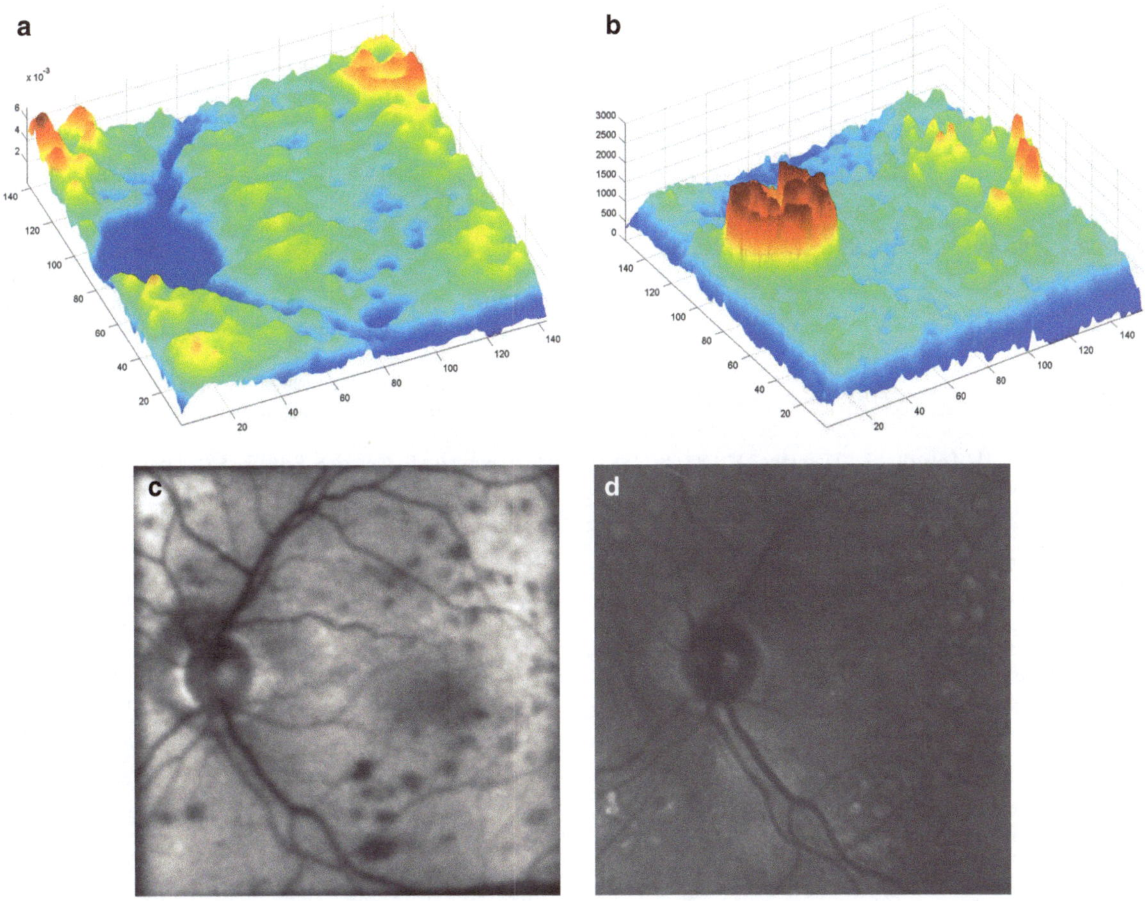

Fig. 10.13 Time-resolved autofluorescence in diabetic retinopathy. **a** Amplitude α1, **b** lifetime τ3 and **c** fluorescence intensity in K1 (490–560 nm)

ocular lens was implanted into his eye. As shown in Fig. 10.13a and c, both the amplitude $\alpha 1$ in the short-wavelength channel and the fluorescence intensity as the sum of all detected photons are reduced at the coagulation spots. That is, the fluorescence of RPE is eliminated, emitting with a short lifetime. In contrast, the long lifetimes of connective tissue are detectable at the coagulation spots (Fig. 10.13b). The force of each laser spot can be evaluated according to the detectable lifetime.

Measurements of dynamic fluorescence open the way for objective estimation of laser therapy in diabetes. As the lifetime $\tau 2$ in the range of 1,000–1,500 ps in the short-wavelength channel is characteristic of unsupplied retinal tissue, its contribution should be reduced after laser coagulation.

Summary for Clinicians

- Time-resolved measurement of endogenous fluorophores in different spectral ranges in combination with selected spectral excitation is a new method for the investigation of cellular metabolism.
- The origination of pathological changes can be determined in a reversible state.
- Individual adapted therapy might be possible on the basis of lifetime measurements.
- Measurement of lifetime is suited to therapy control.

References

1. Schweitzer D, Leistritz L, Hammer M et al (1995) Calibration-free measurement of the oxygen saturation in retinal vessels of men. Ophthalmic Technol V, SPIE 2393: 210–218
2. Feke GT (2006) Laser Doppler instrumentation for the measurement of retinal blood flow: theory and practice. Bull Soc Belge Ophtalmol 302:171–184
3. Leitgeb RA, Schmetterer L, Hitzenberger CK et al (2004) Real-time measurement of in vitro flow by Fourier-domain color Doppler optical coherence tomography. Opt Lett 29(2):171–173
4. Beach JM, Schwenzer KJ, Srinivas S et al (1999) Oximetry of retinal vessels by dual-wavelength imaging: calibration and influence of pigmentation. J Appl Physiol 86(2): 748–758
5. Schweitzer D, Hammer M, Kraft J et al (1999) In vivo measurement of the oxygen saturation of retinal vessels in healthy volunteers. IEEE Trans Biomed Eng 46 (12): 1454–1465
6. Schweitzer D, Lasch A, van der Vorst S et al (2007) Änderung der retinalen Sauerstoffsättigung bei Gesunden und in frühen Stadien der diabetische Retinopathie nach Atmung von 100% Sauerstoff. Klin Monatsbl Augenheilkd 224:402–410
7. Stryer L (1991) Biochemie. Spectrum Akademischer, Verlag GmbH Heidelberg
8. Boettner EA, Wolter JR (1962) Transmission of the ocular media. Invest Ophthalmol 1:776–783
9. La Schiazza O, Bille JF (2008) High-speed two-photon excited autofluorescence imaging of ex vivo human retinal pigment epithelial cells toward age-related macular degeneration diagnostic. J Biomed Opt 13(6):064008
10. American National Standard for the safe use of laser ANSI Z 136.1-2000 (2000) Laser Institute of America, Orlando, FL
11. Schweitzer D, Schenke S, Hammer M et al (2007) Towards metabolic mapping of the human retina. Microsc Res Tech 70:410–419
12. Sionkowska A, Skopinska J, Wisniewski M et al (2007) Spectroscopic studies into the influence of UV radiation on elastin in the presence of collagen. J Photochem Photobiol B Biol 86:186–191
13. Skala MC, Riching KM, Gendron-Fitzpatrick A et al (2007) In vivo multiphoton microscopy of metabolic oxidation-reduction states and fluorescence lifetimes in normal and pre-cancerous epithelia. Proc Natl Acad Sci U S A 104(49): 19494–19499
14. Yagi K, Tanaka F, Nakashima N et al (1983) Picosecond laser fluorometry of FAD of D-amino acid oxidase-benzoate complex. J Biol Chem 258(6):3799–3802
15. Nakashima N, Yoshihara K, Tanaka F et al (1980) Picosecond fluorescence lifetime of the coenzyme of D-amino acid oxidase. J Biol Chem 255 (11):5261–5263
16. König K, Riemann I (2003) High-resolution multiphoton tomography of human skin with subcellular spatial resolution and picosecond time resolution. J Biomed Opt 8 (3): 432–439
17. Schneckenburger H, Wagner M, Weber P et al (2004) Autofluorescence lifetime imaging of cultivated cells using a UV picosecond laser diode. J Fluoresc 14 (5): 649–654
18. Wu Y, Zheng W, Qu J (2006) Sensing cell metabolism by time-resolved autofluorescence. Opt Lett 31(21): 3122–3124
19. Schweitzer D, Jentsch S, Schenke S et al (2007) Spectral and time-resolved studies on ocular structures. In: Schweitzer D, Fitzmaurice M (eds) Diagnostic optical spectroscopy in biomedicine IV. Proceedings of the SPIE, 6628,pp 662807-1–662807-12
20. Schweitzer D, Kolb A, Hammer M et al (2000) Tau mapping of the autofluorescence of the human ocular fundus. SPIE 4164:79–89
21. Goldenberg-Cohen N, Dadon S, Avraham BCR et al (2008) Molecular and histological changes following central retinal artery occlusion in a mouse model. Exp Eye Res 87: 327–333
22. Lakowicz JR (2007) Principles of fluorescence spectroscopy, 3rd edn. Kluwer, Academic, Plenum, New York
23. Becker W (2005) Advanced time-correlated single photon counting techniques. Springer Series in Chemical Physics 81. Springer, Berlin
24. Schweitzer D, Hammer M, Schweitzer F et al (2004) In vivo measurement of time-resolved autofluorescence at the human fundus. J Biomed Opt 9(6)1214–1222

25. Schweitzer D, Quick S, Schenke S et al (2009) Vergleich von Parametern der zeitaufgelösten Autofluoreszenz bei Gesunden und Patienten mit früher AMD. Ophthalmologe 9(6):714–722
26. AREDS Research Group (2001) A randomized, placebo-controlled, clinical trial of high-dose supplementation with vitamins C and E, beta carotene, and zinc for age-related macular degeneration and vision loss: AREDS report No 8. Arch Ophthalmol 119(10):1417–1436
27. Eldred GE, Katz ML (1988) Fluorophores of the human pigment epithelium: separation and spectral characterization. Exp Eye Res 47:71–86
28. Schweitzer D (2010) Quantifying fundus autofluorescence. In: Lois N, Forrester JV (eds) Fundus autofluorescence. Lippincott Williams & Wilkins, Philadelphia
29. Bindewald A, Bird AC, Dandekar SS et al (2005) Classification of fundus autofluorescence patterns in early age-related macular diseases. Invest Ophthalmol Vis Sci 46:3309–3314
30. Birol G, Budzynski E, Wangsa-Wirawan ND et al (2005) Retinal arterial occlusion leads to acidosis in the cat. Exp Eye Res 80:527–533
31. Wakita M, Nishimura G, Tamura M (1995) Some characteristics of the fluorescence lifetime of reduced pyridine nucleotides in isolated mitochondria, isolated hepatocytes, and perfused rat liver in situ. J Biochem 118:1151–1160
32. Wang HW, Gukassyan V, Chen CT et al (2008) Differentiation of apoptosis from necrosis by dynamic changes of reduced nicotinamide adenine dinucleotide fluorescence lifetime in live cells. J Biomed Opt 13(5):054011

Chapter 11

Assessing Diabetic Macular Edema with Optical Coherence Tomography 11

Sebastian Wolf

Core Messages

- Diabetic retinopathy (DR) and diabetic macular edema (DME) are common microvascular complications in patients with diabetes.
- DR and DME are the leading causes of blindness in the working population.
- Diagnosis of DME is based on slit-lamp biomicroscopy and stereo fundus photography.
- Optical coherence tomography (OCT) has been used primarily to analyze macular thickness in DME.
- Structural changes in DME can be assessed by OCT. These include retinal swelling, cystoid macular edema, and subretinal fluid.
- The spectral-domain high-resolution OCT images not only allow to analyze structural changes in DME, but also to analyze the integrity of single retinal layers.
- The presence and integrity of the external limiting membrane (ELM), the photoreceptor inner segment (IS), the outer segment (OS), and the retinal pigment epithelium (RPE) appears to be a good prognostic feature for visual improvement after treatment for DME.

11.1 Diabetic Macular Edema

Diabetes mellitus (DM) is the most common endocrine disease in developed countries. The prevalence ranges between 2 and 5% of the world's population. Diabetic retinopathy (DR) and diabetic macular edema (DME) are common microvascular complications in patients with diabetes. They are the leading causes of blindness in the population aged 20–74 years and responsible for 12% of new cases of blindness each year [1]. As the prevalence of diabetes will double over the next 20 years, DR and DME will continue to cause substantial vision loss unless adequately treated [2].

11.2 Examinations in Diabetic Macular Edema

Diagnosis of DME is traditionally based on slit-lamp biomicroscopy and stereo fundus photography [3, 4]. Additionally, fluorescein angiography is used to evaluate patients with DME to evaluate the extent and origin of fluid leakage as well as the extent of capillary ischemia in the macula [5]. However, these methods are relatively insensitive to determine changes in retinal thickness. More recently, optical coherence tomography (OCT) has been used to analyze DME [6–9]. OCT was introduced into the clinical routine during the past decade as a noninvasive means to assess the posterior pole [10–13]. In the past, OCT has been used primarily to analyze macular thickness in DME [8, 9]: Additionally, OCT in patients with DME has revealed several structural changes in the retina. These include retinal swelling, cystoid macular edema, and subretinal fluid [14, 15]. OCT is an evolving technology. Current advances, e.g., the introduction of Fourier analysis (spectral OCT), made both high resolution and fast scanning speed possible [16–18]. High resolution allows for differentiation of as much as 11 structural characteristics within the retina [19–21].

11.3 Treatment of Diabetic Macular Edema

Currently, laser photocoagulation is the only proven treatment of DME by large-scale studies. The Early Treatment in Diabetic Retinopathy Study (ETDRS) showed that laser photocoagulation reduces the risk of moderate visual acuity loss by about 50% in DME [5]. However, visual acuity improved only in a small percentage of patients and a significant number of eyes did not respond to laser photocoagulation. Other treatment modalities for DME include pars plana vitrectomy, intravitreal triamcinolone acetonide injection, and intravitreal injection of anti-VEGF drugs [22–24]. Especially, intravitreal anti-VEGF treatment appears to be very promising, showing significant visual improvements in several small studies [25].

The response to various treatment modalities for DME is variable. Some patients show excellent visual improvement whereas others show only minimal response. Thus, there is a significant unmet need to develop diagnostic methods that allow identifying prognostic features for the visual outcome after treatment for DME.

11.4 High-Resolution Optical Coherence Tomography in Diabetic Macular Edema

The Spectralis™ HRA + OCT combines high-resolution spectral-domain OCT with an SLO. The system allows for simultaneous OCT scans with high-resolution scanning laser retinal imaging. The instrument uses broadband 870 nm SLD for the OCT channel. The retina is scanned at 40,000 A-scans per second, creating highly detailed images of the structure of the retina. The OCT optical depth resolution is 7 μm, the digital depth resolution is 3.5 μm. The combination of high-resolution scanning laser retinal images and spectral-domain OCT allows for real-time tracking of the eye movements and real-time averaging of scanning laser images and OCT scans, reducing speckle noise of the OCT images [26].

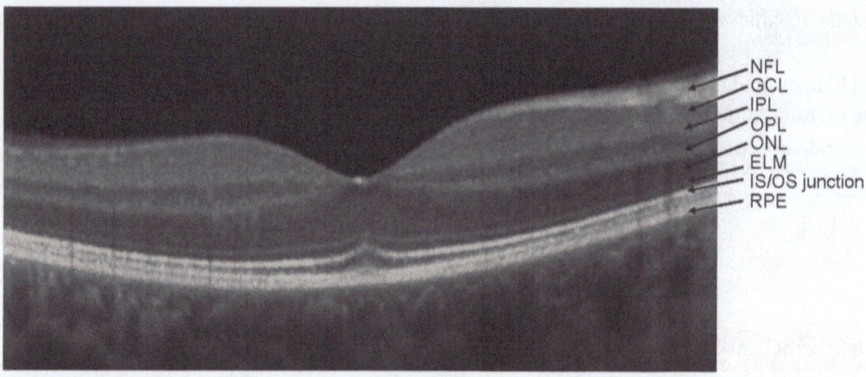

Fig. 11.1 Normal retina as imaged by Spectralis™ HRA + OCT. The ganglion cell layer *GCL*; the inner plexiform layer *IPL*; the inner nuclear layer *INL*; the outer plexiform layer *OPL*; outer nuclear layer *ONL*; external limiting membrane *ELM*; the photoreceptor inner segments *IS*; the outer segments *OS*; and the retinal pigment epithelium *RPE* are marked with *arrows*

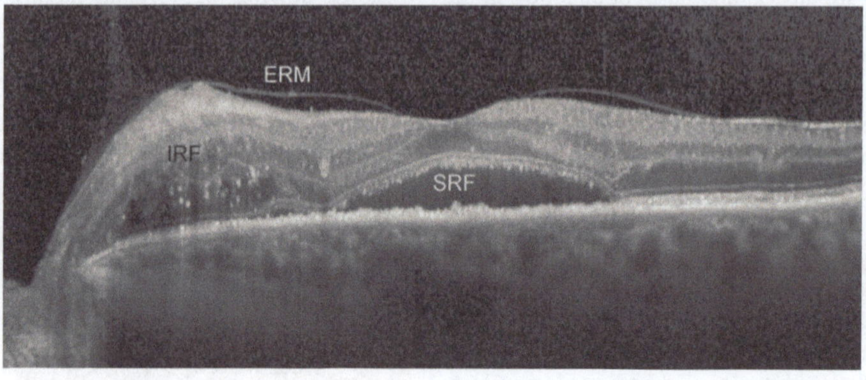

Fig. 11.2 DME as imaged by Spectralis™ HRA + OCT. Note the epiretinal membrane *ERM*; subretinal fluid accumulation *SRF*; and intraretinal fluid accumulation *IRF*

The spectral OCT images allow analyzing the integrity of the retinal layers. In a normal retina imaged by Spectralis™ HRA + OCT, the ganglion cell layer (GCL), the inner plexiform layer (IPL), the inner nuclear layer (INL), the outer plexiform layer (OPL), outer nuclear layer (ONL), the external limiting membrane (ELM), the photoreceptor inner segments (IS), the outer segments (OS), and the retinal pigment epithelium (RPE) can be seen (Fig. 11.1). In patients with DME, high-resolution OCT revealed various pathologic findings. These include epiretinal membranes, subretinal fluid, intraretinal fluid accumulation, and cystoid macular edema (Figs. 11.2 and 11.3).

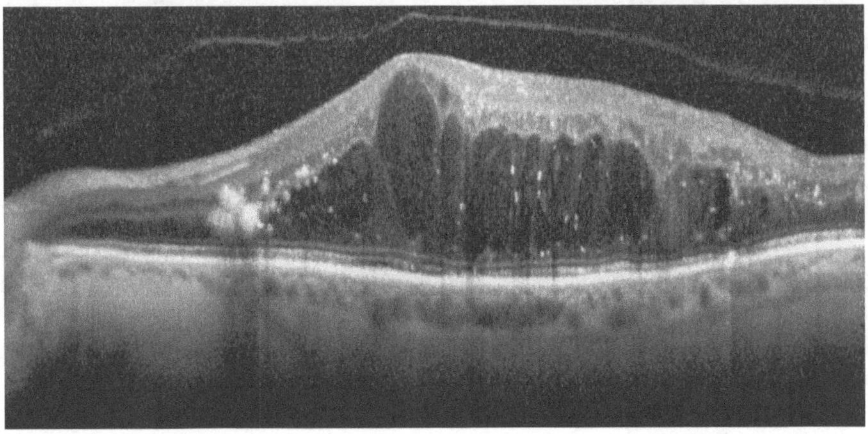

Fig. 11.3 Cystoid DME as imaged by Spectralis™ HRA + OCT. Note the integrity of the outer retinal layers, external limiting membrane, the photoreceptor inner segments, the outer segments, and the retinal pigment epithelium

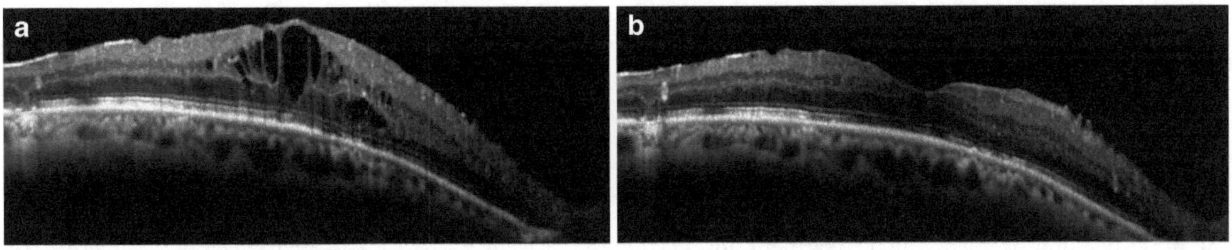

Fig. 11.4 Patients with cystoid macular edema before (**a**) and 4 weeks after (**b**) treatment with intravitreal antiVFGF therapy (ranibizumab). Visual acuity improved from 20/60 to 20/30. Note the normal outer retinal layers at baseline. At the inner surface of the retina, an epiretinal membrane can be seen

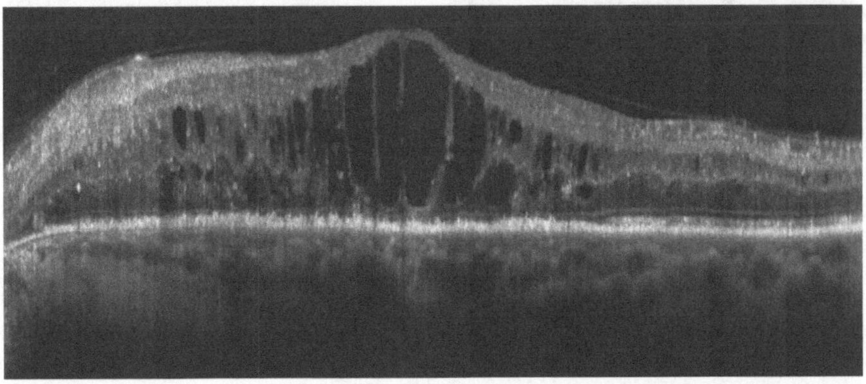

Fig. 11.5 Patient with DME and severe cystoid changes. Note that the outer retinal layers such as the external limiting membrane and photoreceptor layers are severely disturbed. Visual acuity was unchanged in this patient after anti-VEGF therapy

11

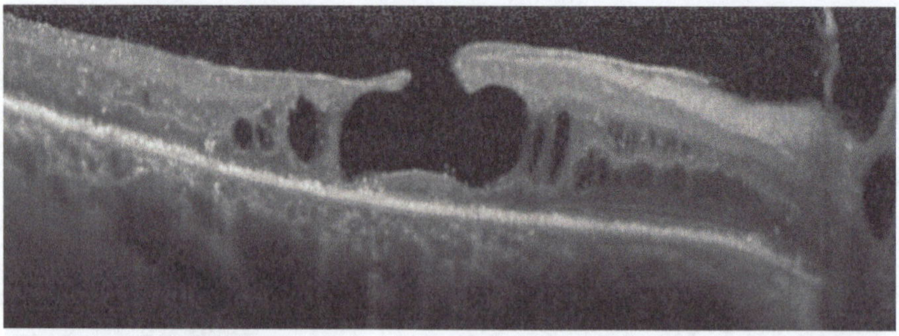

Fig. 11.6 Patient with DME and disrupted inner retinal layers. Additionally, the outer retinal layers are disturbed. Only close to the optic never head (*left*), the outer retinal layers are visible

11.5 Prognostic Features in High-Resolution OCT Scans

High-resolution OCT scans after intravitreal anti-VEGF treatment, in most cases, show a significant reduction in retinal thickness and normalization of the retinal layers (Fig 11.4). In patients with normal appearance ELM, the photoreceptor inner segments, the outer segments, and the RPE improvement of visual acuity after intravitreal anti-VEGF therapy has been observed in most cases. In contrast, patients with disturbed outer retinal layers on high-resolution OCT scans showed only reduction in retinal thickness, but no visual gain after intravitreal anti-VEGF therapy (Fig. 11.5). Additionally, in patients with discontinuity of the inner retinal layers and disturbed outer retinal layers, we were not able to archive anatomical or visual improvements after treatment for DME (Fig. 11.6).

Summary for the Clinician

- High-resolution OCT allows one to identify prognostic features for the visual outcome after treatment for DME.
- In patients with DME, high-resolution OCT shows epiretinal membranes, subretinal fluid, intraretinal fluid accumulation, and cystoid macular edema.
- The integrity of retinal layers can be analyzed with high-resolution OCT scans.
- The presence and integrity of the ELM, the photoreceptor IS, the OS, and the RPE appears to be a good prognostic feature for the visual improvement after treatment for DME.

References

1. Klein R, Moss SE, Klein BEK, Davis MD, DeMets DL (1989) The Wisconsin epidemiologic study of diabetic retinopathy. XI. The incidence of macular edema. Ophthalmology 96: 1501–1510
2. Amos AF, McCarty DJ, Zimmet P (1997) The rising global burden of diabetes and its complications: estimates and projections to the year 2010. Diabet Med 14(Suppl 5):S1–85
3. ETDRS Research Group (1991) Fundus photographic risk factors for progression of diabetic retinopathy. ETDRS Report Number 12. Ophthalmology 98(Suppl):823–833
4. ETDRS Research Group (1991) Grading diabetic retinopathy from stereoscopic color fundus photographs – an extension of the modified Airlie house classification. ETDRS Report Number 10. Ophthalmology 98(Suppl):786–805
5. ETDRS Research Group (1991) Early photocoagulation for diabetic retinopathy. ETDRS Report Number 9. Ophthalmology 98(suppl):766–785
6. Frank RN, Schulz L, Abe K, Iezzi R (2004) Temporal variation in diabetic macular edema measured by optical coherence tomography. Ophthalmology 111(2):211–217
7. Goebel W, Kretzchmar-Gross T (2002) Retinal thickness in diabetic retinopathy: a study using optical coherence tomography (OCT). Retina 22(6):759–767
8. Massin P, Duguid G, Erginay A, Haouchine B, Gaudric A (2003) Optical coherence tomography for evaluating diabetic macular edema before and after vitrectomy. Am J Ophthalmol 135(2):169–177
9. Massin P, Erginay A, Haouchine B, Mehidi AB, Paques M, Gaudric A (2002) Retinal thickness in healthy and diabetic subjects measured using optical coherence tomography mapping software. Eur J Ophthalmol 12(2):102–108
10. Hee MR, Puliafito C, Carlton W, Duker J, Reichel E, Rutledge B, Schuman J, Swanson E, Fujimoto J (1995) Quantitative assessment of macular edema with optical

coherence tomography. Arch Ophthalmol 113(8/95): 1019–1029
11. Hee MR, Puliafito CA, Duker JS, Reichel E, Coker JG, Wilkins JR, Schuman JS, Swanson EA, Fujimoto JG (1998) Topography of diabetic macular edema with optical coherence tomography. Ophthalmology 105(2):360–370
12. Huang D, Swanson EA, Lin CP, Schuman JS, Stinson WG, Chang W, Hee MR, Flotte T, Gregory K, Puliafito CA et al (1991) Optical coherence tomography. Science 254(5035): 1178–1181
13. Kim BY, Smith SD, Kaiser PK (2006) Optical coherence tomographic patterns of diabetic macular edema. Am J Ophthalmol 142(3):405–412
14. Otani T, Kishi S, Maruyama Y (1999) Patterns of diabetic macular edema with optical coherence tomography. Am J Ophthalmol 127(6):688–693
15. Yamamoto S, Yamamoto T, Hayashi M, Takeuchi S (2001) Morphological and functional analyses of diabetic macular edema by optical coherence tomography and multifocal electroretinograms. Graefes Arch Clin Exp Ophthalmol 239(2):96–101
16. Kim KH, Puoris'haag M, Maguluri GN, Umino Y, Cusato K, Barlow RB, de Boer JF (2008) Monitoring mouse retinal degeneration with high-resolution spectral-domain optical coherence tomography. J Vis 8(1):17.1–17.11
17. Sakamoto A, Hangai M, Yoshimura N (2008) Spectral-domain optical coherence tomography with multiple B-scan averaging for enhanced imaging of retinal diseases. Ophthalmology 115(6):1071–1078 e7
18. Srinivasan VJ, Wojtkowski M, Witkin AJ, Duker JS, Ko TH, Carvalho M, Schuman JS, Kowalczyk A, Fujimoto JG (2006) High-definition and 3-dimensional imaging of macular pathologies with high-speed ultrahigh-resolution optical coherence tomography. Ophthalmology 113(11):2054 e1–14
19. Drexler W, Sattmann H, Hermann B, Ko TH, Stur M, Unterhuber A, Scholda C, Findl O, Wirtitsch M, Fujimoto JG, Fercher AF (2003) Enhanced visualization of macular pathology with the use of ultrahigh-resolution optical coherence tomography. Arch Ophthalmol 121(5):695–706
20. Ruggeri M, Wehbe H, Jiao S, Gregori G, Jockovich ME, Hackam A, Duan Y, Puliafito CA (2007) In vivo three-dimensional high-resolution imaging of rodent retina with spectral-domain optical coherence tomography. Invest Ophthalmol Vis Sci 48(4):1808–1814
21. Wolf-Schnurrbusch UE, Enzmann V, Brinkmann CK, Wolf S (2008) Morphologic changes in patients with geographic atrophy assessed with a novel spectral OCT-SLO combination. Invest Ophthalmol Vis Sci 49(7):3095–3099
22. Flynn HWJ, Chew EY, Simons BD, Barton FB, Remaley NA, Ferris FL (1992) Pars plane vitrectomy in the Early Treatment Diabetic Retinopathy Study. ETDRS report number 17. Ophthalmology 99:1351–1357
23. Sutter FK, Kurz-Levin MM, Scherrer M, Barthelmes D, Fleischhauer JC, Helbig H (2007) Intravitreal triamcinolone acetonide for serous retinal pigment epithelial detachments in exudative age-related macular degeneration. Klin Monatsbl Augenheilkd 224(4):297–299
24. Theelen T, Tilanus MA, Klevering BJ (2004) Intraocular inflammation following endotamponade with high-density silicone oil. Graefes Arch Clin Exp Ophthalmol 242(7): 617–620
25. Wolf S, Massin P, Bandello F, Sharp D, Lanzetta P, Larsen M, Wolf-Schnurrbusch U, Gekkieva M, Group RS (2009) Safety and efficacy of ranibizumab treatment in patients with diabetic macular edema: 12-months results of the resolve study. Invest Ophthalmol Vis Sci. 2009;50:ARVO E-Abstract 4331
26. Wolf-Schnurrbusch UE, Ceklic L, Brinkmann CK, Iliev M, Frey M, Rothenbuehler SP, Enzmann V, Wolf S (2009) Macular thickness measurements in healthy eyes using six different optical coherence tomography instruments. Invest Ophthalmol Vis Sci 50:3432–3437

Chapter 12

OCT vs. Photography or Biomicroscopy for Diagnosis of Diabetic Macular Edema

12

Gianni Virgili, Francesca Menchini, and Mariacristina Parravano

Core Messages

- Diabetic macular edema (DME) was defined in Early Treatment Diabetic Retinopathy Study (ETDRS) studies on the basis of central retinal thickening and hard exudates using fundus stereophotography or biomicroscopy (FP/FB). Clinically significant macular edema (CSME) is the more severe form of DME and needs to be treated. Compared with FP/FB, optical coherence tomography (OCT) provides imaging of retinal thickness and morphology, as well as of the vitreoretinal interface.
- Clinical examination using FP/FB is cheap and readily available, but is also a subjective method. When biomicroscopy is used, there is no recording of the amount of thickening, and thus, it cannot reliably monitor CSME except for a gross judgment on its presence or absence.
- Advantages of OCT when compared with FP/FB in patients with DME are its ability to obtain an objective and highly reliable quantitative measure of retinal thickness on a continuous scale, as well as to provide additional morphological details.
- Clinician suspecting CSME requiring treatment can use Stratus central subfield thickness values below 250 μm to rule out CSME, and values above 300 μm to rule in CSME. Thickness values between 250 and 300 μm still suggest CSME, but treatment decision should be based, even more than usual, on patient's symptoms and preferences as well as on other clinical features that an ophthalmologist may use to decide on potential treatment outcome.
- Add 50 μm to the thresholds suggested above when using Cirrus (and possibly other spectral domain) OCT (no CSME: below 300 μm; CSME: above 350 μm); confirmatory research is needed on this correction factor for each spectral-domain device.
- Retinal-thickness measurement should not be a surrogate for visual acuity measurement in patients with DME.
- OCT-based predictors of outcome after photocoagulation, vitrectomy, and intravitreal triamcinolone have been proposed, and the prognosis of cases with subclinical macular edema (i.e., thickening using OCT not found using FP/FB) have been studied in case series and need further investigation.
- Using Stratus OCT, a change in the central subfield thickness exceeding ±11% is likely to represent a true change in a subject if the quality of the scans is acceptable.
- The repeatability of spectral-domain OCTs is expected to be comparable or better than that of the Stratus OCT in patients with DME, but further research is needed.

12.1 Introduction: Diabetic Macular Edema, Fundus Photography, and Optical Coherence Tomography

12.1.1 Incidence and Natural History

In developed countries, diabetic retinopathy (DR) represents the leading cause of blindness in the working age population [1]. It is expected that diabetes mellitus will reach epidemic proportion by the year 2025, with the total number of people with diabetes estimated to rise to 300 millions [2]. Diabetes mellitus and its complications will continue to represent a significant public health challenge. Among diabetes ocular complications, diabetic macular edema (DME) currently represents the major contributor to visual loss. DME can occur at any stage of diabetes and its onset is usually insidious and painless, often leading to a deferred diagnosis. It is characterized by increased vascular permeability secondary to the disruption of the blood–retinal barrier, which leads to intraretinal fluid accumulation.

The risk of developing DME increases with the duration of diabetes: the prevalence is 5% within the first 5 years after diagnosis and 15% at 15 years [3]. If untreated, DME increases the risk of moderate visual loss by 30–50% depending on the level of baseline visual acuity [4]; with current treatment, the risk drops by 50%.

12.1.2 Classification: Early Treatment Diabetic Retinopathy Study Grading

The best validated grading system for DR is the extension of the Airlie House Classification that was developed for the Early Treatment Diabetic Retinopathy Study (ETDRS) [5]. This classification has become the basis for detailed grading of DR and DME, and was used in all the major studies of risk factors and trials of different treatment modalities. It was based on grading seven 30° stereoscopic photographic fields. In the ETDRS classification, macular edema is graded separately: using a grid overlay on one photograph in field 2 (centered on the center of the macula) stereo pair, size, and location of retinal thickening are graded. The ETDRS defined DME as thickening and/or hard exudates within one disc diameter of the center of the macula. When the edema involves or threatens the center of the macula, even if visual acuity is not reduced, it is classified as clinically significant macular edema (CSME). The term CSME represents the threshold level at which laser photocoagulation is recommended and is defined as:

- Retinal thickening at or within 500 µm of the center of the macula
- Hard exudates at or within 500 µm of the center of the macula, if associated with thickening of the adjacent retina
- A zone or zones of retinal thickening one disc area in size, at least part of which is within one disc diameter of the center of the macula

DME grading has a practical application in fundus photographic assessment of DR, where photography substitutes for examination by an ophthalmologist. Comprehensive, regular clinical examination by a trained ophthalmologist, with fundus photography used for documentation only, is the best standard of care. Fundus stereophotography (FP), although validated, is complicated and time-consuming, placing considerable demand on the patients and physicians/photographers, and therefore, its use in everyday clinical practice is unpractical. In clinical setting, fundus biomicroscopy with contact is commonly used and it was found to be in close agreement with stereophotography. However, both methods are relatively insensitive in determining subtle changes in retinal thickness, especially in the absence of hard exudates.

From now on, in this chapter, we will use the acronym FP/FB to refer to fundus photography and fundus biomicroscopy jointly. In fact, while photography is the preferred method for fundus examination in ophthalmic research, biomicroscopy and especially non contact biomicroscopy, is routinely used in clinical practice.

12.1.3 Optical Coherence Tomography and Diabetic Macular Edema

Optical Coherence Tomography (OCT) is a relatively new imaging modality, providing high-resolution, cross-sectional images of the retina, with a resolution of up to 5 µm. It allows in vivo assessment of retinal morphology and thickness, and in the past decade, has gained widespread acceptance as a complementary tool for the diagnosis and management of several macular pathologies, including DME. Retinal thickness by OCT has been recently included in clinical trials assessing the use of different therapeutic modalities for DME: the presence of a minimal retinal thickness (250 or 300 µm according to different trials) constitutes an inclusion criteria, while its change over time is used as a means to assess anatomical efficacy of treatment, which often represents a clinical outcome. According to a previous study [6], normal retinal thickness with OCT 2000 is approximately 130 µm, while the mean central foveal thickness in healthy eyes with Stratus OCT is slightly higher, 182 ± 23 µm (both instruments were manufactured by Carl Zeiss Meditec, Inc.). Studies of CSME (defined according to the ETDRS) with OCT have revealed three basic morphological changes: retinal swelling with sponge-like appearance, cystoid pattern, and serous retinal detachment (see Fig. 12.1) [7]. Compared with FP/FB, OCT provides an objective and quantitative measure of retinal thickness in patients with DME, and it is especially useful in identifying the presence of vitreomacular adherence (see Fig. 12.1) [8].

Summary for the Clinician

- DME was defined in ETDRS studies on the basis of central retinal thickening and hard exudates using FP/FB. CSME is the more severe form of DME and needs to be treated. Compared with FP/FB, OCT provides imaging of retinal thickness and morphology, as well as the vitreoretinal interface.

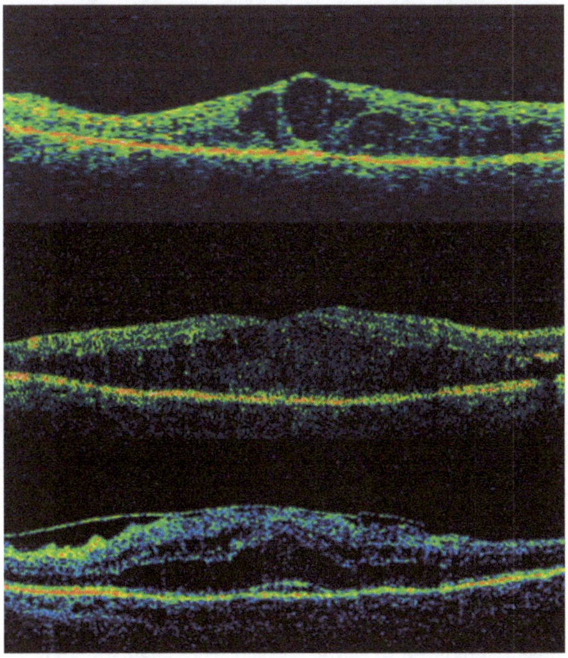

Fig. 12.1 Main Stratus OCT features in eyes with diabetic macular edema: cystoids changes (*top*), sponge-like thickening (*middle*), and edema associated with an adherent posterior hyaloid and a shallow serous retinal detachment (*bottom*)

12.2 Investigation of Diagnostic Accuracy of OCT for Detection of DME

12.2.1 Potential Aims of OCT Testing in Clinical Practice: Diagnostic Accuracy vs. Others

Medical tests are prescribed for several reasons, such as screening, diagnosis, monitoring course of the disease, selecting therapy or following effects of therapy, or determining drug levels or drug effects [9]. Many other factor have been recognized to influence the decision to use a test, including a number of patient's or doctor's characteristics and preferences, let alone the medical–legal value of the test results [10], often making the process of diagnosis subconscious [11].

Clinical research on the use of OCT in patients with DME is evolving together with the technological evolution of these devices, which allow recognizing an increasing number of retinal morphological details. Despite the fact that new information is provided, to be able to use it in practice means that OCT results should be proved to impact on patient outcomes, whether directly or through known predictors of prognosis and treatment effect, such as when the diagnosis of CSME is confirmed.

OCT is currently used in secondary and tertiary ophthalmic care services following biomicroscopic fundus examination and is not used as a screening tool. As biomicroscopy is a part of every ophthalmic examination, it is not meant to replace FP/FB (such as for triage use), but rather to follow (i.e., using it as an add-on test) (see Bossuyt et al., for a methodological reference [12]). In practice, OCT can be used in patients in whom DME or CSME are suspected with the purpose of refining diagnosis, or can be used because of the properties not observed in FP/FB, such as recording retinal thickness to evaluate treatment response.

Among the potential roles of OCT when compared with those of FP/FB in patients with DR, we will discuss the following key issues:

1. Detection or confirmation of DME, or its severe form, CSME, such as when testing is used to rule in disease in people having signs of DR that may be associated with DME, who are referred by primary care professionals;
2. Exclusion of CSME, such as when testing is used to rule out disease in people referred to tertiary care services, e.g., when laser treatment has been suggested but the treating ophthalmologist believes that the presence of CSME is questionable (also medical–legal value in this case);
3. Establishing a baseline measure to monitor response in people who are treated for CSME to integrate imaging methods used in common practice (FP/FB and fluorescein angiography);
4. Other purposes, such as detecting or confirming the presence of a thickened adherent hyaloid, demonstrating chronic changes such a large intraretinal cysts, etc.

Items 1 and 2 refer to diagnostic accuracy, item 3 to monitoring of treatment response, and item 4 to presumed predictive role of some OCT findings in terms of prognosis and treatment response.

12.2.2 Diagnostic Accuracy of OCT for Detection of DME: Are Photography or Biomicroscopy a Valid Gold Standard?

Diagnostic accuracy refers to the ability to correctly diagnose disease, as defined using a gold standard test (or set of tests). The term "reference" standard is preferred to "gold" standard by methodologists because a perfectly valid test does not often exist. This is particularly true for DME which is traditionally defined by means of subjective assessment of retinal thickening using FP/FB. Being a subjective test, the interobserver agreement of FP/FB is substantial, yet far less than perfect, given that Cohen's k was between 0.6 and 0.8 for most retinal lesions in the

ETDRS study [5], a fact that can limit the diagnostic performance of highly reliable OCT devices in a diagnostic test accuracy study. Furthermore, biomicroscopy does not allow recording of retinal thickening and is commonly used only to judge on its presence or absence.

The advantage of OCT when compared with FP/FB in diagnosing CSME is the ability to provide an objective, quantitative, highly reliable (see Appendix) measure of retinal thickness as well as additional morphological details (see last paragraph 2.4.).

In clinical practice, retinal-thickness measurement provided by OCT is always interpreted together with clinical examination, thus, integrating visual acuity and fundus biomicroscopy data. Using biomicroscopy, ophthalmologists can detect hard exudates in the macula which are a key component of the definition of CSME, although not the main finding using OCT. Therefore, the information provided by OCT assessment should always be interpreted together with fundus examination, as opposed to diagnostic test accuracy research, where reciprocal blinding of reference and index test results is a necessary quality item [9].

Summary for the Clinician

- Clinical examination using FP/FB is cheap and readily available, but also a subjective method. When biomicroscopy is used, there is no recording of the amount of thickening and thus, it cannot reliably monitor CSME except for a gross judgment on its presence or absence.
- Advantages of OCT when compared with FP/FB in patients with DME are its ability to obtain an objective and highly reliable quantitative measure of retinal thickness on a continuous scale, as well as to provide additional morphological details.

12.2.3 Diagnostic Accuracy of OCT to Detect CSME Using Time-Domain OCTs: How to Use OCT Retinal Thickness Cut-Offs?

In a meta-analysis including five studies, Virgili et al. [13] found that pooled sensitivity and specificity of OCT for detection of CSME were 0.79 (95% CI: 0.71–0.86) and 0.88 (95% CI: 0.80–0.93), respectively. The prevalence of CSME varied between 19 and 58% in the studies, thus being consistent with patients referred to secondary or tertiary care centers for a moderate to high suspicion of CSME. Two studies used an OCT 2000 and three employed a Stratus OCT. The quality of these studies was often poor or unclear regarding a few methodological quality issues, which were assessed using the QUADAS checklist. Despite these limitations, the authors concluded that OCT devices are sufficiently accurate to diagnose CSME. Furthermore, by graphically inspecting metanalysis results, the authors found a possible threshold effect, i.e., that using values of 230–250 μm to define CSME-favored sensitivity in three studies, while a cut-off of 300-μm-favored specificity in one study. Although this evidence on a threshold effect is sparse, these thickness cut-offs agree with values used to define CSME in studies by the Diabetic Retinopathy Clinical Research Network (http://public.drcr.net).

Central subfield thickness should be preferred to central point thickness [14] and was shown to be relatively unaffected by segmentation errors in fast-map measurements [15], provided that the standard deviation of the center point is <10% of central subfield thickness value [16].

In their review, Virgili et al. [13] used positive and negative likelihood ratios derived from their metanalysis to compute the range of usefulness of OCT to decide upon laser treatment of CSME, taking into account the benefits and making assumptions about adverse outcomes of photocoagulation. In fact, medical decision-making implies an a priori probability of disease which can be increased by positive test results or decreased by negative test results, taking into account the threshold for treatment, and readers can refer to classic evidence-based medicine books regarding this approach [17, 18].

For practical use, we suggest the following decision criteria. If we are rather suspicious, but not sure whether a patient is affected by CSME needing treatment, then finding a central subfield thickness of 300 μm or more with Stratus OCT is confirmatory, while values below 250 μm tend to exclude CSME. We suggest that values between 250 and 300 μm are less strong indicators of CSME presence. In this case, other findings should be considered to decide on laser photocoagulation, emphasizing, even more than usual, patient-reported vision, measured visual acuity, fluorescein angiographic findings, and fundus changes that one might consider to decrease the benefit of photocoagulation, such as an adherent and thickened hyaloid, subretinal fibrosis, or extensive macular ischemia (also see the following paragraph), despite the fact that research on these topics is limited. If the *a priori* suspect of CSME is very low or very high, then there is no point in obtaining an OCT to improve diagnostic accuracy because the test has no power to change such a strong prior belief. However, the test might be used for reasons other than CSME diagnosis, as described in the following paragraph.

Summary for the Clinician

- Clinician suspecting CSME requiring treatment can use Stratus central subfield thickness values below 250 µm to rule out CSME, and values above 300 µm to rule in CSME. Thickness values between 250 and 300 µm still suggest CSME, but treatment decision should be based, even more than usual, on patient's symptoms and preferences as well as on other clinical features that an ophthalmologist may use to decide on the potential treatment outcome.

12.2.4 Do We Expect Any Differences in Retinal Thickness Thresholds Adopted to Define CSME Using Spectral-Domain Compared with Time-Domain OCTs?

An upward adjustment of the thresholds suggested earlier, obtained with the Stratus OCT, may prove necessary for Cirrus and possibly other spectral-domain OCTs. In fact, Wolf-Schnurrbusc et al. [19] found that six spectral-domain OCTs yielded central retinal thickness measurements of 32–77 µm larger when compared with the Stratus OCT in 20 normal subjects, and Forooghian et al. [20] found that central subfield measurements with the Cirrus OCT were larger by 53 µm than the Stratus OCT in 33 patients with DME. Other published research on patients with various retinal conditions suggested similar differences between Stratus and Cirrus OCTs [21–23]. Given the published research, 50 µm should be added to the thresholds suggested earlier to rule in/out CSME when using a spectral-domain OCT, i.e., values below 300 µm would suggest the absence of CSME and values above 350 µm presence of CSME using spectral-domain devices, but confirmatory research is needed for each device. On comparing Stratus and Cirrus OCTs in 25 normal and 25 diabetic subjects, we found that such an overestimate was a function of retinal thickness (unpublished data): a 50 µm was found in normal subjects when compared with no estimated difference at about 550 µm thickness in CSME patients using a linear regression model.

Summary for the Clinician

- Add 50 µm to the thresholds suggested earlier when using Cirrus (and possibly other spectral domain) OCT (no CSME: below 300 µm; CSME: above 350 µm); confirmatory research is needed on this correction factor for each spectral-domain device.

12.3 Use of OCT When Compared with Photography: Beyond Diagnostic Accuracy

12.3.1 Establishing a Baseline Measure to Monitor Response in People who Are Treated for CSME Rather than Simply Assessing its Presence or Absence

Given that OCT is effective to diagnose CSME, its adoption to monitor treatment response seems straightforward. The fact that OCT provides a continuous measure of thickness makes the difference with respect to FP/FB for this purpose. However, while the ETDRS study gave guidance on decision about further photocoagulation based on the presence or absence of CSME, such information is limited regarding the value of, say, a reduction from 400 to 300 µm in a person with diabetic macular thickening a few weeks after antiVEGF injection, to decide about retreatment, which is an issue in ongoing research. Good-quality research on diagnosis–treatment interaction is far less common than that on accuracy, and large multicenter randomized controlled studies designed to compare the diagnostic strategies as a guide to treatment are needed, as summarized in a recently published methodological article [24].

Three aspects should be considered to move beyond diagnostic accuracy. First, a change in measurement well above the instrument reliability should be considered (see Appendix), but this is no longer a problem given the highly reliable OCTs. Second, we should use the diagnostic predictive research based on relatively small (<100 patients), single center cohort studies investigating several predictors of prognosis or treatment outcome, with caution. The results of these studies might not be generalizable to our clinics and would better need confirmation from independent studies. Furthermore, several predictors are typically tested against change in vision in such studies, and there is a high risk of chance findings, especially close to the conventional limits of statistical significance of (p-value 0.05 to 0.01). A few of such studies will be briefly presented in the last paragraph.

Lastly, until research from large multicenter studies will clarify the predictive/prognostic role of OCT in patients with DME, especially regarding treatment response and monitoring, in the following chapter, we review some leading research on the relationship between change in OCT and visual acuity, research conducted by the Diabetic Retinopathy Clinical Research Network [25, 26].

12.3.2 Potential Validity of OCT for Monitoring Treatment Response

A benefit in diagnosing the presence or absence of CSME exists because this has been linked to prognosis (about

30% risk of visual loss in 3 years) and the benefit obtained with laser photocoagulation. Both these types of information were obtained from ETDRS studies conducted many years ago [5, 27].

Construct validity of OCT, specifically its cross-sectional and longitudinal association with visual acuity, has been investigated by the Diabetic Retinopathy Clinical Research Network in patients with CSME included in a randomized study on laser techniques [25]. They found that the cross-sectional correlation of OCT retinal thickness with visual acuity was moderate (correlation coefficient = 0.52), such that the center point thickness alone explains about 27% of the variance of visual acuity. They also found that the longitudinal correlation was modest, as the change in the center point retinal thickness correlation with change in visual acuity at 12 months was 0.40. The authors also provided reference to other studies that obtained similar conclusions. About 7% of patients with retinal thickening gained vision and 26% lost vision despite the fact that thickness decreased at 12 months. Furthermore, the authors could not demonstrate whether considering a lag in this association could improve the correlation, because it did not increase using change in the thickness that occurred months before. This means that OCT retinal thickness still remains the strongest known predictor of visual acuity in patients with DME, but it is not all we need and cannot be a substitute for visual acuity measurement [25].

A follow-up paper on the same cohort re-assessed the correlation of thickness and visual acuity comparing OCT with FP using a seven step ETDRS photographic severity scale of DME [26]. They found a substantial correlation between OCT and FP at baseline (0.67), and a moderate correlation (about 0.5) both cross-sectionally at 12 months and longitudinally (thickness change). Regarding the correlation with visual acuity, OCT did slightly better than FP at baseline (0.57 vs. 0.47, respectively), but FP did worse both at 12 months and considering change (0.53–0.48 vs. 0.29–0.27, respectively). This confirms the expectation that OCT is better than FP to monitor thickness change in DME, although vision is related to factors other than retinal thickness alone.

Summary for the Clinician

- Retinal-thickness measurement should not be a surrogate for visual acuity measurement in patients with DMO.

12.3.3 Candidate Predictors of Visual Outcome Using OCT in Patients with DME

Many other findings are available using OCT in patients with DMO. The diagnostic and predictive role of these features has been mainly studied in case series, and should be considered with caution. The following is a brief description of a series of examples found by inspecting 383 titles retrieved using the key words DME and OCT on PubMed in May 2009.

- The integrity of the photoreceptors' inner and outer layers was associated with visual improvement after vitrectomy for DME in 37 eyes [28].
- The diffuse retinal thickening OCT pattern was associated with a greater reduction in retinal thickening and better visual acuity improvement than the cystoids macular edema or vitreomacular interface abnormalities patterns (see Fig. 12.1) in 70 eyes of 45 patients with CSME, receiving photocoagulation [29].
- Subclinical macular edema, i.e., thickening detected with OCT but not with FP/FB, progressed to CSME in 31% of 153 patients, but OCT thickness increased in 13% of cases and decreased in 11% of cases [30]; according to us, this may be partly due to variability of judgment using FP/FB.

Other candidate features have been investigated within randomized clinical trials, such as:

- Posterior vitreous detachment (PVD) is more common after intravitreal triamcinolone than laser treatment for diffuse DME in 88 consecutive patients in 1 year; eyes with PVD had thinner retina but not better vision [31].

Summary for the Clinician

- OCT-based predictors of outcome after photocoagulation, vitrectomy, and intravitreal triamcinolone have been proposed and the prognosis of cases with subclinical macular edema (i.e., thickening found using OCT, but not found using FP/FB) have been studied mainly in case series and need further investigation.

12.4 Appendix: Reproducibility of OCT Retinal-Thickness Measurement in Patients with DME

12.4.1 How Reproducibility is Reported

Reproducibility relates to how variables are measured in the same subjects under the same condition. Thus, it is commonly measured by test and retest procedures, whether in the same or different sessions and by the same or different observers. A special case of this set of questions is that of agreement between different OCT devices in the same subject.

Three measures of reproducibility are commonly presented: (1) the coefficient of repeatability (CR) or its general form, 95% limits of agreement (LAs) [32]; (2) the coefficient of variation (CV), or the ratio of the measurement error to the mean; and (3) the intraclass correlation coefficient (ICC).

In short, 95% LAs are the limits, exceeding which a measurement taken on the same patient is considered to represent a true change of status. If 95% LAs are centered on the nil value, such as in well done single-session studies on one test, then they can be expressed as CR. For example, the CR of ETDRS chart visual acuity was found to be ± 11 letters (about two lines) in people with late age-related macular degeneration, indicating that a change of 15 letters (three lines) is well beyond chance variability [28].

The CV is similar to the CR, but is expressed as a percentage of the mean measurement. If the CR were expressed as a percent of the mean, it would correspond to $1.96 \times \sqrt{2} \times CV$.

Finally, ICC is the ratio of measurement variability among subjects (between subject variance) to the total variability (between subject variance plus random error), and tells us how well the measurement discriminates the subjects. The ICC is a ratio ranging in value between 0 (representing a totally unreliable measurement) and 1 (implying perfect reliability). As it is independent on the measurement scale, the ICC is useful to compare the measurements using different methods or devices, such as OCT algorithms, volume, and thickness, on the same subject. Values above 0.8 suggest good agreement.

12.4.2 Stratus OCT Reproducibility in Patients with DME

We have reported the results from studies by the Diabetic Retinopathy Research Network, as these are large multicenter studies and are likely to be more generalizable to practice. Stratus OCT coefficient of repeatability was shown to be about ±11% for central subfield thickness by the Diabetic Retinopathy Research Network [16]. They also pointed out that scans with a standard deviation of the center point of ≥10% of central subfield thickness are less reproducible and should be viewed with caution when assessing the validity of an observed change in retinal thickness in patients with DME. Finally, some additional variability between the sessions can be explained by posturing, accounting for a decrease of 6% from 8 A.M. to 4 P.M in the Diabetic Retinopathy Research Network series [33].

12.4.3 Spectral-Domain OCTs Reproducibility

Forooghian et al. [20] showed that both Stratus™ OCT and Cirrus™ OCT scanning systems demonstrated high repeatability on measures of thickness in all subfields in eyes with DME, with respective CRs falling below 18 and 21 μm. For both the devices, ICCs were 0.98 for the central subfield.

Using PubMed, we could not find studies investigating the reproducibility of other OCT devices in patients with DME, but we found a study extracting the CV in normal eyes [21]. Spectral-domain devices yielded CVs comparable or lower than the Stratus OCT (around 3%), with the Spectralis OCT (Heidelberg Engineering, Inc.) yielding the lowest value of 0.5%.

The difference in measurements obtained by time-domain vs. spectral-domain OCT devices can be explained by the different automatic segmentation algorithms used to assess the neuroretinal thickness: while both OCTs identify the inner retinal interface in the inner limiting membrane, for the outer retina limit, spectral-domain OCTs use outer bands corresponding to the retinal pigment epithelium, whereas the Stratus OCT uses the hyper-reflective band corresponding to the junction between the inner and outer photoreceptor segments [19].

Summary for the Clinician

- Using Stratus OCT, a change in the central subfield thickness exceeding ±11% is likely to represent a true change in a subject if the quality of the scans is acceptable.
- The repeatability of spectral-domain OCTs is expected to be comparable or better than that of the Stratus OCT in patients with DME, but further research is needed.

References

1. King H, Aubert RE, Herman WH (1998) Global burden of diabetes, 1995–2025: prevalence, numerical estimates, and projections. Diabetes Care 21:1414–1431
2. National Institute of Health, National Institute of Diabetes and Digestive and Kidney Disease (1995) Diabetes in America, 2nd edn. National Institute of Health, National Institute of Diabetes and Digestive and Kidney Disease, Bethesda
3. Aiello LP, Gardner TW, King GL, Blankenship G, Cavallerano JD, Ferris III FL (1998) Diabetic retinopathy. Diabetes Care 21:143–156
4. Javitt JC, Canner JK, Sommer A (1989) Cost effectiveness of current approaches to the control of retinopathy in type I diabetics. Ophtalmology 96:255–264
5. Early Treatment Diabetic Retinopathy Study Research Group (1991) Fundus photographic risk factors for progression of diabetic retinopathy. ETDRS Report Number 12. Ophthalmology 98:823–833
6. Chan A, Duker JS (2005) A standardized method for reporting changes in macular thickening using optical coherence tomography. Arch Ophthalmol 123:939–943
7. Otani T, Kishi S, Maruyama Y (1999) Patterns of diabetic macular edema with optical coherence tomography. Am J Ophthalmol 127:688–693
8. Otani T, Kishi S (2002) Topographic assessment of vitreous surgery for diabetic macular edema. Am J Ophthalmol 134:214–219
9. Deeks JJ (1999) Using evaluations of diagnostic tests: understanding their limitations and making the most of available evidence. Ann Oncol 10:761–768
10. Whiting P, Toerien M, de Salis I, Sterne JA, Dieppe P, Egger M, Fahey T (2007) A review identifies and classifies reasons for ordering diagnostic tests. J Clin Epidemiol 60:981–989
11. Schmidt HG, Norman GR, Boshuizen HPA (1990) A cognitive perspective on medical expertise: theory and implications. Acad Med 65:611–621
12. Bossuyt PM, Irwig L, Craig J, Glasziou P (2006) Comparative accuracy: assessing new tests against existing diagnostic pathways. BMJ 332:1089–1092
13. Virgili G, Menchini F, Dimastrogiovanni AF, Rapizzi E, Menchini U, Bandello F, Gortana Chiodini R (2007) Optical coherence tomography versus stereoscopic fundus photography or biomicroscopy for diagnosing diabetic macular edema: a systematic review. Invest Ophthalmol Vis Sci 48:4963–4973
14. Diabetic Retinopathy Clinical Research Network (2008) Optical coherence tomography measurements and analysis methods in optical coherence tomography studies of diabetic macular edema. Ophthalmology 115:1366–1371
15. Taban M, Sharma S, Williams DR, Waheed N, Kaiser PK (2009) Comparing retinal thickness measurements using automated fast macular thickness map versus six-radial line scans with manual measurements. Ophthalmology 116:964–970
16. Diabetic Retinopathy Clinical Research Network (2007) Reproducibility of macular thickness and volume using Zeiss optical coherence tomography in patients with diabetic macular edema. Ophthalmology 114:1520–1525
17. Guyatt GH, Rennie D (eds) (2002) Users' guides to the medical literature. A manual for evidence-based clinical practice. AMA Press, Chicago
18. Straus ES, Richardson WS, Glasziou P, Haynes RB (2005) Diagnosis and screening. In: Evidence-based medicine. How to practice and teach EBM. Amsterdam, Elsevier, pp 67–100
19. Wolf-Schnurrbusch UE, Ceklic L, Brinkmann CK, Iliev M, Frey M, Rothenbuehler SP, Enzmann V, Wolf S (2009) Macular thickness measurements in healthy eyes using six different optical coherence tomography instruments. Invest Ophthalmol Vis Sci 50:3432–3437
20. Forooghian F, Cukras C, Meyerle CB, Chew EY, Wong WT (2008) Evaluation of time domain and spectral domain optical coherence tomography in the measurement of diabetic macular edema. Invest Ophthalmol Vis Sci 49:4290–4296
21. Han IC, Jaffe GJ (2009) Comparison of spectral- and time-domain optical coherence tomography for retinal thickness measurements in healthy and diseased eyes. Am J Ophthalmol 147:847–858
22. Kiernan DF, Hariprasad SM, Chin EK et al (2009) Prospective comparison of cirrus and stratus optical coherence tomography for quantifying retinal thickness. Am J Ophthalmol 147:267–75.e2
23. Sayanagi K, Sharma S, Yamamoto T, Kaiser PK (2009) Comparison of spectral-domain versus time-domain optical coherence tomography in management of age-related macular degeneration with ranibizumab. Ophthalmology 116:947–955
24. Lijmer JG, Bossuyt PM (2009) Various randomized designs can be used to evaluate medical tests. J Clin Epidemiol 62:364–373
25. Diabetic Retinopathy Clinical Research Network Study Group (2007) Relationship between optical coherence tomography-measured central retinal thickness and visual acuity in diabetic macular edema. Ophthalmology 114:525–536
26. Diabetic Retinopathy Clinical Research Network Study Group (2008) Comparison of time-domain OCT and fundus photographic assessments of retinal thickening in eyes with diabetic macular edema. Invest Ophthalmol Vis Sci 49:1745–1752
27. Early Treatment Diabetic Retinopathy Study Research Group (1985) Photocoagulation treatment for Diabetic Macular Edema. ETDRS Report Number 1. Arch Ophtalmology 103:1796–1806
28. Sakamoto A, Nishijima K, Kita M, Oh H, Tsujikawa A, Yoshimura N (2009) Association between foveal

photoreceptor status and visual acuity after resolution of diabetic macular edema by pars plana vitrectomy. Graefes Arch Clin Exp Ophthalmol 247:1325–1330

29. Kim NR, Kim YJ, Chin HS, Moon YS (2009) Optical coherence tomographic patterns in diabetic macular edema; prediction of visual outcome after focal laser photocoagulation. Br J Ophthalmol 93:901–905
30. Browning DJ, Fraser CM (2008) The predictive value of patient and eye characteristics on the course of subclinical diabetic macular edema. Am J Ophthalmol 145:149–154
31. Sivaprasad S, Ockrim Z, Massaoutis P, Ikeji F, Hykin PG, Gregor ZJ (2008) Posterior hyaloid changes following intravitreal triamcinolone and macular laser for diffuse diabetic macular edema. Retina 28:1435–1442
32. Bunce C (2009) Correlation, agreement, and Bland–Altman analysis: statistical analysis of method comparison studies. Am J Ophthalmol 148:4–6
33. Diabetic Retinopathy Clinical Research Network (2006) Diurnal variation in retinal thickening measurement by optical coherence tomography in center-involved diabetic macular edema. Arch Ophthalmol 124:1701–1707
34. Early Treatment Diabetic Retinopathy Study Research Group (1991) Grading diabetic retinopathy from stereoscopic color fundus photographs – an extension of the modified airlie house classification. ETDRS report number 10. Ophthalmology 98:786–806
35. Kinyoun J, Barton F, Fisher M, Hubbard L, Aiello L, Ferris F (1989) Detection of diabetic macular edema: ETDRS report number 5. Ophthalmology 96:746–751
36. Patel PJ, Chen FK, Rubin GS, Tufail A (2008) Intersession repeatability of visual acuity scores in age-related macular degeneration. Invest Ophthalmol Vis Sci 49:4347–4352

Chapter 13

Spectral Domain Optical Coherence Tomography for Macular Holes

13

Jerzy Nawrocki and Zofia Michalewska

Core Messages

- Spectral optical coherence tomography (SOCT) offers a 3D mode and has faster scanning times, when compared with time domain OCT. SOCT therefore gives us the opportunity to study retinal pathologies in a more detailed way.
- SOCT enables differentiation between full-thickness macular holes, lamellar macular holes and macular pseudoholes.
- The diameter of the macular hole is the most important factor determining the functional outcome after surgery.
- Spontaneous resolution of full-thickness macular holes is rare.
- Pars plana vitrectomy with internal limiting membrane peeling and air/gas exchange is the treatment of choice for full-thickness macular holes.
- After macular hole repair, different retinal pathological features are present.
- In cases of lamellar macular hole with deteriorated vision or metamorphopsia, surgical treatment should be considered.

13.1 Stages of Full-Thickness Macular Hole in Spectral OCT

Macular hole stages were originally described by Gass [1] and modified by Gaudric et al., who presented a study of macular hole formation documented by optical coherence tomography (OCT) in the 1990s [2].

Stage I macular hole, or impending macular hole, was originally described by Gass as progressive loss of foveal depression with a yellow ring or spot, which Gass explained as detachment of the fovea [47]. In OCT/SOCT, one can see that it is in fact an intraretinal split or cyst, localised in the inner retinal layers and prefoveal vitreous cortex with a centripetally directed tangential force [2, 3]. On SOCT, elevation of the photoreceptor layer can additionally be observed. Visual acuity is often good at this stage, although patients may complain of blurring and metamorphopsia (Fig. 13.1a).

Stage II macular hole, according to Gass, is a full-thickness macular hole with a diameter smaller than 400 μm, with posterior hyaloid still attached to the retinal surface. Gaudric et al. described its OCT appearance as a large opening of the photoreceptor layer and an incomplete opening of the operculum, with posterior hyaloids still attached to the operculum [2]. In SOCT, intraretinal cystoid spaces at the edges of the hole can be noted. Visual acuity deteriorates to a level of 20/40 to 20/100, and metamorphopsia increases. Progression to stage III macular hole can last for several weeks to months (Fig. 13.1b).

Stage III macular hole has a diameter of more than 400 μm. Elevated and slightly thickened retina with cystoid spaces can be observed around the hole. Localised separation of the vitreous cortex is usually noted because of the presence of an operculum, hyperreflective in OCT/SOCT. In addition, as the hole enlarges, discrete white deposits appear on the surface of the retinal pigment epithelium (RPE) at the base of the macular hole that represent nodular proliferations of the RPE cells. Visual acuity ranges from 20/60 to 20/200 (Fig. 13.1c).

Stage IV macular hole, according to Gass, has a diameter of up to approximately one third of the optic disc diameter and is surrounded by elevated retina [1]. Posterior hyaloid detachment can be seen as the Weiss ring. In OCT/SOCT, there is no difference, except in size, between stage III and IV macular holes (Fig. 13.1d).

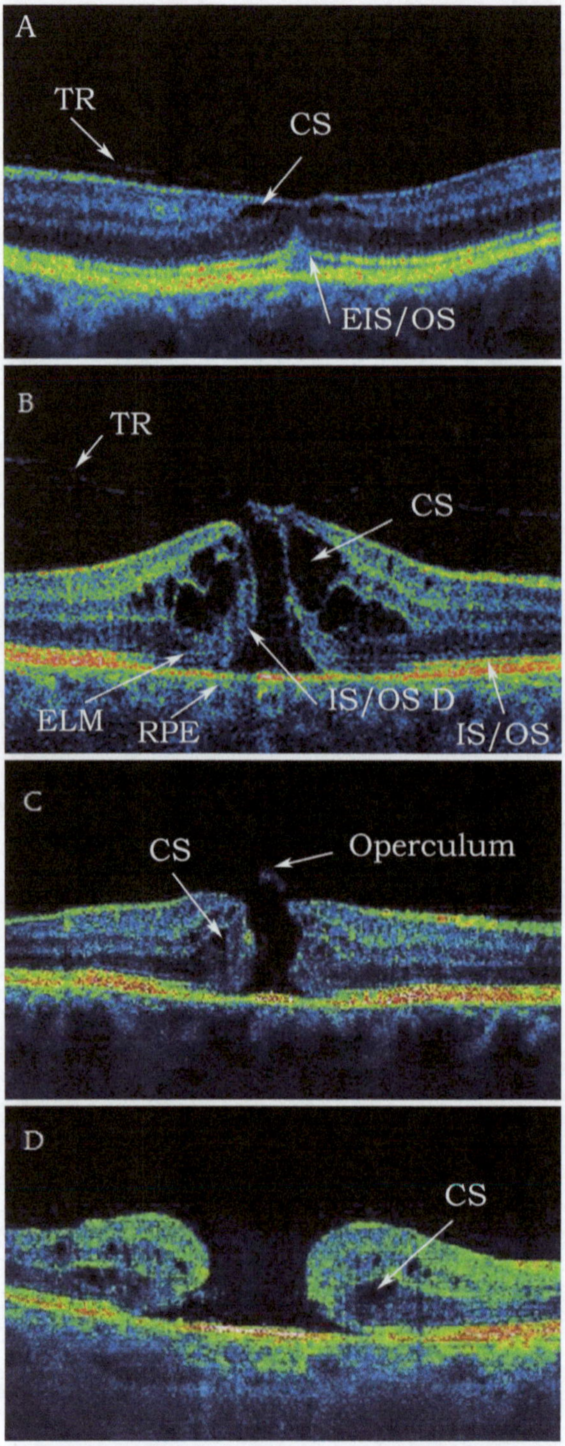

Fig. 13.1 (**a**) Stage I, (**b**) stage II, (**c**) stage III, (**d**) stage IV macular hole (Copernicus HR; Optopol, Zawiercie, Poland). *TR* asymmetric traction, *CS* cystoid space; *E IS/OS* elevation of the hyperreflective line between the inner and outer segments of the photoreceptors, *RPE* retinal pigment epithelium, *IS/OS* hyperreflective line between inner and outer segments of photoreceptors, *ELM* external limiting membrane, *IS/OSD* photoreceptor layer defect

13.2 Clinical Features

The condition is most common in women over 55 years of age and bilateral in 1.2–28.6% of the cases. This wide range, taken from the literature, is probably due to differences in the examination methods used. SOCT data show bilateral appearance of the disease in about 15% of the cases [3].

Macular holes can be asymptomatic in their early stages; the diagnosis can also be delayed in patients with good visual acuity of the fellow eye. Metamorphopsia, central scotoma and decreased visual acuity can also occur.

13.3 Examination

With fundoscopy, stages I–IV, as classified by Gass, can be differentiated (Fig. 13.2a).

With autofluorescence, a round or oval, well-circumscribed, hyperfluorescent area is seen in the foveal region (Fig. 13.2b). The hyperfluorescence is due to the lack of macular pigment in the hole. This allows the excitation light to reach the RPE unimpeded.

With fluorescein angiography, hyperfluorescence is visible in the area of the macular hole (Fig. 13.2c).

With scanning laser ophthalmoscopy, a round or oval hyporeflective area can be observed in the fovea. It can be distinguished from non-full-thickness macular defects when height deviation from the retinal surface is detected on the topography scale (Fig. 13.2d).

OCT and SOCT are the gold standard in the diagnostics of macular holes. They present as full-thickness retinal defects in the fovea (Fig. 13.2e).

Microperimetry and electrophysiology may confirm the diagnosis, but their importance is usually limited to scientific publications.

13.4 Natural History

Spontaneous resolution of stage I macular holes occurs in 40–90% of the cases [4].

Spontaneous closure of idiopathic stage II–IV macular holes is rare. Epidemiological data from before the OCT era described a spontaneous macular hole closure rate of about 33% for stage II and about 14% for stage III macular holes [4]. It is possible that some findings may have been misinterpreted in those times, because, in some cases, diagnosis of the disease (without OCT) may have been incorrect. In our clinic, only four cases of spontaneous resolution of stage II–IV macular holes were noted from approximately 200 cases that were evaluated with SOCT in the last 3 years.

In cases of ocular trauma, it should be considered that the macular hole may close spontaneously during the first few weeks following ocular trauma. Therefore, it is

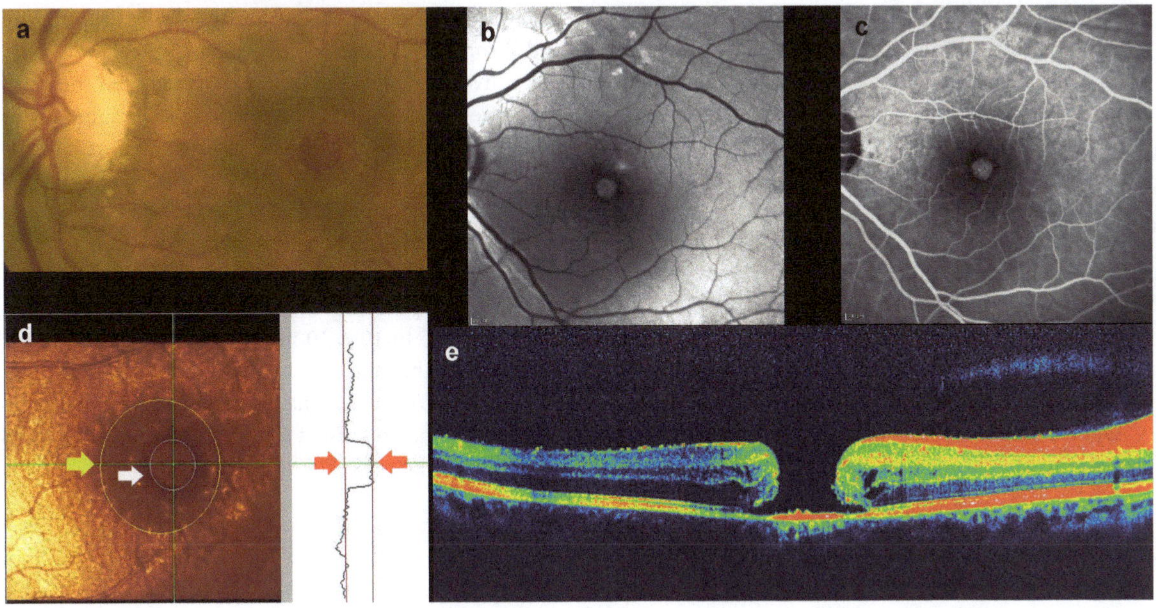

Fig. 13.2 Macular hole. (**a**) Fundus photography. (**b**) Autofluorescence. A hyperfluorescent round region, representing a lack of macular pigment in the hole can be seen (Spectralis; Heidelberg Engineering, Heidelberg, Germany). (**c**) Late phase of fluorescein angiography. A round, well-circumscribed hyperfluorescent region can be noted (Spectralis). (**d**) Scanning laser ophthalmoscopy of the macular hole. The *white circle* and *white arrow* represent the minimal diameter of the macular hole. The *yellow circle* and *yellow arrow* represent the area of edema around the hole. The *red arrows* present the height difference on the topography scale (HRT II; Heidelberg Engineering, Heidelberg, Germany). (**e**) Spectral optical coherence ophthalmoscopy of the macular hole (Spectralis)

advisable to qualify patients for surgery after a few weeks subsequent to the onset of the macular hole.

Summary for the Clinician

- Macular holes can be asymptomatic in the early stages.
- SOCT should be performed if a macular hole is suspected on fundoscopy.
- Because the disease is often bilateral, careful examination of the follow-up of the fellow eye should be a rule.
- Spontaneous resolution is rare; thus, surgery should be proposed for patients with a full-thickness macular hole.
- Post-traumatic macular holes can spontaneously close during the first few weeks after ocular trauma.

13.5 Ultra-High Resolution OCT and Spectral OCT Findings in Macular Holes

Improvements in the quality of OCT may be achieved in two different ways. First, it is possible to use an alternative light source in time domain OCT, e.g. femtosecond laser, which improves the resolution of OCT images up to 3 μm of axial resolution, but does not influence the speed of image acquisition. This method has been presented in the literature as ultra-high resolution OCT. Devices for ultra-high resolution OCT are experimental and have been presented in different papers [5–8].

Another method is the use of Fourier domain or spectral domain OCT (SD-OCT), a new technique in macula examination, which first became available in 2006. SD-OCT changes the method of signal detection and increases the speed of the examination, and improves the image resolution (5–7 μm axial resolution). This method additionally allows serial B- and C-scans of the macular area to be achieved. Various commercially available instruments using this technology have been produced.

Both alternative light source and Fourier domain OCT are combined in the Copernicus HR SOCT (SOCT HR; Optopol, Zawiercie, Poland), which gives us the opportunity both to achieve up to 3 μm of axial resolution and to create serial B- and C-scans of the examined area.

As the resolution of the retinal tissue with ultra-high resolution is similar to that of the commercially available SOCT, this chapter will also present the data published regarding this technology.

Ko et al. presented a multi-case report with images of macular holes examined using ultra-high resolution OCT in 2004. They reported that posterior hyaloid may be attached to the fovea, and on their images, small portions of sensory retina that detached from RPE were visible. Furthermore, small cystic changes were visible in the ganglion cell layer and in the nuclear layer. Enhanced visualisation of fine intraretinal features of the external limiting membrane (ELM) and Henle's fibres from the outer plexiform layer were presented in stage I macular holes. After surgery, Ko et al. also demonstrated resolution of cystic intraretinal spaces and intact photoreceptor inner segments/outer segments (IS/OS) connected to the RPE, as well as some elevation of the outer retina in stage IV macular holes after vitrectomy. These data were confirmed in a case study by Scholda et al. with ultra-high resolution OCT [5–7].

Optical coherence tomography images and ultra-high resolution OCT show an increase in signal from the RPE near the hole, most likely due to the absence of scattering and absorption from the inner retina.

Srinivasan et al. additionally demonstrated the presence of epiretinal membrane formation combined with full-thickness macular hole on ultra-high resolution OCT [8].

SOCT with resolution up to 3 μm allows visualisation of all those findings with commercially available devices. The additional advantage of SOCT over high-resolution OCT is the opportunity to achieve up to 200 B-scans on the surface up to 10 × 10 mm, which allows 3D reconstruction of the macular hole. Additionally, currently available SOCT devices have software that allows the ophthalmologist to present minute details of the vitreous and retinal structures (Fig. 13.3).

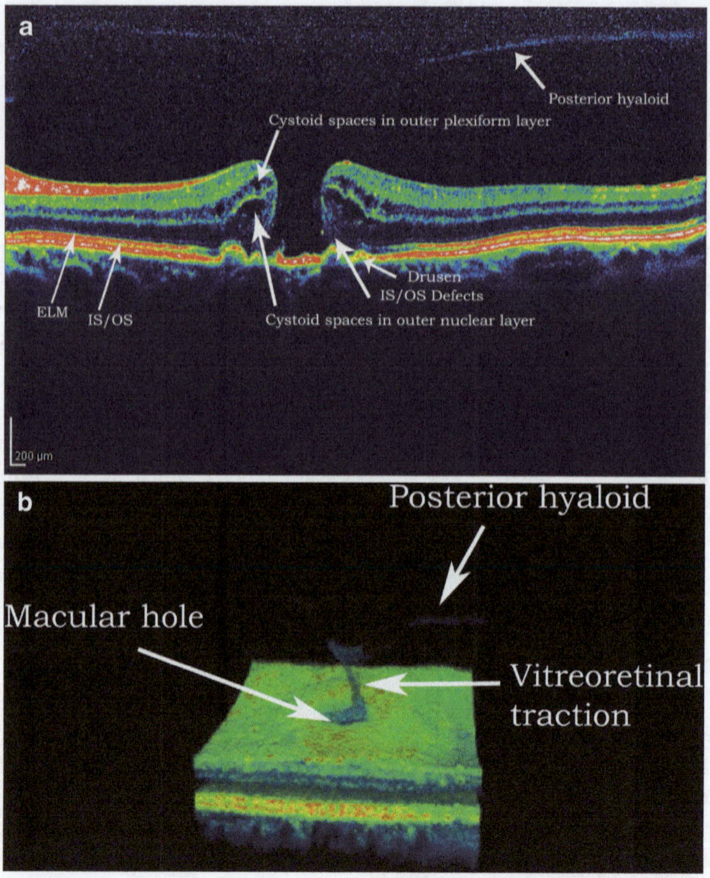

Fig. 13.3 (a) Pathological features of particular retinal layers in a spectral optical coherence tomography (SOCT) image of a macular hole (Spectralis). *ELM* external limiting membrane, *IS/OS* hyperreflective line representing the junction between the inner and outer segments of the photoreceptors. (b) A picture with enhanced visualisation of a macular hole with vitreoretinal traction with 3D OCT (Topcon Company, Tokyo, Japan). (c) Spectral domain OCT (Copernicus HR; Optopol, Zawiercie, Poland) with an axial resolution of 3 μm and maps of particular retinal layers

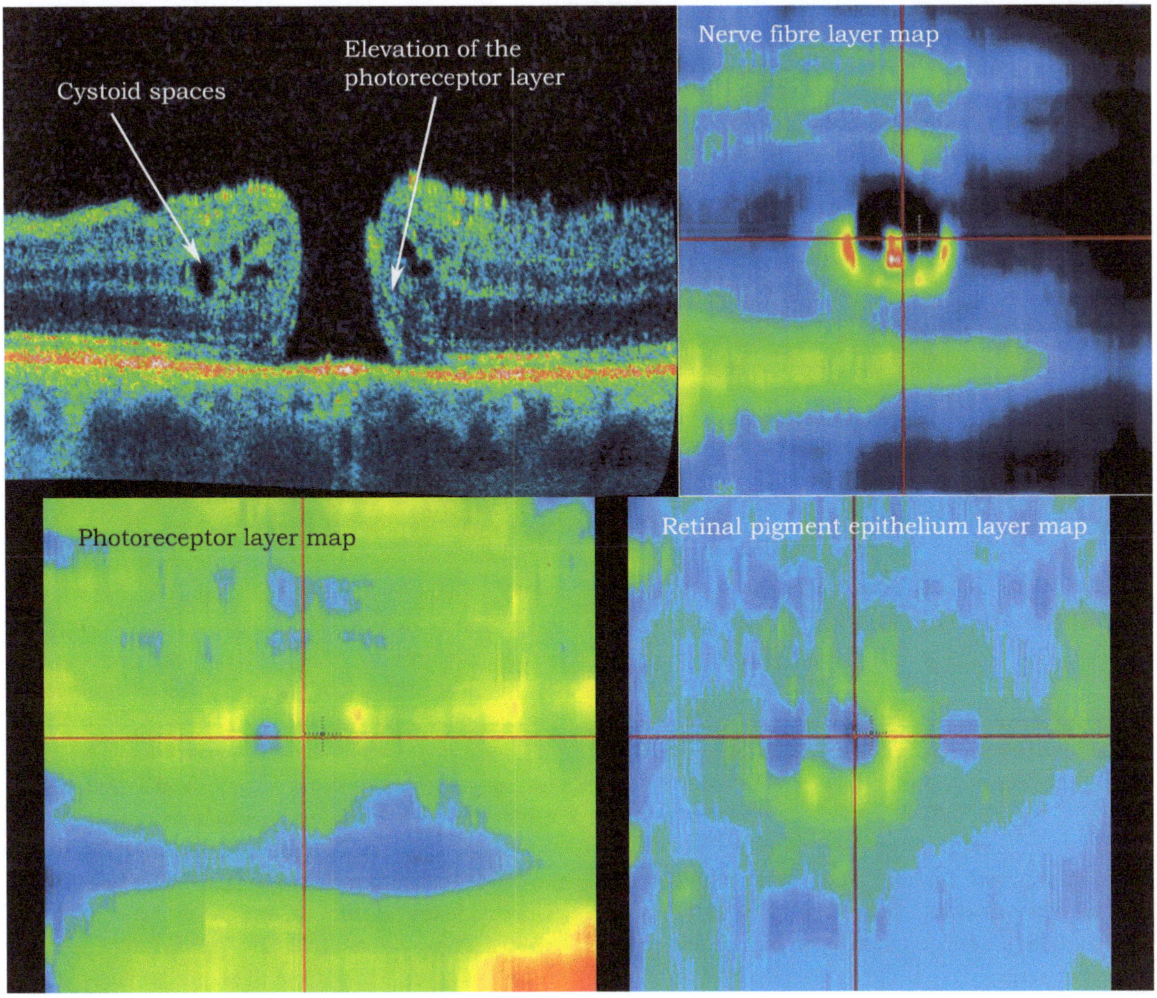

Fig. 13.3 (continued)

Quite recently, the possibility of using a hand-held non-contact SD-OCT system that combines a viewing screen with a movable hand-held scanner connected via a flexible fibre-optic cable to a movable cart holding the SD-OCT system was presented. This device allows good quality SD-OCT B-scans of macular holes in patients who cannot be examined in a sitting position, e.g. children [9].

The size of the macular hole may be an important factor in determining the anatomical and functional outcome after surgery. It may be easily measured with SOCT.

The hole form factor (HFF) may be counted with SOCT, as presented in Fig. 13.4 (HFF = c + d/a). According to Ullrich et al., in all patients with HFF > 0.9, the macular hole was closed following surgical procedure, whereas in eyes with HFF < 0.5, the anatomical success rate was 67%. A better postoperative visual outcome correlated with higher HFF ($p = 0.050$) [10, 11].

The minimum diameter of the macular hole is an important factor determining the visual outcome. Our results showed that all macular holes with a diameter less than 500 μm were closed after surgery, and eyes with a preoperative macular hole area of less than 0.2 mm^2 achieved final visual acuity of more than or equal to 0.3 (Fig. 13.4) [12].

Measurements of macular hole size performed with OCT and HRT showed a difference in size between the two imaging techniques in about 10% of cases. This could be explained by the fact that in some cases, the macular hole is not round but oval. In these cases, measurements performed with time domain OCT may not be adequate, because they are measured in specifically determined planes. Therefore, spectral domain OCT seems to be

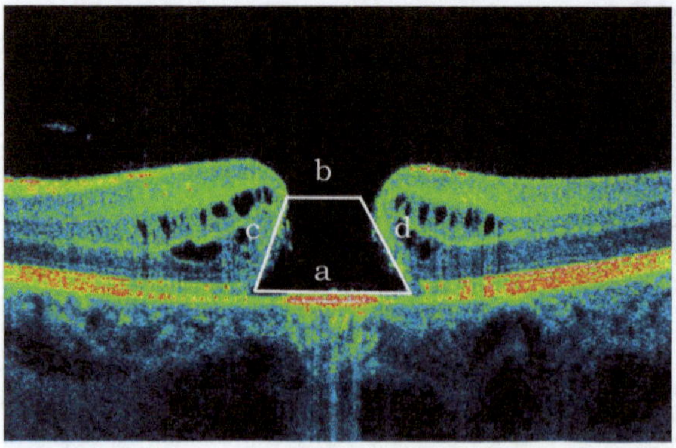

Fig. 13.4 Macular hole in SOCT. Hole form factor = c + d/a. *a* base diameter; *b* minimum diameter; *c* left-arm length; *d* right-arm length (Copernicus HR; Optopol, Zawiercie, Poland)

better suited for the task, because it is able to produce 3D images of the macular region [12].

13.6 Macular Hole Formation

For a long time, macular holes were believed to be secondary to trauma, inflammation, or myopia [13]. In the 1970s, recent posterior vitreous detachment was usually noted in eyes with macular holes, while eyes with pre-existing vitreous detachment very rarely developed a macular hole. This observation led to the conclusion that vitreous traction plays a role in macular hole formation [14].

In the early 1980s, it was suggested that the main cause of macular hole formation was anteroposterior traction exerted by vitreous fibres on the centre of the fovea [15]. This hypothesis was supported by histopathological findings, as it was proven that the vitreous consists of antero-posterior fibres.

In 1995, Gass suggested that most full-thickness macular holes arise from an umbo dehiscence without loss of foveal tissue [1]. Other authors suggested that intraretinal cysts play a role in macular hole formation, due to either a tractional [16] or a degenerative process [17].

Although slit lamp observations and photographic documentation were provided, adequate imaging of the posterior hyaloid detachment and retinal layers was impossible before the OCT era.

Gaudric et al. provided the first data documented by OCT regarding the early stages of macular hole formation due to incomplete posterior hyaloid detachment at the posterior pole, especially around the macula with residual tethering at the fovea. This was described as a trampoline configuration. Eye movements transmit a mechanical force with an oblique vector through the vitreous. The force consists of anterior and tangential vectoral components and may lead to posterior pole vitreous separation. Gaudric et al. also published OCT images of intraretinal cysts, which after rupture, can progress to a macular hole. Some cysts may be secondary to vitreofoveal tractions [2].

Sebag and Sadun hypothesised that age-related liquefaction of the vitreous without vitreomacular dehiscence might provoke tractional forces that may lead to macular holes [18]. Ezra published a study documented by OCT suggesting that failure of normal age-related separation of the cortical vitreous from the posterior pole as a result of an abnormally tenacious attachment to the fovea might lead to macular hole formation [19].

Tornambe recently presented a theory documented by OCT3 on macular hole formation due to vitreous fluid inflow into a cavity in the inner retina which was created by posterior hyaloid traction. His theory explains that separation of the posterior hyaloid can lead to spontaneous closure of some macular holes [20].

Hangai et al. presented, with a prototype of a 3D-OCT, a dynamic interaction of the vitreous and fovea that may play a significant role in macular hole formation. Similar observations were presented earlier for OCT [21, 22]. In the horizontal cross-sections of stage I macular holes, the disrupted parts of the ELM were crown-shaped. An inverted cone-shaped structure was visible over the crowned-shaped parts of the ELM. Additionally, in one case, the authors showed that the macular hole had a flap with a connection not only to the superficial portion of the inner retina, but also to the ELM. This is in agreement with our own observations, which show that asymmetric (dynamic) traction to the fovea initially produces an elevation of hyperreflective lines in SOCT, representing the junction between the inner and outer segments of the photoreceptors (IS/OS) and ELM, which may be visible in relatively healthy structure of the retina, as well as in the presence of intraretinal cysts and traction syndrome [3]. This may also be in agreement with the histopathological examination and the theory of Gass postulating that the Muller cell cones serve as plaque-binding photoreceptor cells in the foveola, and that contraction of the prefoveal vitreous cortex causes disruption of the Muller cell cones resulting in dehiscence of the foveola umbo [23] (Fig. 13.5).

In addition, Hangai et al. presented C-scans of the vitreoretinal interface that demonstrate this dynamic traction on the foveola (Fig. 13.6) [22].

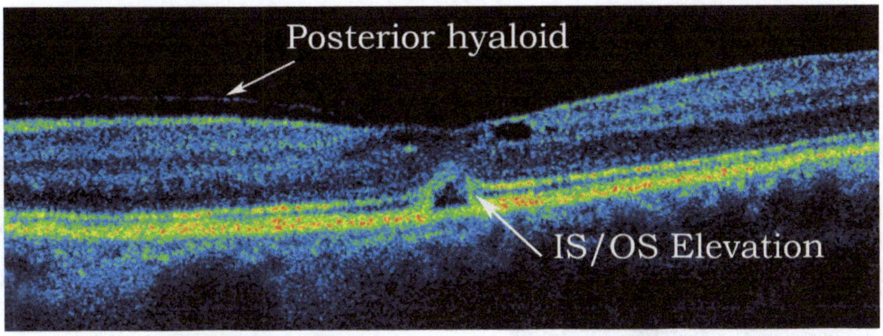

Fig. 13.5 Elevation of the photoreceptor layer and asymmetric vitreous traction occurring in the very early stages (before stage I) of macular hole formation. Only SOCT is capable of imaging this early feature. IS/OS hyperreflective line representing the junction between the inner and outer segments of the photoreceptors (Copernicus HR; Optopol, Zawiercie, Poland)

In conclusion, it seems very probable that vitreoretinal traction directed to the boundary of the Muller cell cone, as described by Gass, produces traction from the inner to the outer layers of the retina, which is possible both with and without cystic spaces in the inner retina, and may produce the elevation of the photoreceptor layer progressing to a full-thickness defect. Additional traction and posterior hyaloid detachment produces internal limiting membrane (ILM) defects and some defects in the Muller cell cone. During this stage, the vitreous may detach without any defects in the retinal structure and self-sealing of the macular hole occurs. However, if structural changes occur, it may also be healed by glial proliferation, but in the majority of cases, the healing process leads to smoothing of the edges of the break, visible as a round macular hole contour.

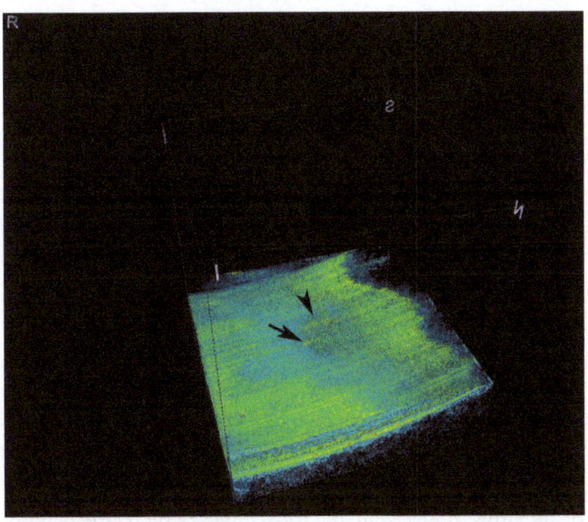

Fig. 13.6 C-scan in the 3D mode of very early-stage macular hole formation. *Black arrows* indicate the subtle crown-shaped appearance, representing elevation of the line showing the junction between the inner and outer segments of the photoreceptors. (Copernicus HR; Optopol, Zawiercie, Poland)

13.7 Postoperative Appearance

Postoperatively, four different types of macular hole closures can be observed. U-shaped closure, describing a normal foveal contour, is usually observed in about half of the cases, and best visual acuity outcome is typical for this group (Fig. 13.7a). V-shaped closure, where by a steep foveal contour has formed, is usually noted in about a quarter of the cases. Visual acuity is usually about 0.3 Snellen lines (Fig. 13.7b). An irregularly closed macular hole, signifying an irregular fovea shape, is seen in about 10% of the cases in the first weeks after surgery. It usually develops into one of the other types of closure (Fig. 13.7c). Thus, different visual acuity outcomes can be associated with this type of closure. A flat/open macular hole, also considered to be a postoperative success because of the stabilisation or slight improvement of vision (about 0.1 Snellen lines), is described as a foveal defect of the neurosensory retina with a flattened cuff of retinal detachment around the hole, and can be postoperatively noted in about 15–30% of the cases (Fig. 13.7d) [24–26].

Additionally, the following retinal abnormalities can be seen on postoperative scans: a linear lack of photoreceptors in the subfoveal area described as a lack of IS/OS line (about 45% of the cases), presented as a lack of tissue in the subfoveal area (Fig. 13.8a), not obligatorily connected to the photoreceptor defects described as a cyst

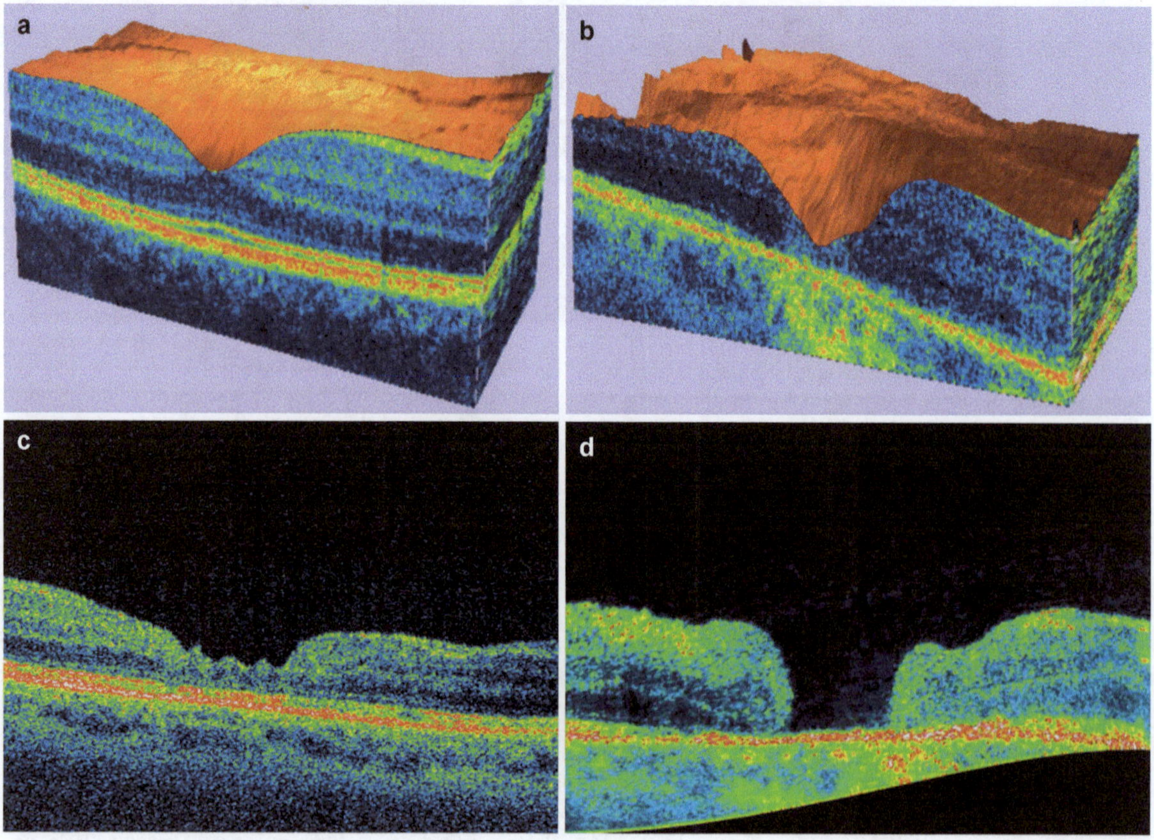

Fig. 13.7 Macular hole closure types (Copernicus HR; Optopol, Zawiercie, Poland) [24]. (**a**) U-shaped closure. (**b**) V-shaped closure. (**c**) Irregular closure. (**d**) Flat/open closure

in the outer retinal layers (Fig. 13.8b); indentation of the outer retinal layer described as nerve fibre layer defects (Fig. 13.8c); photoreceptor layer lesions (Fig. 13.8d); photoreceptor layer irregularities (Fig. 13.8e); and RPE defects (Fig. 13.8f). In about 15% of the cases, no retinal abnormalities were noted on postoperative SOCT scans. In those eyes, visual acuity improved the most. Postoperative functional results have mostly deteriorated when photoreceptor defects or cysts in the outer retinal layers coexist. Chang et al. did not observe any correlation between the size of IS/OS disruption and visual acuity in 17 eyes [27]. Our own observations, confirmed by Inoue et al., in larger groups of patients, demonstrate that the total area of photoreceptor defect in SOCT negatively correlates with the postoperative visual acuity [24,]. However, postoperative central retinal thickness is also a factor influencing postoperative visual acuity. After surgery epiretinal membranes are more often observed in eyes in which no staining was used. It has been suspected that in those eyes, the ILM was not completely removed. If staining is used and the ILM is removed, then no ERM formation in the postoperative period is observed [24]. On the other hand, a complete removal of the internal limiting membrane (with the use of dyes) leads to a higher frequency of the nerve fibre layer defects [24]. It should be taken into consideration that the area of all the above-mentioned defects deteriorates with time, together with an improvement in the visual acuity that can take up to 12 months postoperatively.

In addition, in some rare cases, we can observe paracentral full-thickness retinal defects after macular hole closure after vitrectomy with ILM peeling. Our observations show that small haemorrhages which are usually observed after ILM peeling may be the cause of full-thickness macular defects, and during the follow-up, these defects either decrease in size or disappear. A discussion of these processes will follow in the next chapter [29].

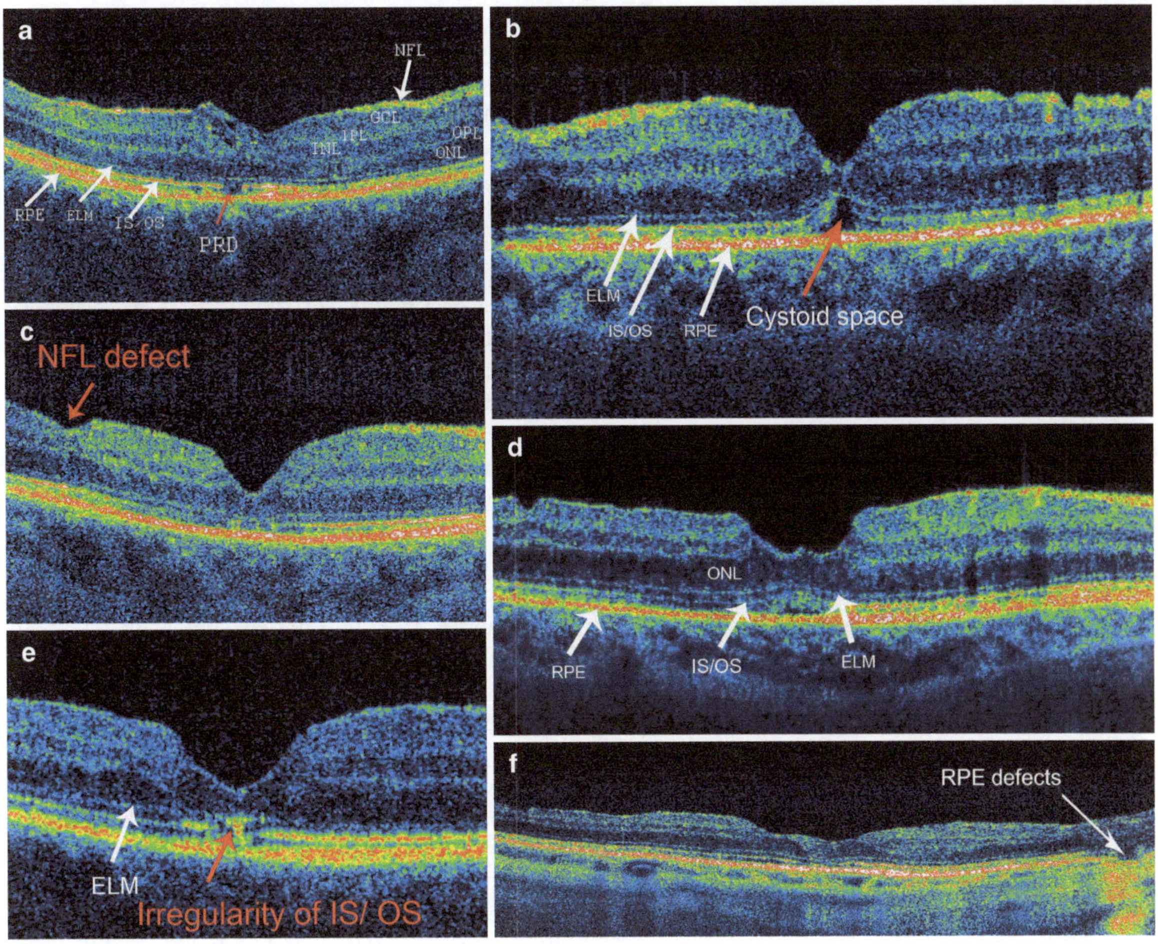

Fig. 13.8 Defects of particular retinal layers in SOCT (Copernicus HR; Optopol, Zawiercie, Poland). (**a**) Photoreceptor defect visible 1 week after surgery for traumatic macular hole in a 25-year-old patient. Initial visual acuity was 0.15. Final visual acuity 9 months after surgery was 0.8. (**b**) A 68-year-old patient with visual acuity of 0.05 before surgery achieved final visual acuity of 0.5. Cysts usually have a tendency to minimise with time. One month after surgery, the cyst diameters in this patient were 573 × 109 μm. After 3 months, it was 307 × 112 μm. (**c**) Nerve fibre defect in a 68-year-old patient. Initial visual acuity was 0.02. Visual acuity 6 months after surgery was 0.3. Photoreceptor defects are visible (462–14 μm). (**d**) Lesion of the photoreceptor layer that is visible 3 months after surgery in a 68-year-old patient. Visual acuity improved from 0.05 before surgery to 0.5. (**e**) Irregularity of the photoreceptor layer observed 6 months after surgery. Initial visual acuity was 0.02. Final visual acuity was 0.3. (**f**) RPE defects visible 12 months after surgery in a 68-year-old patient. Visual acuity improved from 0.02 to 0.4. Photoreceptor defects were observed in this patient. *NFL* nerve fibre layer, *GCL* ganglion cell layer, *IPL* inner plexiform layer, *INL* inner nuclear layer, *OPL* outer plexiform layer, *ONL* outer nuclear layer, *ELM* external limiting membrane, *IS/OS* hyper-reflective line representing the junction between the inner and outer segments of the photoreceptors, *RPE* retinal pigment epithelium, *PRD* photoreceptor layer (IS/OS) defect [24]

13.8 Theory of Macular Hole Closure After Vitrectomy

SOCT images are most helpful to detect the possible mechanism of macular hole closure. First, we can draw some conclusions from the presented cases of spontaneous macular hole closure, as demonstrated by SD-OCT. Currently, these are very rare cases, and are usually macular microholes. However, our own observations show that it is even possible in cases of large macular holes. They may close after spontaneous posterior hyaloid detachment in cases where the edges of the macular hole have some extensions, that is, before the contour of the macular hole becomes oval in shape. In such situations, some cell migration may be responsible for macular hole closure [30].

Bridging of retinal tissue over the macular hole illustrates the probable initial phase of the macular hole closure process with a small overhang of the inner part of the neurosensory retina. The macular hole healing process may comprise glial proliferation of Muller cells, which has already been described in histopathological papers [31, 32].

Eckardt et al. demonstrated with SD-OCT that macular hole closure appears within 24 h of surgery in 54.5% of the cases and in 48 h in 75.7%. Such fast closure of the macular hole after vitrectomy with ILM peeling may support the theory that ILM peeling is a type of refreshment of the edges of the macular hole, and allows for a similar situation to that observed in spontaneous macular hole closure, which is additionally supported by the gas bubble that provides a surface for cell migration so that the macular hole can close. According to Eckardt et al., if the macular hole does not close during the first 3 days, it will not close later on and will require repeated surgery [33].

The healing process does not end with macular hole closure. In the postoperative period, restoration of two hyperreflective lines, which are believed to be the ELM and the IS/OS junction, is observed [27, 34, 35]. Lee et al. presented three cases of restoration of the photoreceptor layer after macular hole surgery [34]. Chang et al. observed that 6 out of 7 eyes with macular hole closure had a decrease in the IS/OS defect size after the hole was closed. Visual acuity showed a trend towards improvement, but the improvement was not correlated with the change in the size of the IS/OS boundary defect [33]. Sano described 28 cases of healing of the IS/OS line. The visual outcomes were significantly better in eyes with a continuous IS/OS line than in those with a disrupted IS/OS line [35].

Summary for the Clinician

- Elevation of the photoreceptor layer combined with asymmetric posterior hyaloid traction on the fovea can be considered an early step in macular hole formation.
- After successful surgery, various defects of the retinal layers in the fovea can be noted. Some of them may be influenced by surgical procedures.
- Visual acuity improves up to 12 months after surgery, as does the appearance of the fovea in SOCT.

13.9 Surgical Considerations

Vitrectomy as a method of treatment for macular holes was introduced in 1990–1991 by Kelly and Wendel [36]. During the 1990s, different adjuvants were used to improve the results of surgery. By the end of the 1990s and the beginning of the 21st century, the increasing role of ILM peeling combined with vitrectomy and gas injection was observed. Various dyes are being used to improve the quality of ILM peeling. This kind of treatment is nowadays considered a standard procedure for the treatment of macular holes.

As this chapter is designed to present the diagnostics of macular hole with SOCT, surgical methods will not be widely presented or discussed. However, we recently presented a new method of treating large macular holes [37]with the use of an inverted ILM flap to cover the macular hole and to improve the closure rate of large macular holes. Postoperative SOCT examination after the use of the inverted ILM flap technique gave us the opportunity to demonstrate macular hole closure in those eyes. As can be seen, the ILM serves as a scaffold for tissue migration or proliferation with the aim of closing the macular hole. Without the use of SOCT, it would not be possible to observe this process. This mechanism may explain how full-thickness retinal defects close. Without a histopathological examination of the eyes after macular hole closure with the inverted ILM flap technique, one cannot be sure whether this process is due to glial proliferation or movement of the retinal cells [37]. Histopathological studies of the eyes operated on with vitrectomy but without ILM peeling show that glial proliferation (Muller cells) may be responsible for the healing process [31, 32]. A regeneration process of the photoreceptor cells, initiated by Muller glial proliferation, was recently described in zebrafish, and the same mechanism may take place in the above described situation. (Figs. 13.9, 13.10) [38].

Summary for the Clinician

- Vitrectomy with ILM peeling and gas injection is the method of choice in the treatment of macular holes.
- Spectral OCT demonstrates the mechanism of macular hole closure.

13.10 Lamellar Macular Hole and Macular Pseudohole

The 1970's, Gass described pseudomacular hole formation, as being caused by spontaneous contraction of an epiretinal membrane surronding but not covering the foveal area, and which may produce a biomicroscopic appearance simulating a full-thickness macular hole [39, 40]. Usually,

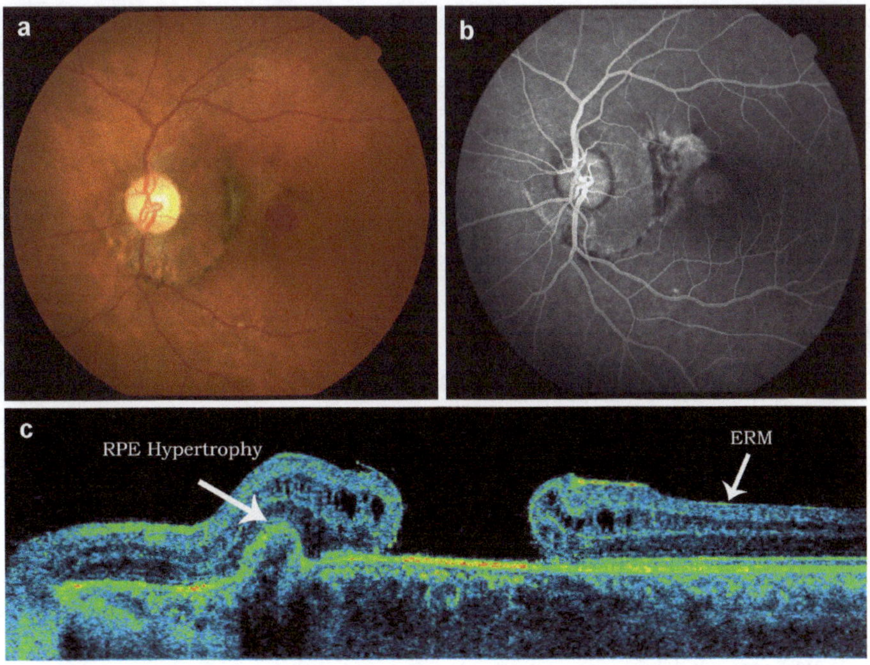

Fig. 13.9 The images show an extremely large macular hole with a minimum diameter of 1,268 × 1,958 μm, which was operated on using the inverted internal limiting membrane (ILM) flap technique and air injection [37]. (**a**) Fundus view. (**b**) Fluorescein angiography (Topcon Company, Tokyo, Japan). (**c**) Spectral domain OCT (Copernicus; Optopol, Zawiercie, Poland) demonstrates preoperative view of a macular hole. *RPE* retinal pigment epithelium, *ERM* epiretinal membrane

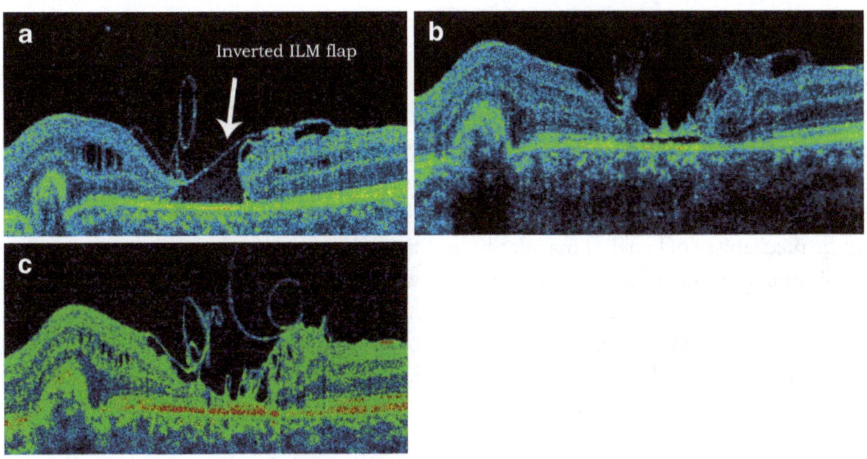

Fig. 13.10 (**a**) Spectral OCT picture demonstrates closure of the macular hole presented in Fig. 13.9 with the inverted ILM flap only. (**b**) However, the next picture, 1 month later, demonstrates that the ILM flap serves as a scaffold for tissue migration or proliferation along the ILM to close the macular hole. (**c**) Further closure is visible after 3 months (Copernicus HR; Optopol, Zawiercie, Poland) [37]

these patients have no or very few complaints and visual acuity is normal or almost normal.

Haouchine et al. confirmed this observation with OCT [41]. Differential diagnosis of macular pseudoholes (Fig. 13.11a) from lamellar macular holes (Fig. 13.11b) may be difficult, but it is possible on the basis of OCT, which shows the lack of dehiscence of the inner foveal retina from the outer foveal retina in the pseudoholes.

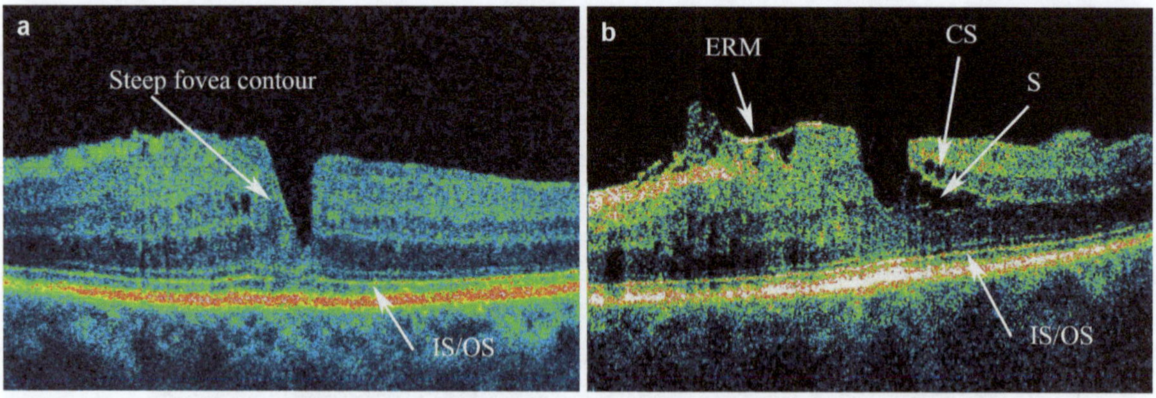

Fig. 13.11 (**a**) Macular pseudohole. Note the irregular foveal contour with normal central macular thickness. (**b**) Lamellar macular hole. Note the cystoid spaces. *ERM* epiretinal membrane, *CS* cystoid spaces, *S* dehiscence of the inner from the outer retinal layer in the fovea, *IS/OS* intact photoreceptor layer (Copernicus HR; Optopol, Zawiercie, Poland)

Other criteria such as a irregular foveal contour and a break in the inner fovea, as well as the absence of full-thickness foveal defects, may be observed in both entities.

The pathogenesis of lamellar macular holes is not known. It was originally described by Gass as a macular lesion resulting from macular edema [42]. It was believed to be the result of an abortive process in macular hole formation [2, 43].

A number of authors have observed that in the majority, if not all, cases of lamellar macular holes and pseudoholes, epiretinal membranes are present around the fovea [44–46]. There are no cases in which we have been able to visualise development of a full-thickness macular hole during the follow-up observations of lamellar macular holes with SOCT (unpublished data). The authors therefore suggest that the mechanism of lamellar macular hole formation might be similar to that of a macular pseudohole working by contraction of the epiretinal membranes. This should be classified as a subtype of epiretinal membrane formation rather than a full-thickness macular hole. Furthermore, in SOCT, the very small difference between the macular pseudoholes and lamellar macular holes may lead to the suggestion that they might not be two different diseases. Most of the information regarding these diseases was presented before SOCT was available. The 3D imaging mode in SOCT can be presented for a single patient; one B-scan showing a macular pseudohole and the next few scans showing what appears to be a lamellar macular hole. Some authors also believe that lamellar macular holes may be a subtype of macular pseudoholes [46]. An interesting question is why, in some cases, an epiretinal membrane covers the whole macular area and in other cases, the fovea remains free of epiretinal membrane formation.

13.11 Clinical Features

Visual acuity ranges from 0.1 to 1.0 (mean 0.43) [46]. There is metamorphopsia, but usually a good visual prognosis.

13.11.1 Examination of Lamellar Macular Holes and Pseudoholes

With fundoscopy, crinkling of the inner retinal surface surrounding the hole and the punched-out appearance in the area of the hole are observed. As the slit beam is moved across the hole, there is usually a light reflex, which is the evidence of retinal tissue at the base of the hole. The foveal reflex is usually absent [39]. Only 28–37% of lamellar macular holes are correctly diagnosed on clinical examination [41, 46].

With autofluorescence, slight irregular hyperfluorescence in the fovea can be noted (Fig. 13.12a).

Fluorescein angiography is usually normal or slightly irregular; hyperfluorescence can be present (Fig. 13.12b).

With scanning laser ophthalmoscopy, a hypofluorescent macular region with visible retinal striae, representing epiretinal membranes with no height deviation from the retinal surface on the topography scale is observed (Fig. 13.12c) [44].

With SOCT, in lamellar macular holes, an irregular fovea contour with break in the inner fovea and

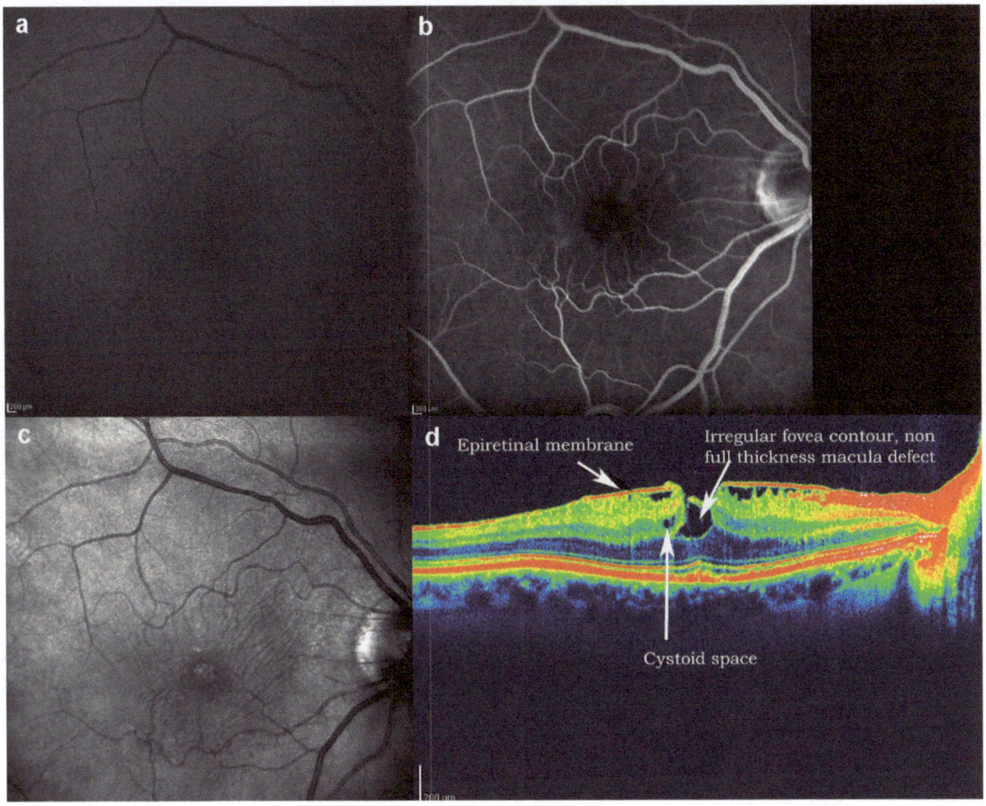

Fig. 13.12 (**a**) Autofluorescence of a lamellar macular hole (*LMH*). (**b**) Late phase of fluorescein angiography of LMH. (**c**) Scanning laser ophthalmoscopy of LMH. (**d**) SOCT of the lamellar macular hole (Spectralis; Heidelberg Engineering, Heidelberg, Germany)

dehiscence of the inner from the outer retinal layer in the fovea is observed. Absence of a full-thickness foveal defect with intact foveal photoreceptors can be noted. Additionally, near the fovea cystoid spaces are present. In most, if not in all cases, epiretinal membranes coexist. Posterior hyaloid detachment is present in about 50% of the cases (Fig. 13.12d).

13.12 Treatment

Some authors suggest that treatment of lamellar macular holes improves visual acuity. On the other hand, full-thickness macular hole formation after vitrectomy has been noted [46]. Currently, there is a lack of evidence-based studies presenting indications for surgery of lamellar macular holes.

Spectral OCT allows presentation of the normalisation of the foveal structure after vitrectomy with ILM peeling for lamellar macular holes or pseudoholes.

The authors of this chapter usually advise surgery if vision deteriorates between consecutive visits.

Summary for the Clinician

- Appearance of lamellar macular holes in SOCT:
  - An irregular foveal contour
  - Break in the inner fovea
  - Dehiscence of the inner from the outer retinal layer in the fovea
  - Absence of a full-thickness foveal defect
  - Intact foveal photoreceptors in most cases
  - Cystoid spaces near to the fovea
  - In most if not in all cases, epiretinal membranes coexist
- Appearance of macular pseudoholes in SOCT:
  - Steep foveal contour
  - Normal central macular thickness
  - Absence of a full-thickness foveal defect
  - No cystoid spaces or dehiscence of the inner from the outer retinal layers
  - Epiretinal membrane in most if not in all cases
- Vitrectomy with ILM peeling can be considered as a surgical treatment in selected cases.

References

1. Gass JD (1995) Reappraisal of biomicroscopic classification of stages of development of a macular hole. Am J Ophthalmol 119:752–759
2. Gaudric A, Haouchine B, Massin P et al (1999) Macular hole formation: new data provided by optical coherence tomography. Arch Ophthalmol 117:744–751
3. Michalewska Z, Michalewski J, Sikorski BL et al (2009) A study of macular hole formation by serial spectral optical coherence tomography. Clin Exp Ophthalmol. 37: 373–383
4. Guyer DR, de Bustros S, Diener-West M, Fine SL (1992) Observations on patients with idiopathic macular holes and cysts. Arch Ophthalmol 110:1264–1268
5. Ko TH, Fujimoto JG, Duker JS et al (2004) Comparison of ultrahigh- and standard-resolution optical coherence tomography for imaging macular hole pathology and repair. Ophthalmology 111:2033–2043
6. Ko TH, Fujimoto JG, Schuman JS et al (2005) Comparison of ultrahigh- and standard-resolution optical coherence tomography for imaging macular pathology. Ophthalmology 112:1–15
7. Scholda C, Wirtitsch M, Hermann B et al (2006) Ultrahigh resolution optical coherence tomography of macular holes. Retina 26:1034–1041
8. Srinivasan VJ, Wojtkowski M, Witkin AJ et al (2006) High-definition and 3-dimensional imaging of macular pathologies with high-speed ultrahigh-resolution optical coherence tomography. Ophthalmology 113:1–14
9. Scott AW, Farsiu S, Enyedi LB et al (2009) Imaging the infant retina with a hand-held spectral-domain optical coherence tomography device. Am J Ophthalmol 147:364–373
10. Desai VN, Hee MR, Puliafito CA (1999) Optical coherence tomography of macular holes. In: Madreperla SA, McCuen BW (eds) Macular hole: pathogenesis, diagnosis and treatment. Butterworth-Heinemann, Oxford, pp 37–47
11. Ullrich S, Haritoglou C, Gass C et al (2006) Macular hole size as a prognostic factor in macular hole surgery. Br J Ophthalmol 86:390–393
12. Michalewska Z, Michalewski J, Nawrocki J (2007) Diagnosis and evaluation of macular hole with the HRT 2 retina module. Ophthalmologe 104:881–888
13. Collins ET (1900) Unusual changes to the macular region. Trans Ophthalmol Soc U K 20:196–197
14. Aaberg TM (1970) Macular holes: a review. Surv Ophthalmol 15:139–162
15. Avila MP, Jalkh AE, Murakami K et al (1983) Biomicroscopic study of the vitreous in macular breaks. Ophthalmology 90:1277–1283
16. Reese AB, Jones IS, Cooper WC (1967) Macular changes secondary to vitreous tractions. Am J Ophthalmol 64: 544–549
17. Asrani S, Zeimer R, Goldberg M, Zou S (1988) Serial optical sectioning of macular holes at different stages of development. Ophthalmology 105:66–77
18. Sebag J, Sadun AA (2004) Reflections. Graefes Arch Clin Exp Ophthalmol 242:811–813
19. Ezra E (2001) Idiopathic full thickness macular hole: natural history and pathogenesis. Br J Ophthalmol 85:102–109
20. Tornambe PE (2003) Macular hole genesis: the hydration theory. Retina 23(3):421–424
21. Chan A, Duker JS, Schuman JS, Fujimoto JG (2004) Stage 0 macular holes: observations by optical coherence tomography. Ophthalmology 111:2027–2032
22. Hangai M, Ojima Y, Gotoh N et al (2007) Three-dimensional imaging of macular holes with high-speed optical coherence tomography. Ophthalmology 114:763–773
23. Gass JD (1999) Müller cell cone, an overlooked part of the anatomy of the fovea centralis: hypotheses concerning its role in the pathogenesis of macular hole and foveomacular retinoschisis. Arch Ophthalmol 117:821–823
24. Michalewska Z, Michalewski J, Cisiecki S et al (2008) Correlation between foveal structure and visual outcome following macular hole surgery: a spectral optical coherence tomography study. Graefes Arch Clin Exp Ophthalmol 246:823–830
25. Imai M, Iijima H, Gothoh T, Tsukashara S (1999) Optical coherence tomography of successfully repaired idiopathic macular holes. Am J Ophthalmol 128:621–627
26. Kang SW, Ahn K, Ham DI (2003) Types of macular hole closure and their clinical implications. Br J Ophthalmol 87: 1015–1019
27. Chang LK, Koizumi H, Spaide RF (2008) Disruption of the photoreceptor inner segment-outer segment junction in eyes with macular holes. Retina 28:969–975
28. Inoue M, Watanabe Y, Arakawa A et al (2009) Spectral-domain optical coherence tomography images of inner/outer segment junctions and macular hole surgery outcomes. Graefes Arch Clin Exp Ophthalmol 247:325–330
29. Michalewska Z, Michalewski J, Nawrocki J (2009) Paracentral retinal defects after vitrectomy for macular hole and their evolution over time. Retin Cases Brief Rep doi: 10.1097/ICB.0b013e31819f1ffa
30. Michalewska Z, Cisiecki S, Sikorski B et al (2008) Spontaneous closure of stage III and IV idiopathic full-thickness macular holes-a two-case report. Graefes Arch Clin Exp Ophthalmol 246:99–104
31. Madreperla SA, Geiger, GL, Fumata M et al (1994) Clinicopathologic correlation of a macular hole treated by cortical vitreous peeling and gas tamponade. Ophthalmology 101:682–686
32. Rosa RH Jr, Glaser BM, de la Cruz Z, Green WE (1996) Clinicopathologic correlation of an untreated macular hole and a macular hole treated by vitrectomy, transforming

growth factor- beta 2 and gas tamponade. Am J Ophthalmol 122:853–863
33. Eckardt C, Eckert T, Eckardt U et al (2008) Macular hole surgery with air tamponade and optical coherence tomography-based duration of face-down positioning. Retina 28: 1087–1096
34. Lee JE, Seung UL, Jea SY et al (2008) Reorganization of photoreceptor layer on optical coherence tomography concurrent with visual improvement after macular hole surgery. Korean J Ophthalmol 22:137–142
35. Sano M, Shimoda Y, Hashimoto H, Kishi S (2009) Restored photoreceptor outer segment and visual recovery after macular hole closure. Am J Ophthalmol 147:313–318
36. Kelly NE, Wendel RT (1991) Vitreous surgery for idiopathic macular holes. Results of a pilot study. Arch Ophthalmol 109:654–659
37. Michalewska Z, Michalewski J, Nawrocki J (2009) Macular hole closure after vitrectomy: the inverted flap technique. Retina Today 3:73–74
38. Thummel R, Kassen SC, Enright JM et al (2008) Characterization of Muller glia and neuronal progenitors during adult zebrafish retinal regeneration. Exp Eye Res 87: 433–444
39. Allen AW Jr, Gass JD (1976) Contraction of a perifoveal epiretinal membrane simulating a macular hole. Am J Ophthalmol 82:684–691
40. Gass JD (1977) Stereoscopic atlas of macular diseases and treatment, 2nd edn. Mosby, St Louis
41. Haouchine B, Massin P, Tadayoni R (2004) Diagnosis of macular pseudoholes and lamellar macular holes by optical coherence tomography. Am J Ophthalmol 138: 732–739
42. Gass JD (1975) Lamellar macular hole: a complication of cystoid macular oedema after cataract extraction: a clinicopathologic case report. Trans Am Ophthalmol Soc 73: 231–250
43. Tanner V, Chauhan DS, Jackson TL et al (2001) Optical coherence tomography of the vitreoretinal interface in macular hole formation. Br J Ophthalmol 85: 1092–1097
44. Michalewska Z, Michalewski J, Nawrocki J (2009) Vergleich von SOCT und Laser-Scanning-Ophthalmoskopie bei der Differenzierung der durchgreifenden von den lamellären und Pseudo-Makulaforamina. Ophthalmologe doi: 10.1007/s00347-009-1985-2
45. Michalewski J, Michalewska Z, Cisiecki S, Nawrocki J (2007) Morphologically functional correlations of macular pathology connected with epiretinal membrane formation in spectral optical coherence tomography (SOCT). Graefes Arch Clin Exp Ophthalmol 245:1623–1631
46. Witkin AJ, Ko TH, Fujimoto JG (2006) Redefining lamellar holes and the vitreomacular interface: an ultrahigh-resolution optical coherence tomography study. Ophthalmology 113:388–397
47. Gass JD (1988) Idiopathic senile macular hole: its early stages and pathogenesis. Retina 23:629–639

Chapter 14

Combined Spectral-Domain Optical Coherence Tomography/Scanning Laser Ophthalmoscopy Imaging of Vitreous and the Vitreo-Retinal Interface

14

Jerry Sebag and Michelle Y. Wang

Core Messages

- Vitreous is not a space but an important ocular structure that maintains transparency, provides shock absorption, and plays a role in ocular physiology. The *vitreo-retinal interface* is the site of much pathology that leads to blindness.
- The outermost layer of vitreous is known as the posterior vitreous cortex. Hyalocytes are mononuclear phagocytes, which reside in a single layer embedded within the posterior vitreous cortex. As members of the reticulo-endothelial system, hyalocytes function as sentinel cells.
- During aging, there is dissociation of collagen from hyaluronan (HA) resulting in fibers and liquefied vitreous, a process known as synchisis. Concurrent weakening of vitreous adhesion to retina allows for collapse (syneresis) of the liquefied vitreous away from the retina, a phenomenon known as posterior vitreous detachment (PVD).
- Anomalous PVD occurs when there is synchisis (gel liquefaction) without sufficient dehiscence at the vitreo-retinal interface to allow for innocuous syneresis and PVD.
- The consequences of anomalous PVD vary depending on where the posterior vitreous cortex most firmly adheres to the retina and posterior pole, and where the vitreous is most liquefied. In the periphery, anomalous PVD causes retinal tears and detachments. At the macula, anomalous PVD causes vitreo-macular traction syndrome, if the attached posterior vitreous cortex is intact and has full thickness.
- Vitreoschisis occurs when during anomalous PVD there is a split in the posterior vitreous cortex, leaving the outermost layer of vitreous attached to the macula. The split can either occur anterior or posterior to the level of hyalocytes.
- Anomalous PVD with vitreoschisis anterior to the hyalocytes leaves these cells attached to the macula. These cells mediate inward (centripetal) tangential traction and macular pucker (MP). There are very few cases of vitreo-papillary adhesion (VPA) in MP.
- Anomalous PVD with vitreoschisis posterior to the level of hyalocytes and persistent adhesion of vitreous to the optic disc results in outward (centrifugal) tangential traction and macular holes (MHs).
- Pharmacologic vitreolysis is a new modality to treat disorders of the vitreo-retinal interface using agents that liquefy vitreous, known as "liquefactants," and agents that weaken vitreo-retinal adhesion, known as "interfactants." The former agents induce synchisis, while the latter agents allow innocuous syneresis. There are agents that have both properties.

14.1 Introduction

Recent years have seen an increased appreciation for the role of vitreous in retinal disease, especially maculopathies. This is primarily due to an improved understanding of vitreous biochemistry and structure, especially as relating to the vitreo-retinal interface. The changes that occur with aging, which result in posterior vitreous detachment (PVD), are now better understood, enabling an appreciation of how anomalous PVD causes disease and vision loss.

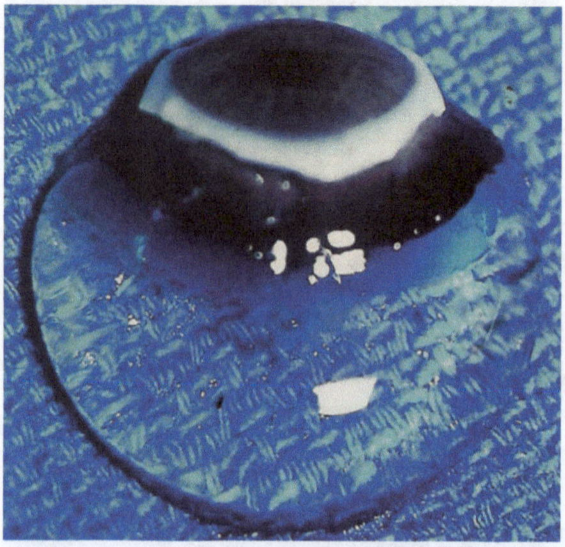

Fig. 14.1 Human vitreous. Vitreous body of a 9-month-old child dissected of the sclera, choroid, and retina, still attached to the anterior segment. Although the specimen is fresh, unfixed, and situated on a surgical towel in room air, the vitreous maintains its shape, because in youth the vitreous body is nearly entirely gel. [Specimen courtesy of the New England Eye Bank]

"Designed" to be invisible (Fig. 14.1), vitreous has long been very difficult to evaluate in both research and clinical settings. However, the advent of improved imaging modalities such as spectral-domain optical coherence tomography combined with scanning laser ophthalmoscopy (SD-OCT/SLO) has enabled confirmation that vitreo-macular interface pathology is a significant cause of many macular disorders. This has in turn made possible more precise clinical diagnoses and routinely successful therapeutic interventions.

This chapter briefly discusses the biochemistry and anatomy of vitreous and the vitreo-retinal interface and more extensively the role of vitreous in the pathogenesis of premacular membrane formation with macular pucker (MP), macular holes (both full-thickness, MH; and lamellar, LH), exudative age-related macular degeneration (AMD), and the vitreo-macular traction syndrome (VMTS). Since it is fundamental to an understanding of these disorders, the unifying concept of anomalous PVD is described.

14.2 Vitreous Biochemistry

Vitreous is an extended extracellular matrix composed mostly of water (98%) and a network of collagen fibrils stabilized by hyaluronan (HA), whose hydrophilic properties keep the collagen fibrils separated far enough to minimize light scattering and maintain vitreous transparency [1–3]. Vitreous collagen is composed of 75% type II collagen, 15% type XI collagen, and 10% type V/XI hybrid collagen [1, 2, 4]. Type IX collagen may be particularly important as it is situated on the fibril surface and thus mediates interactions between the collagen fibrils and other extracellular components of vitreous [5]. Most important of these is HA, a long unbranched polymer of repeating disaccharides (glucuronic acid β-1, 3-*N*-acetylglucosamine) linked by β 1–4 bonds. HA renders vitreous its viscoelastic properties, but it also inhibits cell migration and proliferation, contributing to the maintenance of transparency.

14.3 Vitreo-Retinal Interface Anatomy

The innermost layer of the retina is the internal limiting lamina, mostly comprising type IV collagen. The peripheral shell of vitreous, known as the posterior vitreous cortex, consists of densely packed collagen fibrils [3], as well as a high concentration of HA. Immunohistochemical studies [6] have shown that the outer layer of vitreous has a lamellar structure (Fig. 14.2). Embedded within the posterior vitreous cortex are hyalocytes [Fig. 14.3]. These oval-shaped mononuclear phagocytes are situated 20–50 μm from the internal limiting lamina of the retina in a single layer. Hyalocytes are possibly responsible for HA

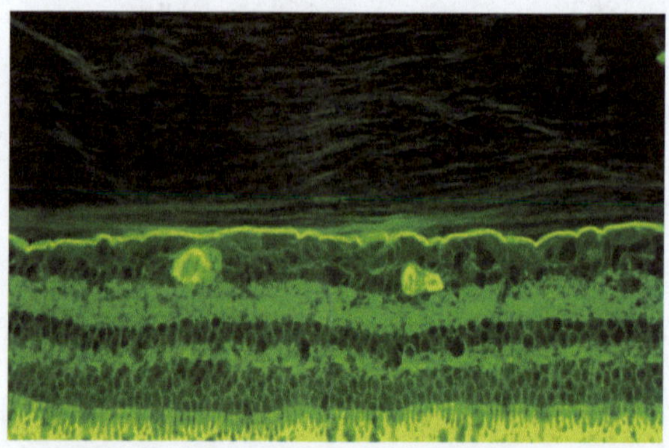

Fig. 14.2 Lamellar structure of posterior vitreous cortex. This immunofluorescence micrograph of the vitreo-retinal interface shows that the posterior vitreous cortex (above the intensely stained internal limiting lamina) appears lamellar in structure. This lamellar organization predisposes to splitting into separate layers during pathological processes such as the anomalous posterior vitreous detachment (PVD). (Courtesy Dr. Greg Hageman, University of Iowa)

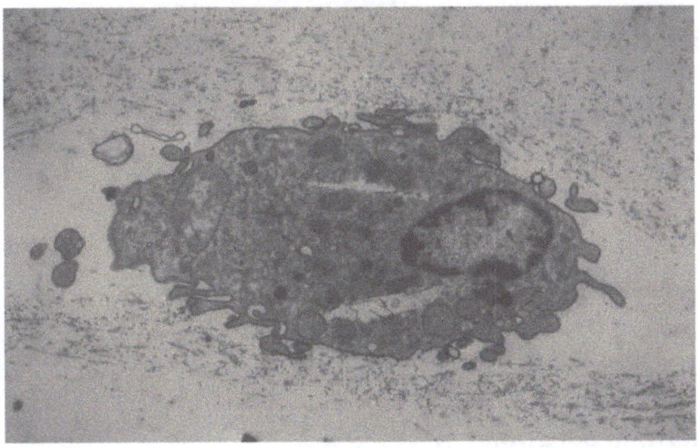

Fig. 14.3 Ultrastructure of human hyalocyte. A mononuclear cell is seen embedded within the dense collagen fibril network of the vitreous cortex. (x 1670). (Courtesy Craft and Albert, Harvard Medical School, Boston [7]

synthesis [8, 9] and probably important in a variety of proliferative as well as tractional vitreo-retinal disorders [3–5, 10, 11].

While it was previously believed that vitreous is directly attached to the retina, it is now thought that vitreo-retinal adhesion is mediated by an extracellular matrix "glue" composed of fibronectin, laminin, chondroitin sulfate, heparin sulfate, opticin, and other constituents [4, 10].

14.3.1 Age-Related Changes

In youth, vitreous is a solid, transparent gel that firmly adheres to the retina in a fascial (as opposed to focal) manner [12]. Homogeneous distribution of collagen and HA results in little or no light scattering (Fig. 14.1). In the adult, vitreous liquefies while collagen fibrils aggregate into bundles of parallel fibers [13] that insert into the vitreous base and the posterior vitreous cortex [14, 15]. During aging, there is dissociation between vitreous collagen fibrils and HA resulting in the simultaneous breakdown of the gel and an increase in the liquid volume. By ages 80–90, more than half of the gel has liquefied (synchisis), which destabilizes the vitreous body and predisposes to collapse (syneresis). If there is concurrent and sufficient weakening of vitreo-retinal adhesion, then there is complete separation of the posterior vitreous cortex away from the retina beginning posteriorly and extending peripherally with displacement of liquid vitreous between the posterior vitreous cortex and the retina, known as PVD.

14.4 Anomalous Posterior Vitreous Detachment (PVD)

PVD occurs without complications when there is sufficient weakening of vitreo-retinal adhesion to permit innocuous separation of vitreous from the retina. Insufficient weakening of vitreo-retinal adhesion to allow dehiscence at the vitreo-retinal interface during collapse (syneresis) of the liquefied vitreous body results in anomalous PVD [3]. The consequences of anomalous PVD are variable, depending on where vitreous is most firmly adherent to the retina, and perhaps also depending on where the gel vitreous is most liquefied and unstable (Fig. 14.4).

Both genetic and acquired causes can lead to an imbalance between the degree of vitreous liquefaction and vitreo-retinal adhesion. Inborn errors of collagen metabolism that underlie disorders such as Marfan's, Ehlers-Danlos, and Stickler's syndromes result in considerable gel liquefaction at an early age when vitreo-retinal adherence is still strong. Anomalous PVD in these cases results in large posterior tears that are typical of these conditions. Myopic vitreopathy [16] is also characterized by vitreous liquefaction at a relatively young age when anomalous PVD causes an increased incidence of rhegmatogenous retinal detachment that is directly proportional to the degree of myopia [5, 16].

Anomalous PVD can have a variety of untoward effects on the macula, depending on whether or not there is persistent vitreo-papillary adhesion (VPA) and whether the vitreous, which remains attached to the retina, is of full-thickness or partial-thickness (Fig. 14.4). If there is persistent attachment to the optic disc, the vector of forces may be more tangential resulting in conditions such as macular holes (MHs). If there is no persistent attachment to the optic disc, the vector of forces may be more axial resulting in conditions like the vitreo-macular traction syndrome.

In cases of anomalous PVD with a split in the posterior vitreous cortex, known as vitreoschisis, the outermost layer of the split posterior vitreous cortex remains attached to the macula [6, 11]. The exact level of the split within the cortex might also be important. If the split occurs in the anterior region of the posterior vitreous cortex, hyalocytes will remain in the layer of vitreous that is still attached to the inner retina while the remainder of the vitreous collapses anteriorly. The result is a relatively thick, hypercellular membrane that is attached to the macula. The hyalocytes in these membranes can produce a considerable degree of tangential contraction mediated by the collagen fibers of the posterior vitreous cortex. If the split occurs in the posterior region of the posterior vitreous cortex (sometimes called the "hyaloid"), then only a thin, hypocellular sheet of vitreous will remain

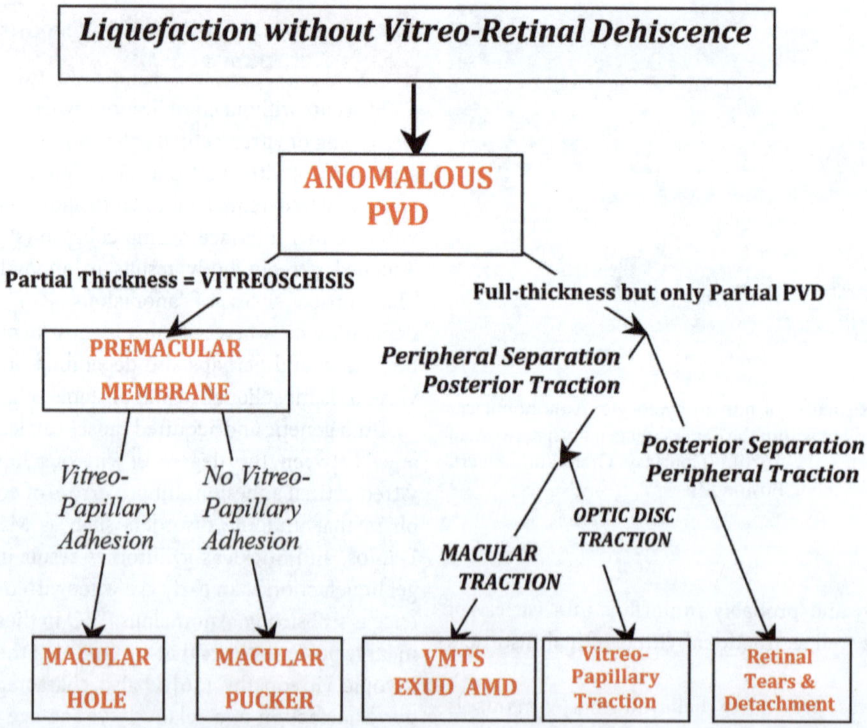

Fig. 14.4 The unifying concept of anomalous PVD. This flowchart demonstrates the various possible manifestations of anomlaous PVD. When gel liquefaction and weakening of vitreo-retinal adhesion occur concurrently, the vitreous separates away from the retina without untoward sequelae. If the separation of vitreous from retina is full-thickness (no splitting of either vitreous or the internal limiting lamina of the retina) but incomplete, there can be different topographic forms of partial PVD (*right side of flowchart*). Posterior separation with persistent peripheral vitreo-retinal attachment can induce retinal breaks and detachments. Peripheral vitreo-retinal separation with persistent full-thickness attachment of vitreous to the retina posteriorly can induce traction on the macula, known as the VMTS. This phenomenon also appears to be highly associated with exudative AMD, while total PVD appears to promote dry AMD. Persistent attachment to the optic disc can induce vitreo-papillopathies and also contribute to neovascularization and vitreous hemorrhage in ischemic retinopathies.
If during PVD, the posterior vitreous cortex splits (vitreoschisis), there can be different effects, depending on the level of the split (left side of flowchart). Vitreoschisis anterior to the level of the hyalocytes leaves a relatively thick, cellular membrane attached to the macula. Inward (centripetal) contraction of this membrane induces macular pucker (MP). If the split occurs at a level posterior to the hyalocytes, the remaining premacular membrane is relatively thin and hypocellular. Persitent vitreo-papillary adhesion (VPA) can produce outward (centrifugal) tangential traction from the fovea and induce a macular hole (MH)

adherent to the macula. This may or may not be pathogenic, depending on whether or not there is persistent vitreous attachment to the optic disc [17].

14.5 Spectral-Domain OCT (SD-OCT)

As previously mentioned, imaging vitreous has been a challenge in the past because it is "designed" to be invisible [4, 18, 19]. Since its development over 15 years ago, optical coherence tomography (OCT) has become a widely used imaging modality for retinal disorders. This optical signal acquisition device allows high-resolution cross-sectional structural imaging of the eye analogous to ultrasound B-scan imaging. The principle of OCT is based on low coherence interferometry, which uses diode laser light in the near-infrared spectrum (810 nm) to illuminate the retina. By comparing the reflected light from the retina and the light from the reference mirror, images of the retina can be created. In the time domain, OCT/SLO has provided useful insights into vitreo-retinal interface pathology by imaging in the coronal plane [20]. However, all time-domain OCT instruments have had insufficient resolution to extensively image the vitreo-retinal interface longitudinally.

In spectral domain OCT (SD-OCT), a spectrometer in the detection arm of the interferometer measures the interference pattern in the spectrum of reflected light, which is converted to depth information by Fourier analysis. A higher sensitivity and faster speed of acquisition allow for detection of weaker signals, and higher-resolution imaging of the vitreo-retinal interface is made possible.

14.5.1 SD-OCT/SLO

In the scanning laser ophthalmoscope (SLO), a single wavelength of laser light is used to illuminate the retina one spot at a time, enabling dynamic inspection in vivo, features tremendous depth of field, and offers real-time recording of findings. While the SLO has improved visualization of pre-papillary and pre-macular vitreous, it has not enhanced visualization of the vitreo-retinal interface, probably due to limited resolution.

The spectral domain OCT/SLO (SD-OCT/SLO) combines the longitudinal scans of the retina and the vitreo-retinal interface obtained by OCT with surface imaging of the retina acquired by SLO. Because there is point-to-point correspondence between the two imaging modalities, combining both the OCT and the SLO enables integration of the OCT scans with the retinal surface landmarks and enhanced visualization of the vitreo-retinal interface. Imaging in the coronal (so-called "en face") plane enables a unique perspective, since it provides the same orientation as during ophthalmoscopy and fundus photography, but with much higher resolution.

14.6 Vitreo-Maculopathies

Changes at the vitreo-retinal interface can subject the macula to both untoward physiologic and pathologic effects, which may eventually evolve into serious maculopathies.

14.6.1 Macular Pucker (MP)

MP is characterized by an avascular, fibrocellular, premacular membrane that causes folds and striae in the inner retina underneath the membrane. A milder form, sometimes called cellophane maculopathy, is characterized by a thin, transparent membrane, which is usually asymptomatic as it does not produce distortion of the inner retina. MP, on the other hand, features contraction of the premacular membrane with irregular distortions of the underlying macula and retinal vasculature. MP is bilateral in 20–30% of cases [21–23] and is usually found in individuals over 50. The incidence in women is higher than that in men. Presenting symptoms include metamorphopsia and loss of visual acuity.

PVD is present in approximately 90% of cases, suggesting a role in the etiology of pre-retinal membrane formation and MP. One hypothesis describes that PVD produces breaks in the inner retina that allow the migration of glial cells from the retina, which form the premacular membranes. While this may occur, it is not necessary to invoke a break in the retina as the source of cells that migrate and proliferate at the vitreo-retinal interface. Matrix metalloproteinases are synthesized and released by cells, enabling them to migrate across structures like the internal limiting lamina of the retina. An alternate hypothesis states that the PVD in patients with MP is anomalous, insofar as there can be splitting of the posterior vitreous cortex, known as vitreoschisis (Fig. 14.5) [6, 11].

In MP, the plane of this split is most likely anterior to the level of the hyalocytes, leaving these cells embedded within a relatively thick premacular membrane. As members of

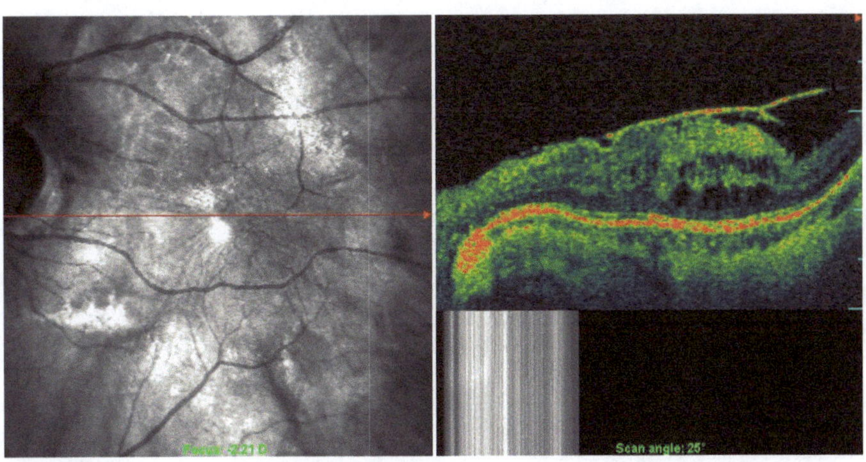

Fig. 14.5 Combined OCT/SLO of vitreoschisis in MP. The SLO image to the left demonstrates MP. A split in the posterior vitreous cortex is demonstrated in the OCT image to the right. Note the outer layer of the split still remains adherent to the retina, which has many folds as a result of centripetal (*inward*) tangential traction

the reticulo-endothelial system, hyalocytes act as "sentinel cells" and are responsible for antigen processing as well as eliciting monocyte migration from the circulatory system. Glial and RPE cells are exposed to the cytokines and growth factors elaborated by hyalocytes and also participate (perhaps as innocent bystanders) in the process of proliferative vitreo-retinal membrane formation [24]. This most likely accounts for the hypercellularity of premacular membranes in MP. Hyalocytes have also been shown to be capable of inducing membrane contraction [25], another important component in the pathophysiology of MP. Thus, following anomalous PVD with vitreoschisis, the remnant hyalocytes can induce cell migration and proliferation as well as collagen contraction, all important features of macular MP.

Recent studies using OCT/SLO detected multifocal retinal contraction in nearly half of eyes with MP (Fig. 14.6) [20]. In this investigation, multifocal retinal contraction was associated with more intraretinal cysts and macular edema than unifocal MP, suggesting that multifocality may cause greater retinal damage, possibly due to greater amounts of tangential traction. Another feature that has been found to be associated with the formation of intraretinal cysts in MP is VPA (Fig. 14.7). In that study [17], a higher incidence of intraretinal cysts was found in eyes with MP and VPA (80%) when compared with those having MP without VPA (4.3%), suggesting that VPA may

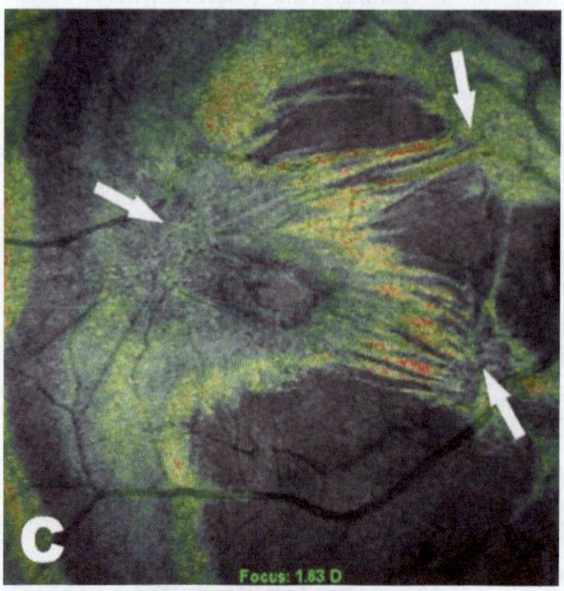

Fig. 14.6 Multifocal retinal contraction in MP. The coronal plane OCT image shows three centers of retinal contraction. Studies have shown that nearly half of eyes with MP have multifocality on coronal plane imaging. The number of contraction centers also appears to correlate with the degree of retinal damage, possibly secondary to greater tractional force

contribute to intraretinal cyst formation by providing an anchor for the forces of tangential traction on the macula.

14.6.2 Macular Hole (MH)

Macular hole (MH) is characterized by a full-thickness defect of the neural retina in the center of the macula. Most cases are unilateral, but 10–20% of patients can be affected bilaterally. Presenting symptoms include central visual distortion, central scotomas, and loss of visual acuity. The prevalence of MH has been reported to be 1:3,300, usually affecting patients in the 6th and 7th decades of life [26]. The incidence in women is twice as high as in men [27]. SD-OCT/SLO is particularly helpful in identifying and staging MH as it provides precise in vivo measurement of MH diameter as well as accurate characterization of the vitreo-macular interface.

The cause of MH is not known. Gass described four stages based on biomicroscopic observations [28–30]. In a stage 1 MH, the retina is believed to be intact without neural retinal defect or vitreo-foveal separation. Oblique vitreous traction on the fovea has been speculated to be the initial mechanism. Stage 1 MH can be further divided into stage 1a and stage 1b, the former characterized by a small central yellow spot representing cystic changes within the fovea [31]. Tangential vitreous traction on the fovea may cause elevation of the fovea, foveal detachment, and an increase in the xanthophyllic pigment. A yellow ring in the foveal area with a bridging interface characterizes stage 1b MH. An MH progresses to stage 2 when the vitreofoveal separation occurs. Recently, it has been proposed that perifoveal vitreous detachment is the primary pathogenic event in MH formation [32]. A stage 2 MH is characterized by a central or eccentric full thickness retinal defect (100–300 μm) with or without an overlying pseudo-operculum. Unlike stage 1 MH, most stage 2 holes will advance to stage 3 as a result of persistent vitreo-foveal traction. Stage 3 MH is characterized by a central round full-thickness retinal defect (350–600 μm) associated with a gray ring surrounding the hole (previously believed to be a cuff of subretinal fluid), yellow deposits, and cystic changes. A stage 4 MH is distinguished from a stage 3 MH by a complete PVD.

Recent studies have identified vitreoschisis (Fig. 14.8) in 53% of eyes with MH. The vectors of force that induce tangential vitreo-retinal traction most likely result from anomalous PVD, but there may also be a contribution from persistent adhesion of vitreous to the optic disc. Studies [17] have shown that VPA is far more prevalent in MH (87.5%) than lamellar hole (LH) (36.4%) and MP (17.9%), suggesting that persistent adhesion at the disc

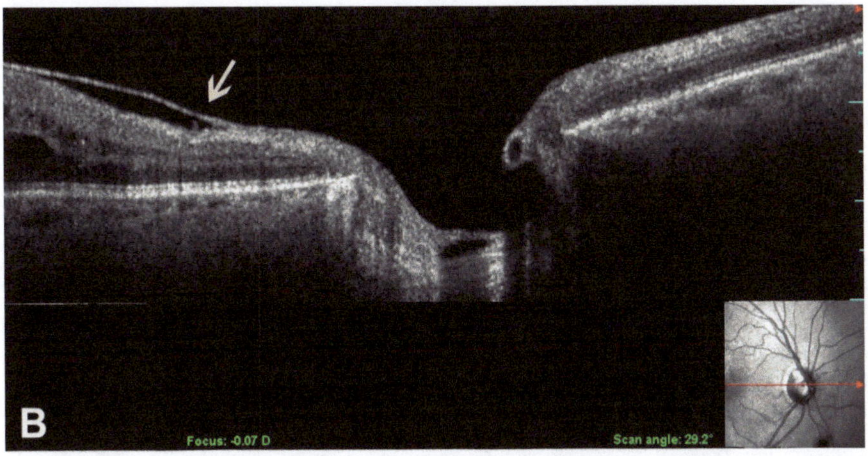

Fig. 14.7 VPA in MP. The presence of VPA in MP has been associated with a higher incidence of intraretinal cysts, most likely due to tangential traction exerted by the persistent adhesion of vitreous to the optic disc. The longitudinal OCT/SLO image demonstrates persistent vitreous attachment at the margin of the optic disc

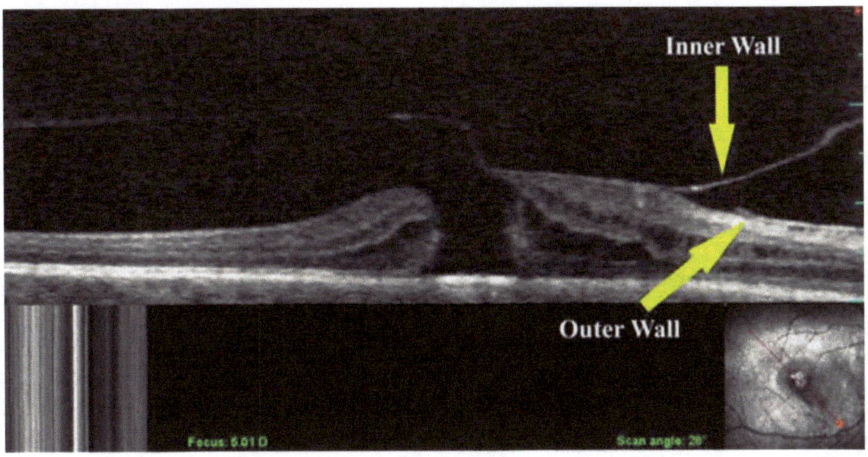

Fig. 14.8 Vitreoschisis in MH. Studies have shown that about half of patients with MH have vitreoschisis. In this OCT/SLO scan of an eye with a stage 3 MH, the inner wall is anterior and the outer wall is posterior, attached to the inner surface of the retina (*arrow*)

may contribute to the hole formation. While anomalous PVD with vitreoschisis may be the initial event in the pathophysiology of both MH and MP, VPA could influence the vector of forces and subsequent course of pathology. Persistent traction at the disc provides an anchor for outward (centrifugal) tangential traction, resulting in central retinal dehiscence and MH development (Fig. 14.9). In the absence of VPA, inward (centripetal) tangential traction is more likely and will result in MP.

In recent years, vitrectomy with membrane peel and air-fluid exchange has become a successful treatment for MH, with a very high (85–100%) reported closure rate [33, 34]. Intraoperative findings and histological analyses have determined that these membranes are thin and hypocellular. This is consistent with the hypothesis that if anomalous PVD and vitreoschisis play a role in MH pathogenesis, then the split most likely occurs posterior to the level of the hyalocytes embedded in the posterior vitreous cortex [11]. These cells separate away from the retina along with the anterior portion of the posterior vitreous cortex, leaving the thinner, hypocellular portion attached to the macula. Persistent attachment of vitreous to the optic disc (found in 87.5% of cases) somehow influences the tangential forces that open a dehiscence in the central macula (Fig. 14.9).

Another interesting feature that was demonstrated by coronal plane imaging with combined OCT/SLO was that 40% of subjects with MH also have eccentric MP. Thus, the level of the split, which occurs during anomalous PVD with vitreoschisis, may not be the same in all MP

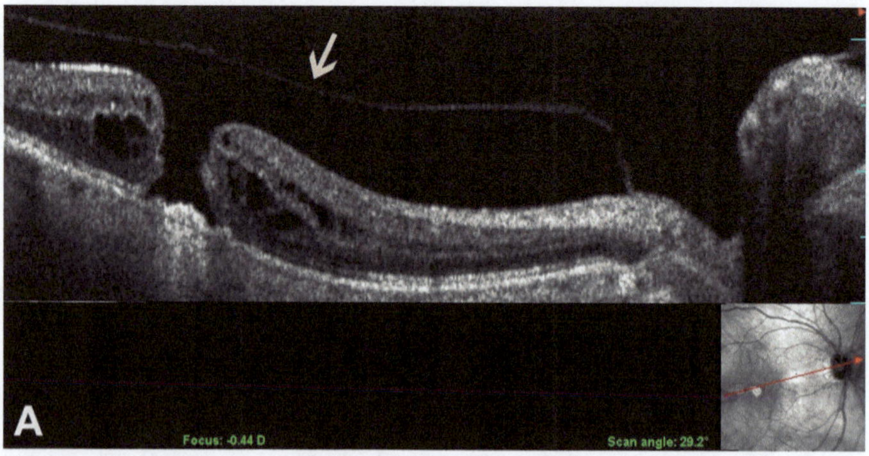

Fig. 14.9 VPA in MH. Persistent VPA has been shown to play a role in MH formation, possibly by providing ananchor for a centrifugal tangential traction. The detachment of posterior vitreous cortex (arrow) and persistent adhesion to the optic disc are shown

can develop. Studies [11] have shown that the membranes inducing pucker in eyes with MH are smaller in diameter and farther from the center of the macula than eyes with MP alone.

14.6.2.1 Lamellar Hole (LH)

LH is characterized by a thin, irregular fovea and avulsion of inner layers of the central macula. SD-OCT/SLO has proven useful in the diagnosis of LHs, which have characteristic configuration on the longitudinal scans (Fig. 14.10). Clinically, patients may retain relatively good visual acuity but in some instances surgery is indicated for distortions and loss of visual acuity.

LH is believed to result from an abortive process of MH formation, although this is by no means certain. Foveal cysts are believed to be the precursors of either full-thickness MH or LH. Indeed, a recent study [17] confirmed the presence of intraretinal cysts in both MH and LH. Interestingly, a higher prevalence of cysts was found in MH (100%) than LH (54.5%) and MP (17.9%). Similar to what was previously described for MP, VPA seems to play a role in the formation of cysts in LH as well. LH with VPA had cysts in 50% of cases, while LH without VPA only had cysts in only 20% of cases.

Based on all the aforementioned findings, it would appear that VPA is important in some, but not all vitreomaculopathies. Indeed, these diseases can be grouped according to the prevalence of VPA (in descending order) as: MH with cysts (87.5%), MP with cysts (80%), LH with cysts (50%), LH without cysts (20%), and MP without cysts (4.3%) (Fig. 14.11) [17]. Regarding intraretinal cysts, there appears to be a similar distribution with 100% prevalence in MH with VPA, 80% in MP with VPA, 75% in LH with VPA, 42.9% of LH without VPA, and 4.3% of MP without VPA (Fig. 14.12) [35]. Thus, VPA appears to be an important factor in the pathophysiology of vitreomaculopathies, probably by influencing the vector of forces at the vitreo-retinal interface.

14.6.3 Age-Related Macular Degeneration (AMD)

The etiology of AMD is multifactorial. Risk factors include age, family history, ethnicity, cardiovascular diseases, hypertension, and cigarette smoking. AMD can be subdivided into two patterns: (a) atrophic, dry, or nonexudative AMD and (b) neovascular, wet, or exudative AMD. Dry AMD is by far the most common type, characterized by drusen and geographic atrophy. Wet AMD is characterized by neovascularization with edema and sometimes hemorrhage, causing severe vision loss. While it is known that neovascularization arises from the choriocapillaris through breaks in the Bruch's membrane, the stimuli and true cause(s) for exudative AMD are not known.

Recent studies [36] employing ultrasound and OCT have shown that persistent vitreo-macular adhesion is more prevalent in exudative AMD (Fig. 14.13), whereas a higher prevalence of complete PVD was found in eyes with dry AMD. This suggests that vitreo-macular adhesion may be a risk factor for choroidal neovascularization and exudative changes in AMD, whereas PVD may be protective against exudative AMD. Subsequent studies confirmed these findings [37, 42] and determined that these phenomena are only important during active AMD and not in end stages such as geographic atrophy and disciform macular scarring. Furthermore, these studies showed that genetics

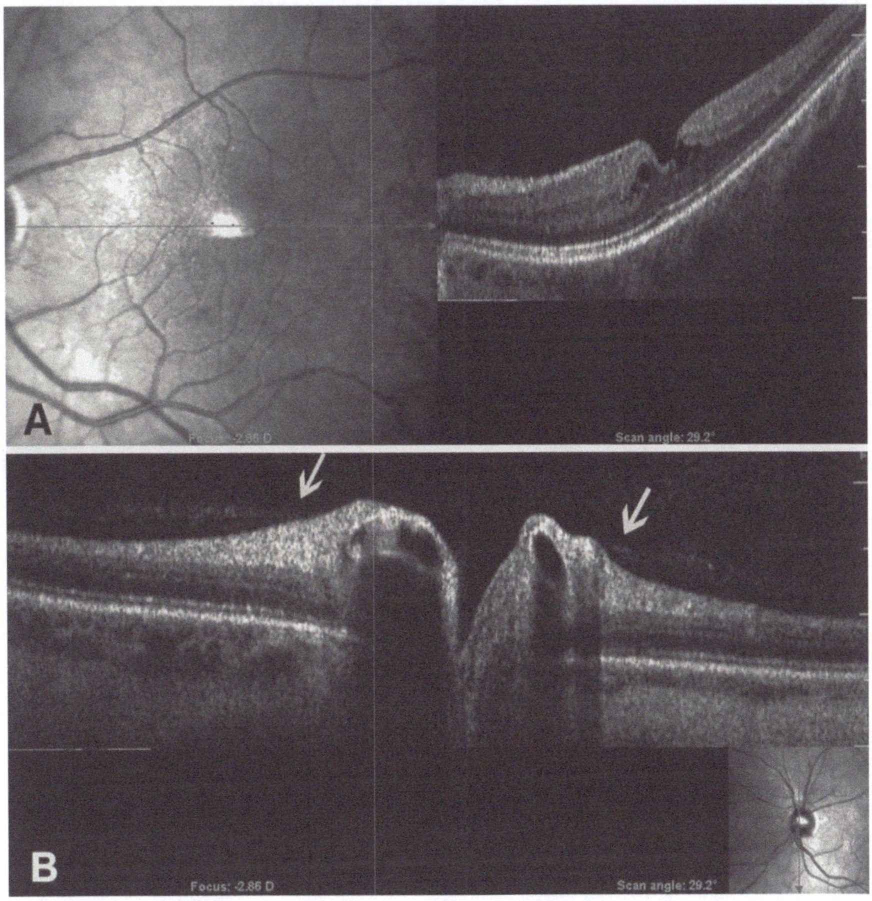

Fig. 14.10 SD-OCT/SLO imaging of lamellar hole (LH). Combined spectral domain OCT/SLO imaging of LH demonstrates intraretinal cysts (**a**) and vitreous adhesion to the margins of the optic disc (**b**)

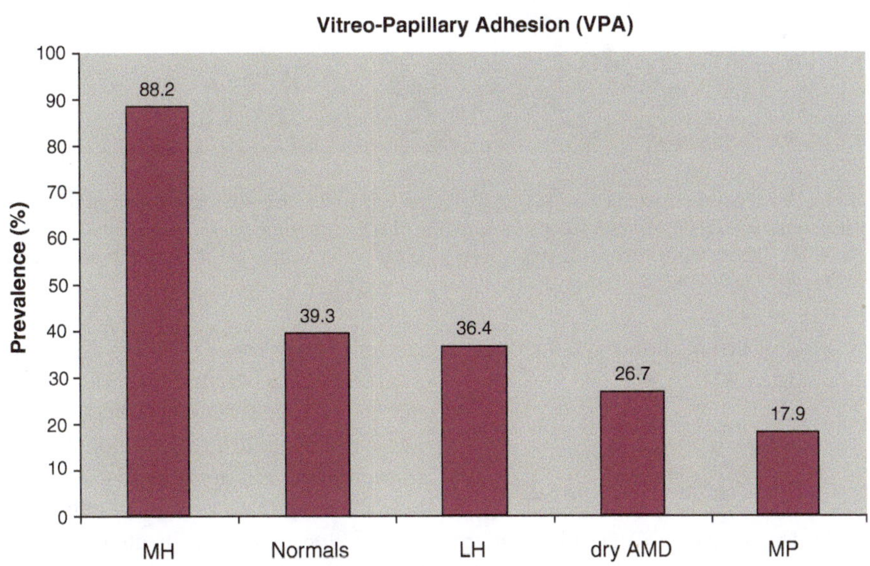

Fig. 14.11 The prevalence of VPA in vitreo-maculopathies. The prevalence of VPA is highest in MH with cysts, followed by MP with cysts, LH with cysts, LH without cysts, and lowest in MP without cysts. Hence, VPA appears to play an important role in certain vitreo-maculopathies but not others

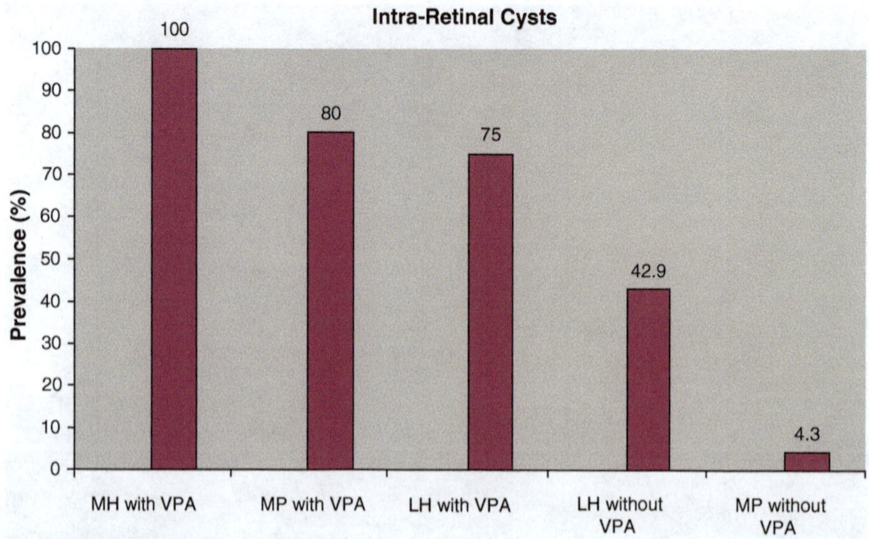

Fig. 14.12 The prevalence of intraretinal cysts in vitreo-maculopathies. The prevalence of intraretinal cysts is highest in MH with VPA, followed by MP with VPA, LH with VPA, LH without VPA, and MP without VPA. That the prevalence distribution of intraretinal cysts in various vitreo-maculopathies is similar to that of VPA suggests that VPA may influence the vectors of tractional force and cyst formation

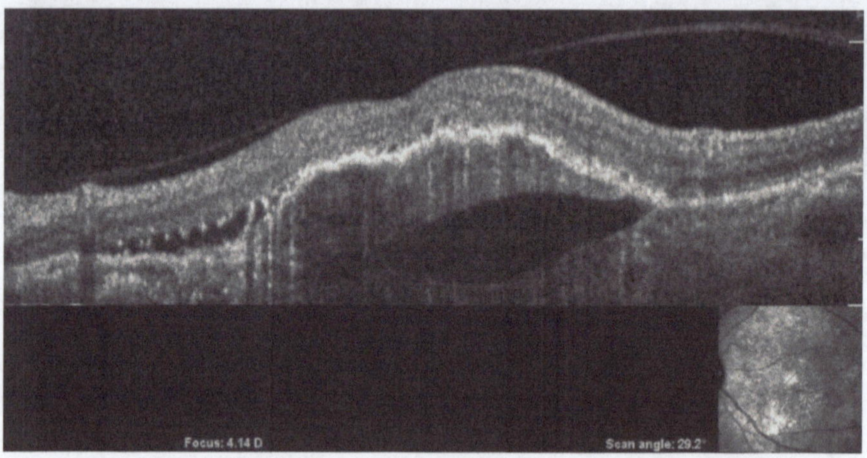

Fig. 14.13 Vitreo-macular adhesion in exudative AMD. A higher prevalence of vitreo-macular adhesion was found in exudative age-related macular degeneration (AMD) when compared with dry AMD, suggesting that vitreo-macular adhesion may be a risk factor for exudative AMD. The posterior vitreous cortex is seen attached to the macula in the area of choroidal neovascularization in this SD-OCT/SLO scan

and environmental factors do not appear to influence the role of vitreous in exudative AMD.

14.6.4 Vitreo-Macular Traction Syndrome (VMTS)

VMTS is characterized by anomalous PVD with persistent vitreous adhesion to the macula, resulting in macular thickening, edema, and decreased visual acuity. VMTS is more prevalent in women than in men, and usually occurs in the sixth and seventh decade of life. Spontaneous resolution may occur following complete PVD, but cell proliferation has been implicated as a possible mechanism that may hinder PVD [38]. VMTS is distinguished from MP in that there are no corrugations in the retina, since the traction is axial and not tangential. At times, this axial traction is so severe that it elevates the central retina (Fig. 14.14). Presenting symptoms are predominantly decreased central vision with less metamorphopsia than in patients with MP. The other distinguishing feature is that VMTS features full-thickness vitreous attachment to the macula, in contrast to MP where vitreoschisis splits the posterior vitreous cortex

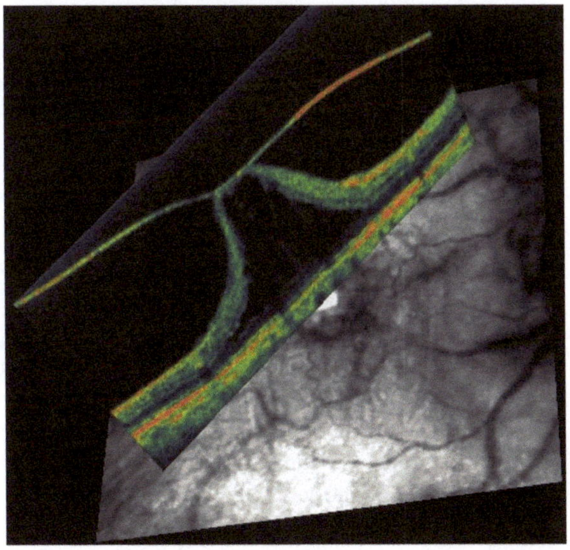

Fig. 14.14 Posterior vitreous adhesion in VMTS. Vitreomacular traction syndrome (VMTS) results from peripheral PVD with persistent (anomalous) vitreous adhesion to the macula. There is full-thickness (i.e., no vitreoschisis) posterior vitreous adhesion to the macula inducing such significant traction that the result is a tractional retinal detachment

leaving the outer layer of the vitreous cortex (partial thickness) still attached to the macula.

There is a broad, full-thickness posterior vitreous adhesion in VMTS, while a more focal adhesion is found in the vitreo-foveal traction syndrome (VFTS). In both instances, there is peripheral vitreo-retinal separation but persistent adhesion at the macula. The tractional forces are primarily antero-posterior, inducing retinal thickening with edema in the VMTS and a central cyst in the VFTS. There is most likely no role for vitreoschisis or VPA in VMTS or VFTS, although VPA has not been studied in this group of individuals.

Summary for the Clinician

- Owing to its *intended* transparency, vitreous has been difficult to image and thus overlooked as important in retinal disease. Recent advances in the understanding of vitreous biochemistry, structure, and aging have forged the unifying concept of anomalous PVD. Combined SD-OCT/SLO has enabled imaging of the vitreo-retinal interface and elucidated the pathogenic mechanisms of vitreomacular disorders, including vitreoschisis. This enhanced understanding will improve current surgical therapeutics and in the future replace surgery with pharmacologic vitreolysis.

14.7 Conclusion

Anomalous PVD is a unifying concept of vitreo-retinal diseases that brings together conditions that were previously considered disparate in origin. This perspective not only contributes to our understanding of the pathogenic mechanisms in vitreo-retinal disorders, but could also influence therapeutic approaches. The advent of SD-OCT/SLO has enabled in vivo visualization of various diseases, and thus our understanding of pathophysiology is increasingly elucidated, and better treatments are being developed. One of the most exciting of these new modalities is pharmacologic vitreolysis [39–41, 43]. To date, this approach has been largely used as a surgical adjunct, but the future will see more preventative applications in high-risk individuals. For example, pharmacologic vitreolysis may be an effective way to lower the risk of exudative changes by inducing innocuous liquefaction of the gel and concurrent dehiscence at the vitreo-macular interface. Future studies using SD-OCT/SLO and other advanced imaging technologies will hopefully identify individuals at risk of other vitreo-retinopathies as candidates for prophylactic PVD with pharmacologic vitreolysis.

References

1. Bishop PN (2000) Structural macromolecules and supramolecular organization of the vitreous gel. Prog Retin Eye Res 19:323–344
2. Scott JE, Chen Y, Brass A (1992) Secondary and tertiary structures involving chondroitin and chondroitin sulphate in solution, investigated by rotary shadowing electron microscopy and computer simulation. Eur J Biochem 209:675–680
3. Sebag J (2004) Anomalous posterior vitreous detachment: a unifying concept in vitreo-retinal disease. Graefes Arch Clin Exp Ophthalmol 242:690–698
4. Sebag J (1992) The vitreous. In: Hart WM Jr (ed) Adler's physiology of the eye. Mosby, St. Louis, pp 268–347
5. Sebag J, Yee KM (2009) Vitreous – from biochemistry to clinical relevance. In: Tasman W, Jaeger EA (eds) Duane's ophthalmology. Lippincott Williams & Wilkins, Philadelphia, Chapter 16
6. Sebag J (2008) Vitreoschisis. Graefes Arch Clin Exp Ophthalmol 246:329–332
7. Sebag J (1989) The vitreous – structure, function and pathobiology. Springer, New York
8. Nishitsuka K, Kashiwagi Y, Tojo N et al (2007) Hyaluronan production regulation from porcine hyalocyte cell line by cytokines. Exp Eye Res 85:539–545
9. Sebag J, Hageman GS (2000) Vitreo-retinal interface. In: Sebag J, Hageman GS (ed) Interfaces. Fondazione G.B. Bietti, Rome, pp 41–58

10. Green WR, Sebag J (2001) Vitreous and the vitreo-retinal interface. In: Ryan SJ (ed) Retina. Mosby, St. Louis, pp 1882–1960
11. Sebag J, Gupta P, Rosen RR et al (2007) Macular holes and macular pucker: the role of vitreoschisis as imaged by optical coherence tomography/scanning laser ophthalmoscopy. Trans Am Ophthalmol Soc 105:121–129
12. Sebag J (1991) Age-related differences in the human vitreoretinal interface. Arch Ophthalmol 109:966–971.
13. Sebag J, Balazs EA (1989) Morphology and ultrastructure of human vitreous fibers. Invest Ophthalmol Vis Sci 30: 1867–1871
14. Sebag J (1987) Ageing of the vitreous. Eye 1:254–262
15. Sebag J (1987) Age-related changes in human vitreous structure. Graefes Arch Clin Exp Ophthalmol 225:89–93
16. Nguyen N, Sebag J (2005) Myopic vitreopathy – significance in anomalous PVD and vitreo-retinal disorders. In: Midena E (ed) Myopia and related diseases. Ophthalmic Communications Society, New York, pp 137–145
17. Wang MY, Nguyen D, Hindoyan N, Sadun AA (2009) Vitreo-papillary adhesion in macular hole and macular pucker. Retina 29:644–650
18. Sebag J (2004) Seeing the invisible: the challenge of imaging vitreous. J Biomed Opt 9:38–46
19. Sebag J (2008) To see the invisible: the quest of imaging vitreous. Dev Ophthalmol 42:5–28
20. Gupta P, Sadun AA, Sebag J (2008) Multifocal retinal contraction in macular pucker analyzed by combined optical coherence tomography/scanning laser ophthalmoscopy. Retina 28:447–452
21. Miyazaki M, Nakamura H, Kubo M et al (2003) Prevalence and risk factors for epiretinal membranes in a Japanese population: the Hisayama Study. Graefes Arch Clin Exp Ophthalmol 241:642–646
22. Roth AM, Foos RY (1971) Surface wrinkling retinopathy in eyes enucleated at autopsy. Trans Am Acad Ophthalmol Otolaryngol 75:1047–1058
23. Wise GN (1975) Clinical features of idiopathic preretinal macular fibrosis. Am J Ophthalmol 79:349–357
24. Kita T, Hata Y, Kano K et al (2007) Transforming growth factor-beta2 and connective tissue growth factor in proliferative vitreoretinal diseases: possible involvement of hyalocytes and therapeutic potential of Rho kinase inhibitor. Diabetes 56:231–238
25. Hirayama K, Hata Y, Noda Y et al (2004) The involvement of the rho-kinase pathway and its regulation in cytokine-induced collagen gel contraction by hyalocytes. Invest Ophthalmol Vis Sci 45:3896–3903
26. Ezra E (2001) Idiopathic full thickness macular hole: natural history and pathogenesis. Br J Ophthalmol 85:102–108
27. Tashimo A, Mitamura Y, Ohtsuka K et al (2003) Macular hole formation following ruptured retinal arterial macroaneurysm. Am J Ophthalmol 135:487–492
28. Gass JD (1988) Idiopathic senile macular hole: its early stages and pathogenesis. Arch Ophthalmol 106:629–639
29. Gass JD (1995) Reappraisal of biomicroscopic classification of stage of development of a macular hole. Arch Ophthalmol 119:752–759
30. Johnson RN, Gass JD (1988) Idiopathic macular holes: observations, stages of formation, and implications for surgical intervention. Ophthalmology 95:917–924
31. Kokame GT (1995) Clinical correlation of ultrasonographic findings in macular holes. Am J Ophthalmol 119:441–451
32. Johnson MW, Van Newkirk MR, Meyer KA (2001) Perifoveal vitreous detachment is the primary pathogenic event in idiopathic macular hole formation. Arch Ophthalmol 119:215–222
33. DaMata AP, Burk SE, Foster RE et al (2004) Long-term follow-up of indocyanine green assisted peeling of the retinal internal limiting membrane during vitrectomy surgery for idiopathic macular hole repair. Ophthalmology 111:2246–2253
34. Smiddy WE, Feuer W, Cordahi G (2001) Internal limiting membrane peeling in macular hole surgery. Ophthalmology 108:1471–1478
35. Sebag J, Wang MY, Nguyen D et al (2009) Vitreo-papillary adhesion in macular diseases. Trans Am Ophthalmol Soc 107 (in press)
36. Krebs I, Brannath W, Glittenberg C et al (2007) Posterior vitreomacular adhesion: a potential risk factor for exudative age-related macular degeneration? Am J Ophthalmol 144:741–746
37. Robison CD, Krebs I, Binder S et al (2009) Vitreomacular adhesion in active and end-stage age-related macular degeneration. Am J Ophthalmol 148:79–82
38. Smiddy WE (2009) Vitreomacular traction syndrome. In: Yanoff M, Duker JS (eds) Ophthalmology. Mosby, Philadelphia, pp 691–695
39. Sebag J (1998) Pharmacologic vitreolysis. Retina 18:1–3
40. Sebag J (2002) Is pharmacologic vitreolysis brewing? Retina 22:1–3
41. Sebag J (2005) Molecular biology of pharmacologic vitreolysis. Trans Am Ophthalmol Soc 103:473–494
42. Lee SJ, Lee CS, Koh HJ (2009) Posterior vitreomacular adhesion and risk of exudative age-related macular degeneration: paired eye study. Am J Ophthalmol 147:621–626
43. Sebag J (2009) Pharmacologic vitreolysis – premise and promise of the first decade. Retina 29:871–874

Chapter 15

Choroidal Imaging with Optical Coherence Tomography

15

Richard Spaide

Core Messages

- Commercially available contact b-scan ultrasonography units and conventional optical coherence tomography (OCT) techniques do not image the choroid well.
- If an OCT instrument is positioned closer to the eye, an inverted image is obtained that has more information from the deep choroid. Image averaging with the aid of eye tracking can improve additional improvement in the signal-to-noise ratio. This technique is known as Enhanced Depth Imaging OCT or EDI OCT.
- The subfoveal choroidal thickness in normals is about 350 μm in the young, and decreases to 250 μm in elderly people.
- Some people develop extremely thin choroids. These people have a variety of visual complaints and have what has been termed age-related choroidal atrophy (ARCA). These patients seem to have a higher glaucoma risk.
- Eyes with high myopia have choroidal thinning that varies inversely with age and amount of myopia.
- The same imaging EDI OCT technique allows visualization of the contents of pigment epithelial detachments (PEDs), which appear to have fibrovascular material filling portions or all of the space within the PED.

The choroid is an integral structure in the eye that accounts for most of the ocular blood flow [1], participates in many disease processes, and yet defies current methods of clinical examination. Commercially available contact b-scan ultrasonography can provide evidence of choroidal thickening in some disease states, but has an axial resolution of about 0.5 mm and a much lower lateral resolution. Fluorescein angiography has difficulties because of light scattering and absorption by the pigment in the retinal pigment epithelium (RPE) and choroid and by blood in the choroid. Indocyanine green (ICG) angiography is helpful in examining the vascular structures in the choroid but does not supply any cross-sectional information. Optical coherence tomography (OCT) is used to obtain cross-sectional images of the retina, but imaging of the choroid is limited in most individuals because of light scattering and absorption, as well as depth-dependent roll-off in sensitivity and resolution with increased depth imaging for spectral-domain (SD) OCT instruments. Increased visualization of the choroid is possible in albinism and the ability to visualize the depth of the choroid using OCT has been used in a grading system of ocular albinism [2]. Imaging of the choroid in nonalbinotic individuals is possible with research OCT devices that use light sources deeper in the infrared region [3]. As the consequence of the wavelength used, these instruments may have comparatively reduced resolution for retinal visualization, which may ultimately limit the clinical appeal. A new, simple, method of imaging the choroid using a conventionally available OCT device has been devised that exploits several inter-related factors to improve image quality [4].

15.1 Enhanced Depth Imaging Optical Coherence Tomography

The method of obtaining OCT sections of the choroid using conventional SD OCT is easy, but the explanation of how it works is a bit more complex. The method is to push the OCT instrument closer to the eye so that an inverted image is obtained. The inverted image contains more information from deeper depths than does the noninverted image obtained further away from the eye. The best image is obtained by keeping the inverted image as close to the top of the screen as is practical. To improve the image appearance, we can average many images together. This is best accomplished when using a device that has eye tracking, so the same location is sampled from one scan to the next. The image can be used as is, but for presentation purposes, it is re-inverted so that the orientation matches the conventional OCT sections. For the purposes of identification, this method of imaging of the choroid has been termed enhanced depth imaging optical coherence tomography (EDI OCT) [8]. An area of 5 by 30° is usually visualized with seven sections each comprised of 100 averaged scans. There are two important caveats; keep the scan image close to the top of the screen and keep the image straight. It is slightly more difficult to keep the image straight with the EDI OCT technique than with the conventional method of OCT imaging.

> **Summary for the Clinician**
>
> - The method of EDI OCT is easy. Push the instrument close enough to the eye to obtain an inverted image.
> - A useful scanning protocol is seven sections each comprised of 100 averaged scans obtained within a volume of 5 by 30°.
> - Keep the image near the top of the screen and keep the image straight.

15.2 Mechanism of Enhanced Depth Imaging

In SD OCT, the eye is illuminated with light from a broad band source. Backscattered light is combined with that from a reference arm to generate an interference signal. The depth information of the reflective source is frequency encoded such that the interferometric signals have a higher frequency with the greater path length mismatch (i.e., greater depth of origin in the object space). The information from the interferometric fringes is obtained by using a dispersive detector in which a grating is used to spread out the various frequencies onto a linear CCD (charge coupled device) detector [4–6]. Deeper objects show a larger group delay, which results in a higher frequency of the interferogram (Fig. 15.1). The magnitude and time delay of the reflection is obtained from the Fourier transform of the interferogram [4–6]. There is a decreasing sensitivity to detect signals originating from deeper depths because of decreasing visibility of higher fringe frequencies. The signal generated decreases exponentially such that the depth where a falloff of ½ is expressed by

$$\frac{\ln(2)}{\pi}\,\frac{\lambda_0^2}{\delta_s\lambda}$$

where λ_0 is the center wavelength and

$$\delta_s\lambda$$

is the full-width half-maximum spectral resolution, which is equal to one-half of the coherence length [7].

The resolved image of a reflection from an infinitely thin reflector in the object space has a finite width, as related to the axial point spread function of the OCT instrument. In reality, the Fourier transform output produces two images, one being the inverted mirror image of the other. Using convention OCT instruments, one of the equivalent images is picked to display, one in which the inner surface of the retina faces up. The magnitude of the detected reflection from elements in the object space is dependent on the path length mismatch between the sample arm and the reference arm (Fig. 15.1). Objects capable of producing equivalent reflection will not produce the same detected reflections if they differ in depth with deeper objects producing lower signals (Fig. 15.2). There are other related factors as to why images from deeper depths have poorer image quality. The interferogram is not sampled evenly in k-space and the analog to digital conversion limits the dynamic range of the signal [8]. These factors contribute to decreasing sensitivity and resolution with increasing group delay that is not amenable to postprocessing [8].

Most commercial OCT instruments image a depth of approximately 2 mm, although the image quality varies substantially over that range because of the falloff of sensitivity as shown in Fig. 15.2. In presenting the image, histogram stretching and other image processing techniques function to increase the gain on the acquired signal. This is analogous to turning up the volume of a radio when listening to a distant radio station. The radio sounds louder and so does the signal, but increasing the volume increases static as well. The ratio of signal to noise is not altered by changing the volume control. In a similar sense, increasing the brightness of the image also increases the apparent noise in Fig. 15.2d. The peak sensitivity of SD OCT instruments is conventionally located in the posterior vitreous. This affords high sensitivity to detecting vitreous abnormalities, particularly vitreoretinal interface abnormalities. However, the sensitivity to signals originating from the choroid is decreased.

A strategy to overcome these limitations would be to push the instrument closer to the eye so that the peak sensitivity would be located at the outer sclera border (Fig. 15.3). Potentially confounding images from the orbit

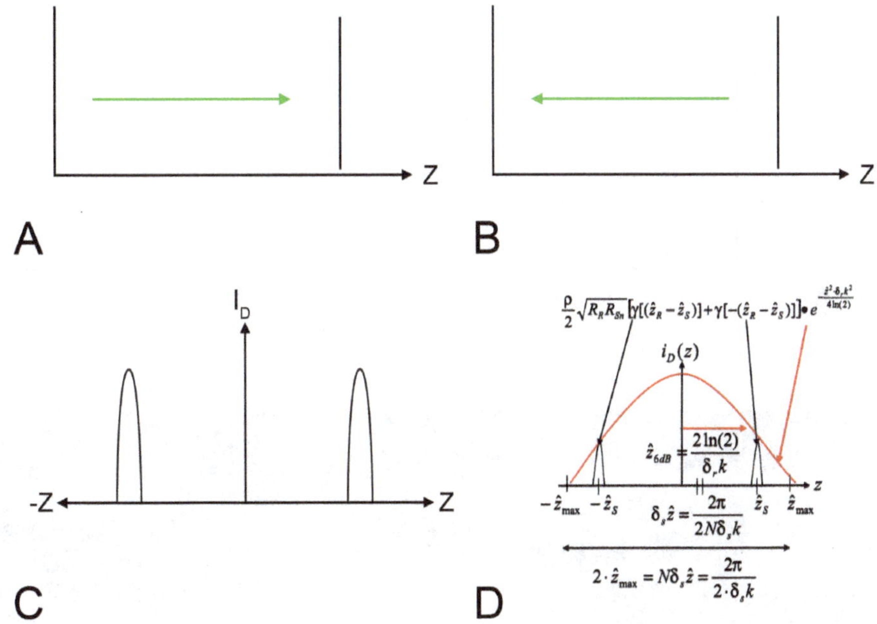

Fig. 15.1 Production of depth-resolved signal. (**a**) In the sample arm, light is directed to potential reflectors, as shown by the line, and the reflected light returns to the detector. (**b**) The detected light is compared with light from a reference arm and the reflectivity and position in depth of the reflector is determined from Fourier analysis of the interferometric fringes. (**c**) The output of the Fourier transform is the mirror image version of the same image, with one being inverted (as denoted by the *negative sign*). In practice, only one of the two mirror images is shown. (**d**) The sensitivity of spectral-domain image detection varies with object depth as shown. The *red curve* shows the maximal signal level that could be detected from a reflector as a function of depth. The interferometric signal is determined from the cross-correlation between the field of the reference arm (R_R) and the sample arm (R_{Sn}), the difference between the optical path length of the reference arm ($\hat{z}_R$) and the sample arm ($\hat{z}_S$), *N* is the number of samples, δ_s is the thickness of the sample, and k is the wavenumber. (**d**) is derived from Fig. 2.9 in ref [7].

are not imaged, presumably because of the exponential decrease in light penetration as would be expected from the Beer-Lambert law, but from the even more prominent loss of coherence information from not only light loss, but light scattering. By placing the peak sensitivity closer to the region of the choroid, a relative gain in sensitivity is obtained when compared with the conventional mode of imaging. The contents of the eye would create the mirror images as previously described. However, the OCT instrument appears to only show the inverted image. The signal-to-noise ratio is further enhanced with image averaging. For noise that follows a random Poisson distribution, such as shot noise or thermal noise, the reduction in noise is related to the square root in the number of images averaged. The reduction in other forms of noise, specifically speckle noise, is more complicated. Speckle noise originates from the same source as the signal, namely subwavelength reflectors within the tissue. If these subwavelength reflectors are spaced such that the reflected light reaching the detector varies in phase, there is a potential to create interference. So, the reflectors are both the cause of signal and speckle, and what is called speckle "noise" is a consequence of coherence imaging. Microscopic changes in any positioning, even with eye tracking, create slightly different patterns of speckle noise, which are consequently reduced by averaging.

Summary for the Clinician

- The sensitivity of SD OCT instruments decreases with increasing depth within the image
- The peak of sensitivity is conventionally placed in the posterior vitreous for conventional OCT imaging
- In EDI OCT, the peak of the sensitivity curve is placed within the sclera. The choroid is imaged at the higher portions of the sensitivity curve
- Noise can be reduced by image averaging

15.3 Imaging the Choroid

It is possible to obtain images of the choroid with conventional OCT imaging, but the quality is generally poor. This is particularly true for OCT devices that do not have

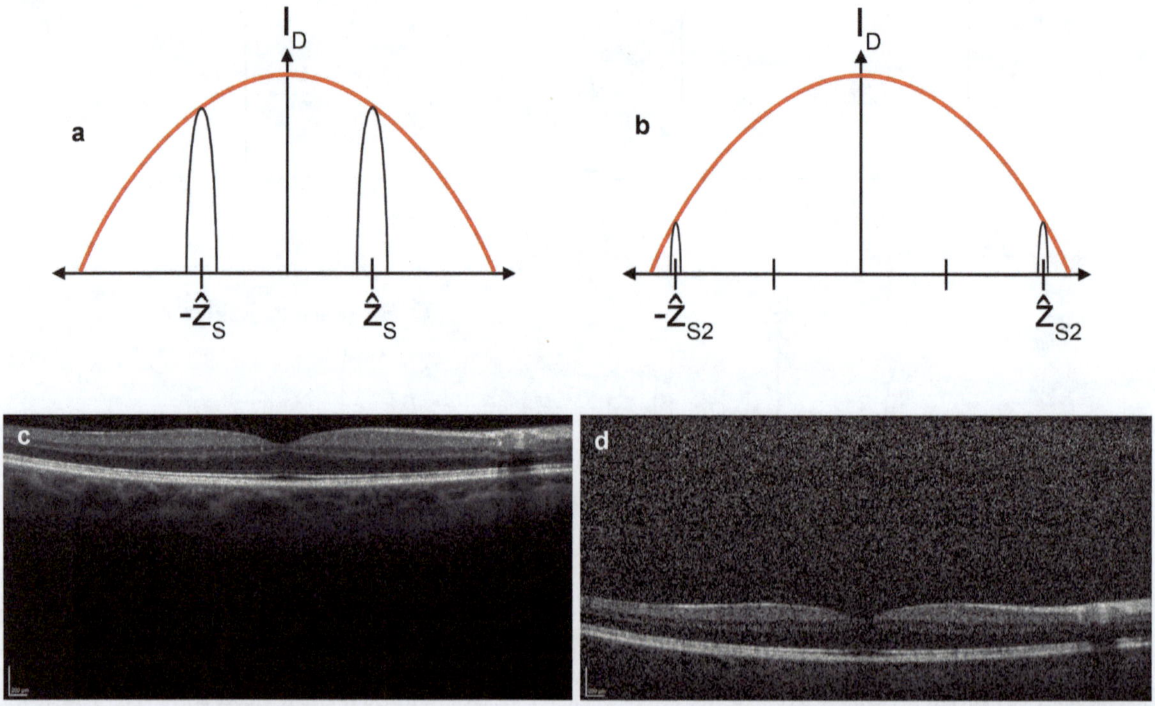

Fig. 15.2 Relationship between location and sensitivity. (**a**) Following the convention of Fig. 15.1d, the peak signal produced by a reflector displaced by distance z is shown by the symmetrically located curves at $-\hat{z}_S$ and $-\hat{z}_{S.B.}$ If the same reflector was located at a greater distance so that the mismatch in the optical path length between the reference arm was larger, the maximal detected signal would be represented by the curves at $-\hat{z}_{S2}$ and $-\hat{z}_{S2}$. Note the difference between (**a**) and (**b**) even though the reflector is the same. (**c**) This relationship can be illustrated by (**c**) and (**d**). In (**c**), the image is placed close to the top of the scanning region and consequently, the image is obtained near the top of the curve shown in (**a**). (**d**) If the image is placed near the bottom of the imaging area, the image is closer to the base of the curve as in (**b**). Because the image processing software incorporated in the OCT device tries to compensate for the weak signal by increasing the gain, the image has much more noise

eye tracking and therefore, cannot adequately perform image averaging. The increase in signal-to-noise ratio provided by the shift in the peak of the sensitivity curve coupled with the increase provided by the large number of averaged frames enables the full thickness of the choroid to be imaged without difficulty (Fig. 15.4). Since the outer edge of the choroid can be imaged similar to the posterior surface of the RPE and Bruch's membrane complex, measurements of the choroidal thickness are possible. Many of the early studies have focused on the subfoveal choroidal thickness, but other regions of the eye are measurable as well.

Measurement of the subfoveal choroidal thickness was shown to be reproducible [8]. The measurement in one eye was very similar to that found in the other eye. Later investigation of normal, nonmyopic eyes found a significant correlation between age and choroidal thickness (Fig. 15.5) [10].This study of 54 eyes found that the choroidal thickness was greatest in the subfoveal location (Fig. 15.6). The thickness of the choroid decreased rapidly in the nasal direction and less so in the temporal direction. The subfoveal choroidal thickness was 287 (standard deviation [±] 76) microns, which decreased to 145 ± 57 μm at 3 mm nasal to the fovea and 261 ± 77 μm at 3 mm temporal to the fovea. The choroidal thickness showed a negative correlation with age for the subfoveal location ($r = -0.424$; $p = 0.001$; Fig. 15.7) and at each extrafoveal location, which were measured at 0.5 mm intervals from the fovea, 3 mm nasal to 3 mm temporal. Regression analysis showed that subfoveal choroidal thickness decreased by 1.56 μm for each year of age. The decrease in thickness per year of age was 1.34 μm at 3 mm nasal to the fovea, while the constant was 210 μm. The slope of the fitted line therefore, approximated that of the subfoveal region, while there was a difference in the offset because of the inherent thinness of the more nasal measurements. Over the course of an 80-year lifespan, an average person would be expected to lose a greater proportion of the choroidal thickness of 3 mm nasal to the fovea than in the subfoveal location [10].

The choroid is a highly vascular structure with blood flow and thickness varying in relation to the intraocular

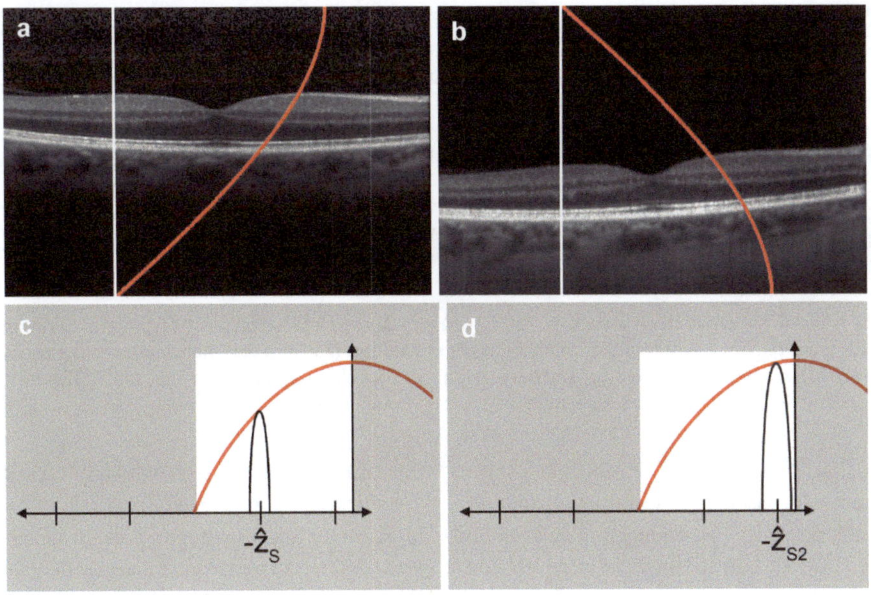

Fig. 15.3 Effect of using the inverted image. (**a**) In a conventionally acquired OCT image, the peak of the sensitivity curve is well within the vitreous cavity. The sensitivity curve (in *red*) is rotated 90° with increasing sensitivity represented by a greater distance from the baseline (represented by the *white line*). (**b**) If the OCT instrument is pushed closer to the eye in order to obtain an inverted image, the peak of the sensitivity curve is placed near or at the back of the sclera. The choroid is very near the peak of the sensitivity curve. For the purpose of illustration, the image was inverted to match the orientation of conventional OCT scans. (**c**) In the inverted image, the size of the curve at $-\hat{z}_S$ (the only one of the two shown by the OCT instrument as illustrated by the grayed-out region outside the inverted portion of the curve) is similar to that in Fig. 15.2a. (**d**) Note the size of the curve at $-\hat{z}_{S2}$ as compared with that in Fig. 15.2b. The relative difference in sensitivity of the deeper signal contributes to the increased signal-to-noise ratio from the choroid of the inverted image. On the other hand, note that the relative brightness of the inner retinal components, such as the nerve fiber layer, is lower in the inverted image as compared with the conventional image in (**c**)

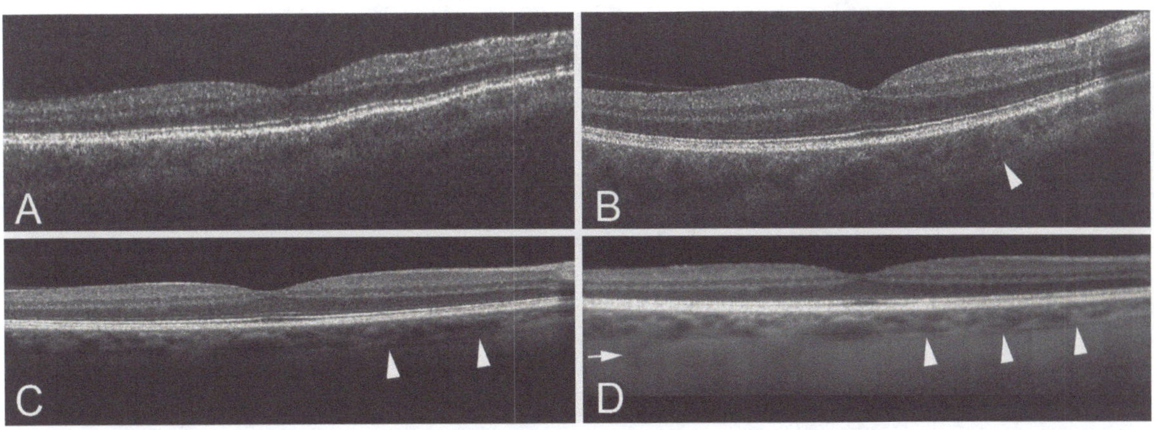

Fig. 15.4 Comparative Optical Coherence Tomography (OCT) sections through the fovea of the same individual taken with various optical coherence tomographic instruments: (**a**) Stratus OCT, (**b**), Cirrus OCT, (**c**), Heidelberg Spectralis. (**a**) With the Stratus OCT, details from the choroid are lost in noise. (**b**) Some choroidal details are visible, including a linear hyporeflective line (*arrowhead*). (**c**). With the Heidelberg Spectralis used in a normal fashion, more choroidal details are visible, including better visualization of the hyporeflective line (*arrowheads*). (**d**) The choroidal image taken with the enhanced depth imaging technique. Note the clarity and delineation of the hyporeflective line, which appears to be in the suprachoroidal space. The *arrow* points to a vessel coursing through the sclera. The scaling for vertical height varies among the instruments [8]

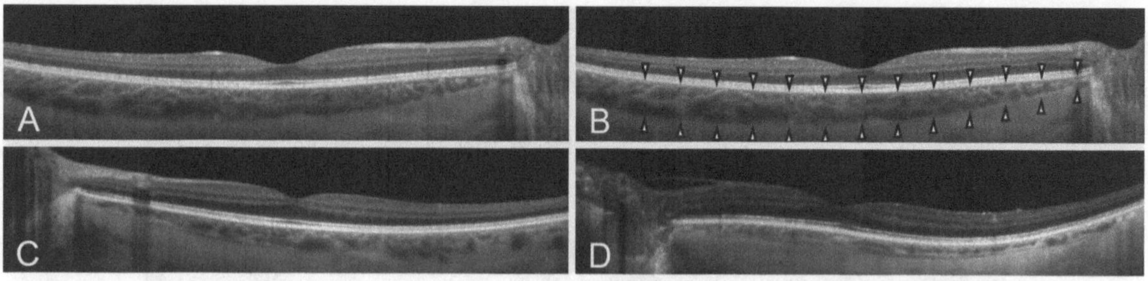

Fig. 15.5 (**a**) The choroid is seen in cross-section on OCT scan of a 31-year-old subject. (**b**) (*Top right*) Choroidal thickness was measured vertically from the basal aspect of the retinal pigment epithelium (RPE) to the outer border of the choroid (*arrowheads*) [9]. Representative OCT scans of 61-year-old (**c**) and 67-year-old (**d**) eyes showing decreasing choroidal thickness with increasing age (From Margolis and Spaide [10]; used with permission)

pressure, perfusion pressure [11], endogenous nitric oxide production [12], vasoactive secretory production of choroidal ganglion cells [13], endogenous circulating catecholamines [14–16], and its intrinsic vasomotricity [17]. After death, all of these functions fail or cease to exist. Fixation of tissue as part of histologic analysis causes shrinkage, thus affecting any measured thicknesses. As such, histology can provide an estimate of sorts, but not an accurate measurement of the thickness of the choroid *post mortem*. Histologic measurement, of course, cannot measure in vivo thickness, which in turn is different than the thickness *post mortem*. A study involving the histologic evaluation of autopsy eyes, in which the refractive error was not stated, found a yearly decrease in choroidal thickness of 1.1 μm/year, which was fairly similar to what was found by EDI OCT, 1.56 μm [18]. The constant of the regression equation was 193.5 μm in the histology study[18] vs. 366 μm in the EDI OCT study, which probably relates not only to shrinkage from the processing required to examine the histology, but to the loss of blood

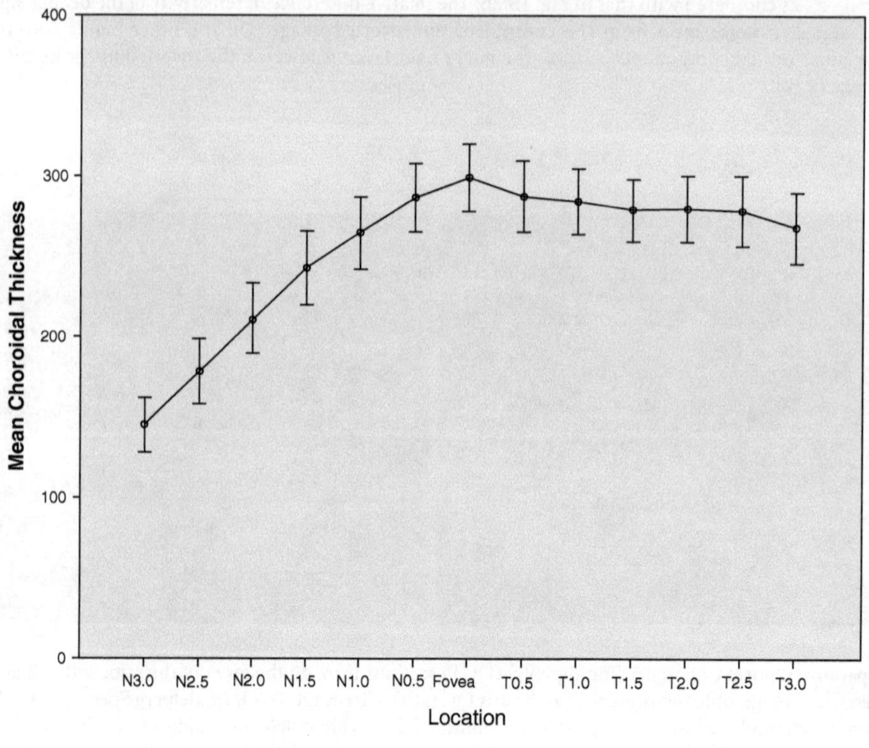

Fig. 15.6 The mean choroidal thickness measured at different locations across a horizontal section through the fovea at 500 μm intervals from 3 mm nasal to the fovea to 3 mm temporal. The error bars represent 1 standard deviation. (From Margolis and Spaide [10]; used with permission)

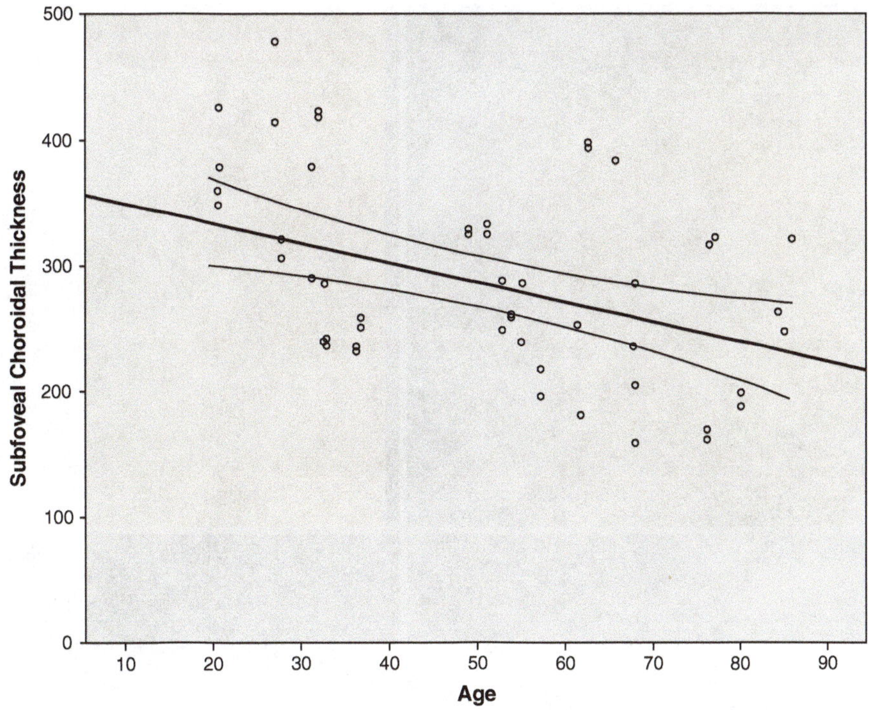

Fig. 15.7 Scatter plot of the subfoveal choroidal thickness with age. The subfoveal choroidal thickness (in μm) = 366–1.56*age in years ($p = 0.001$). The trend line is shown with 95% confidence intervals. (From Margolis and Spaide [10]; used with permission)

pressure inflating the vascular structure of the autopsy eyes. There are several possible reasons for the decreases in choroidal thickness with age, including loss of the choriocapillaris, a decrease in the diameter of the choriocapillary vessels, decrease in luminal diameter of blood vessels, and in some cases, a diminution of the middle layer of the choroids [18–20].

15.4 Age-Related Choroidal Atrophy

A relatively common condition affecting the choroid in older adults is age-related choroidal atrophy or ARCA [21]. The choroid becomes increasingly thin in people with age, but people with ARCA have an exaggerated thinning of the choroid such that they have recognizable fundus changes associated with characteristic visual complaints. It is common for patients with ARCA to have numerous visual complaints, despite what seems to be relatively good Snellen acuities. These complaints frequently involve difficulty reading. Ophthalmic examination of the fundus in these patients shows several common findings: the larger choroidal vessels are easily discerned, many of the visible choroidal vessels do not appear to be red, but are yellow or white, there are few visible vessels of any size in the central macula, there may be pigment aggregates in the macular region, there can be peripapillary atrophy despite the absence of myopia, and there often is mild optic nerve pallor (Figs. 15.8 and 15.9). The EDI OCT shows marked loss of thickness of the choroid in these patients. There appears to be loss of the choroidal vessels such that the remaining larger choroidal vessels can fill the entire thickness of the choroid. Given that ARCA happens in older adults, it is not surprising that some of these may also have concurrent late age-related macular degeneration (AMD). Choroidal neovascularization (CNV) in ARCA patients does not appear to be as aggressive, and seems to show a longer-term response per injection of anti-VEGF agents than does CNV in other forms of AMD (Figs. 15.10 and 15.11).

Summary for the Clinician

- The mean subfoveal choroidal thickness in a group of normal eyes was 287 μm
- The mean choroidal thickness at 3 mm nasal to the fovea was 145 μm
- The choroidal thickness showed a statistically significant inverse correlation with age at all measured positions

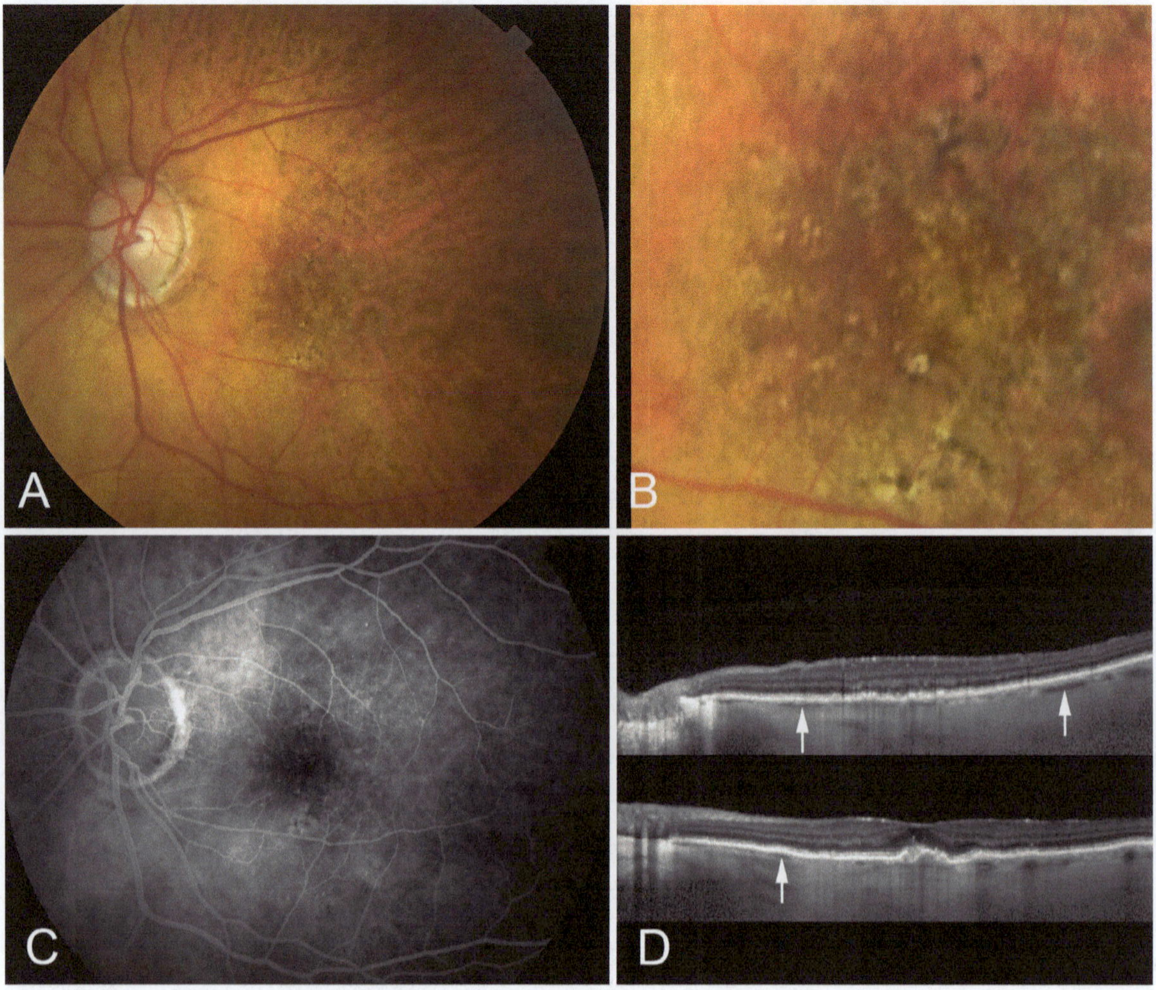

Fig. 15.8 This 82-year-old was referred because she was thought to have choroidal neovascularization (CNV). (**a**) Her color photograph shows the hallmarks of age-related choroidal atrophy (ARCA). Note the slight optic nerve pallor, the peripapillary atrophy present even though she was emmetropic, and the tigroid fundus appearance with some of the choroidal vessels adopting a *yellowish* appearance. (**b**) Note the paucity of vessels except for a few red choroidal vessels. (**c**) The fluorescein angiogram did not show any neovascularization. (**d**) In two EDI OCT sections, note the thinness of the choroid and how the full thickness of the choroid appears to be filled with the remaining large choroidal vessels (*arrows*)

Histopathologic analysis of the eyes with what has been termed "senile choroidal sclerosis" has shown atrophy of the choroid with the loss of small and medium vessels to the point that Bruch's membrane was immediately contiguous with the sclera in areas, and the remaining larger vessels of the choroid occupied the full-thickness of the remaining choroid in others [22]. There was a loss of the expected pigmented cells in the choroid with clumping of preserved pigmented cells in various regions in the choroid. In a series of patients with ARCA, approximately 1/3 had glaucoma [21]. The prelaminar portion of the optic nerve is supplied by the choroid. The contribution of vascular abnormalities to the development and progression of glaucoma is not known, but it is conceivable that patients with poor blood supply to the optic nerve may be at higher risk for glaucoma, all other things being equal. An association suggested in an older publication was that patients with choroidal sclerosis may develop a particular type of glaucoma called "senile sclerotic glaucoma" [23], a term used at the time of publication of that article. The use of EDI OCT allows for actual quantification of choroidal changes and may help elucidate the interaction between the choroid and glaucoma in the future.

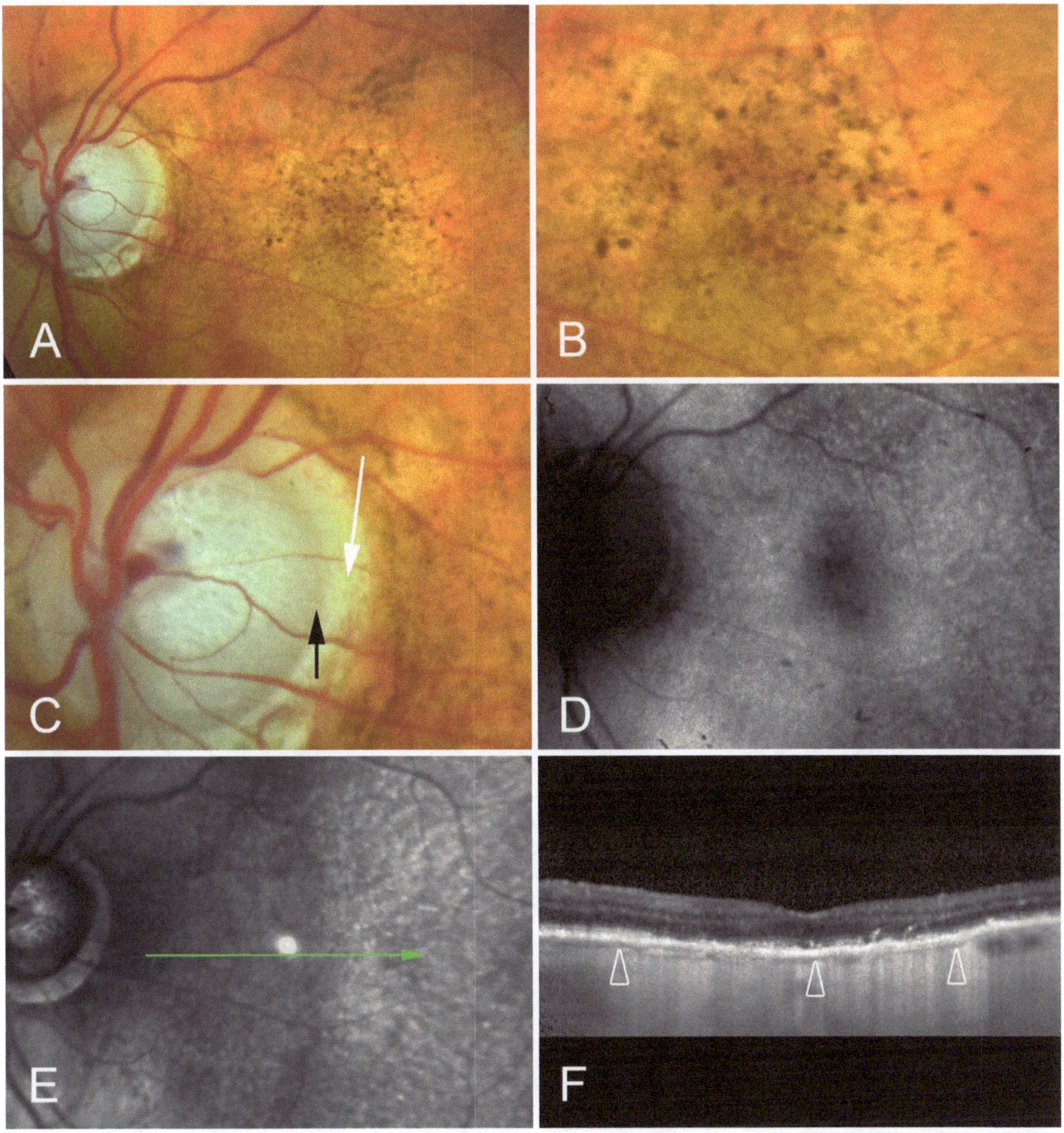

Fig. 15.9 ARCA with associated macular and optic nerve changes. (**a**) The patient had 20/80 best-corrected visual acuity and a diagnosis of low-tension glaucoma. A higher magnification of the macula (**b**) showed focal areas of hyperpigmentation with intervening areas of pigment rarefaction. Note the paucity of visible choroidal vessels. (**c**) The optic nerve showed disc pallor with thinning of the rim (*black arrow*), and only a few visible choroidal vessels in the beta-zone of parapapillary atrophy (*white arrow*). (**d**) The fundus autofluorescence photograph shows a relatively preserved autofluorescence profile, indicating an intact retinal pigment epithelial layer. (**e**) The infrared scanning laser ophthalmoscopic image documents the enlarged optic nerve cupping and reticular pseudodrusen in the posterior pole. The *green arrow* shows the site of the optical coherence tomographic scan. (**f**) Enhanced depth imaging optical coherence tomography (EDI OCT) shows the choroid to be very thin (*open arrowheads*); the subfoveal choroidal thickness was 45 μm. (From Spaide [21]; used with permission)

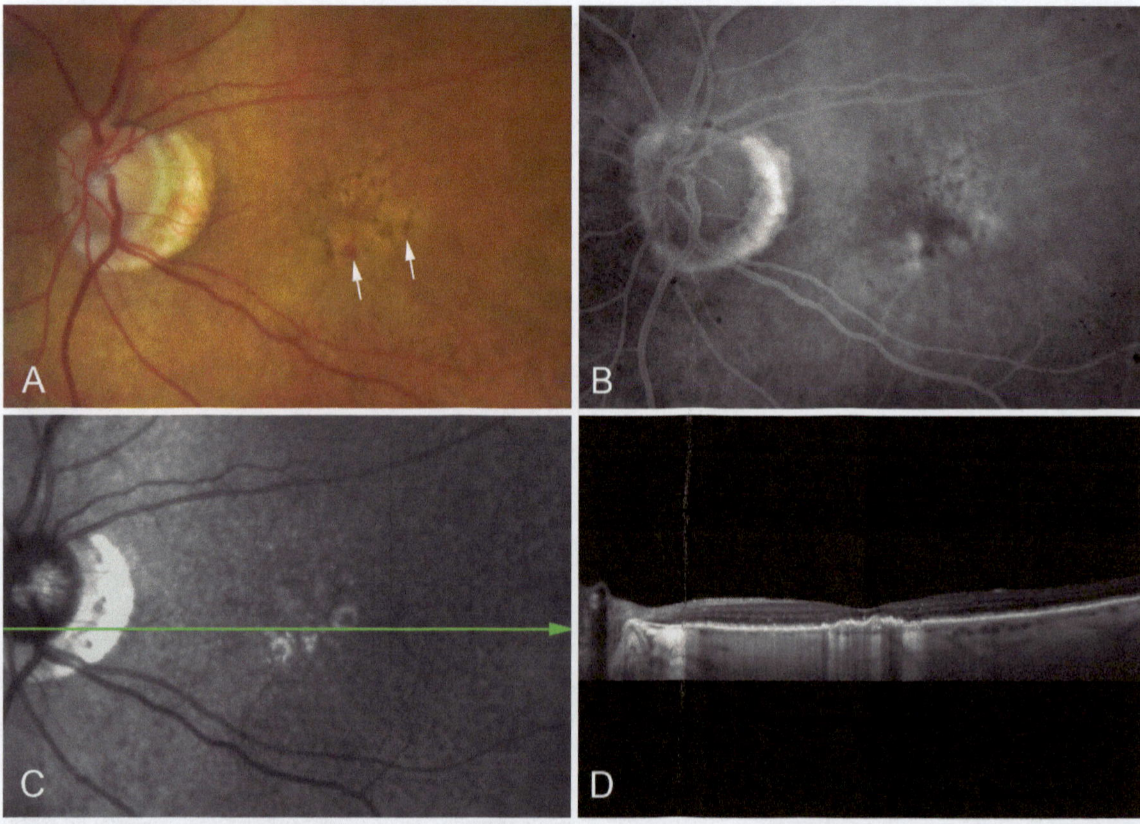

Fig. 15.10 ARCA with CNV. This 90-year-old presented with new onset CNV in the left eye. (**a**) Note the two small hemorrhages (*arrows*). (**b**) The fluorescein angiogram shows occult CNV. (**c**) The infrared scanning laser ophthalmoscopic image shows reticular pseudodrusen in the posterior pole and reflective figures in the central macula that do not seem to correspond to any feature visible in the color photograph. (**d**) There is an elevation of the RPE centrally and a thin choroid. (Spaide [21]; used with permission)

Summary for Clinicians

- Some patients have remarkable thinning of the choroid with advanced age
- These patients can have numerous complaints despite relatively good visual acuity measurements
- This condition is known as age-related choroidal atrophy or ARCA, and is common
- Patients with ARCA can develop late AMD
- Patients with ARCA seem to have a high prevalence of glaucoma

15.5 Choroid in High Myopia

High myopia associated with excessive and progressive elongation of the globe results in a variety of fundus changes that lead to visual impairment, including lacquer cracks in Bruch's membrane, CNV, and chorioretinal atrophy [7, 9, 23–35]. There is evidence that axial elongation of the globe leads to reduced retinal function [7, 9, 24, 28, 32, 36]. If the visual dysfunction in the absence of CNV was solely due to retinal stretching, visual function would be expected to correlate with the amount of myopia, regardless of the patient's age. However, visual function tends to be normal in highly myopic young people, irrespective of the amount of myopia and worsens with age [31, 34, 35]. Histologic studies of older eyes have demonstrated choroidal thinning in high myopia, with a lack of vessels in some areas and pronounced thinning of the choriocapillaris in others [23, 29]. Animal models of myopia reported decreased choriocapillaris density and diameter [26]. Studies using ICG angiography [37, 38], color Doppler ultrasonography [39], and ocular pulse amplitude [40] have also shown that choroidal circulation is decreased in myopic eyes. As the choroid supplies oxygen and nutrition to the retinal pigment epithelial cells and the outer retina [41], compromised choroidal circulation may account, in part, for the retinal dysfunction and vision loss that is seen in high myopia.

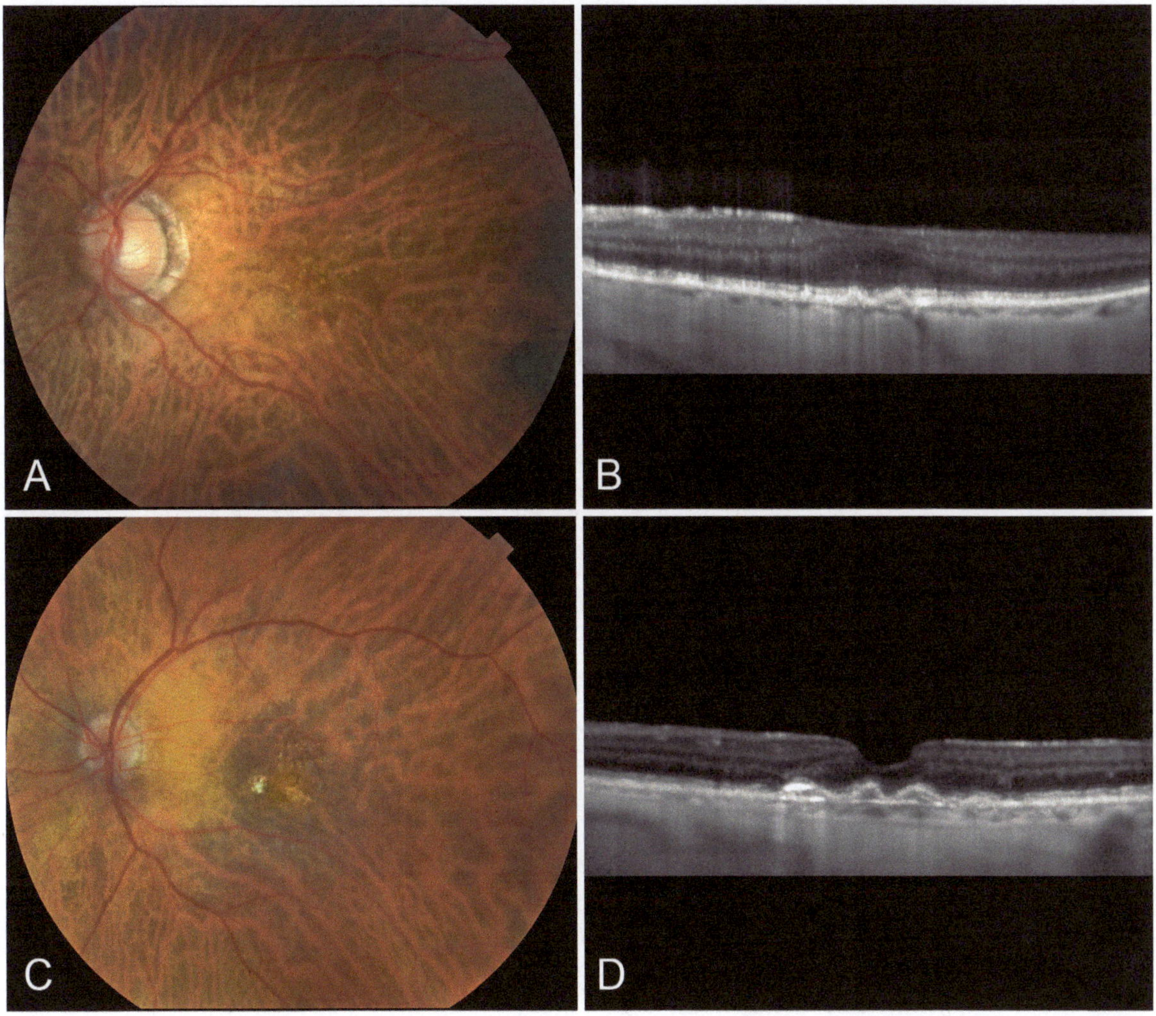

Fig. 15.11 CNV in eyes with ARCA. (**a**) This 80-year-old patient had CNV diagnosed 3 years earlier when she had a subretinal hemorrhage and fluorescein angiographic findings of occult CNV. She had one injection of intravitreal bevacizumab and had a complete resolution of her exudative manifestations. She had a diagnosis of glaucoma. (**b**) The EDI OCT shows minimal thickening at the level of the RPE and a subfoveal choroidal thickness of 49 μm. The visual acuity was 20/30. (**c**) This 83-year-old had a diagnosis of occult CNV made by fluorescein angiography years previously but, because of no signs of exudation, never had treatment. Two years previously, the patient finally developed subretinal bleeding and was treated with three doses of intravitreal bevacizumab. Note the lack of visible scarring. (**d**) The subfoveal choroidal thickness was 85 μm. The visual acuity was 20/40. (Spaide [21]; used with permission)

A group of 31 patients (55 eyes) with a mean age of 59.7 ± years and a mean refractive error of −11.9 ± 3.7 diopters was evaluated with EDI OCT [18]. The mean subfoveal choroidal thickness was 93.2 (±62.5) μm, and was negatively correlated with age ($p = 0.006$) (Fig. 15.12), refractive error ($p < 0.001$) (Fig. 15.13), and history of CNV ($p = 0.013$). Regression analysis suggested that subfoveal choroidal thickness decreased by 12.7 μm for each decade of life, and by 8.7 μm for each diopter of myopia. The choroid in areas of peripapillary atrophy was exceedingly thin or not visualizable, as would be expected, but the choroid in pigmented areas adjacent to the peripapillary atrophy was markedly attenuated in thickness (Figs. 15.14 and 15.15). Glaucoma was present in 21.8% of the eyes. A prior history of CNV was present in 19 eyes. For those with no history of CNV, a linear regression of explanatory variables with subfoveal choroidal thickness as the dependent variable reduced to a model containing age in years and refraction in spherical equivalent diopters. For those with CNV, linear regression did not find any significant explanatory variables associated with subfoveal choroidal thickness.

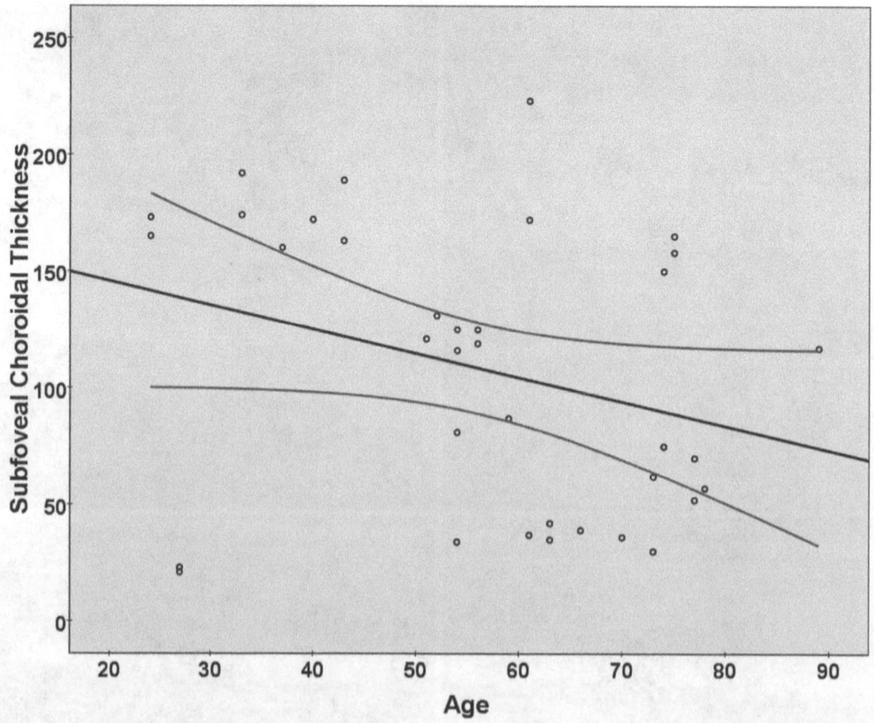

Fig. 15.12 Scatter plot of mean subfoveal choroidal thickness vs. age in highly myopic eyes. The gray lines are the 95% confidence interval for the trend line (*black*). (From Fujiwara et al. [42])

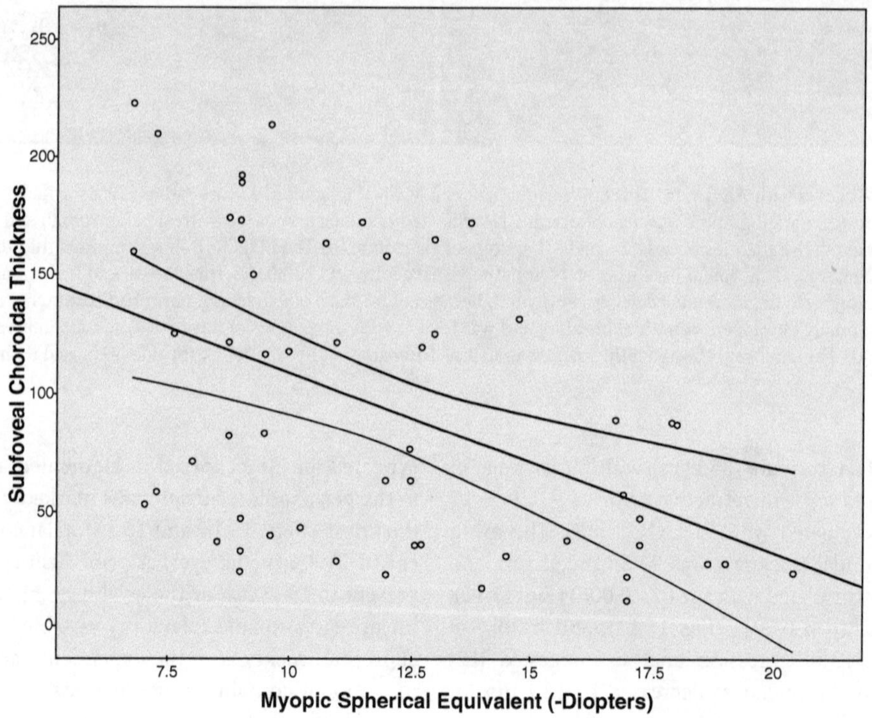

Fig. 15.13 Scatter plot of mean subfoveal choroidal thickness vs. diopters spherical equivalent refractive error in highly myopic eyes. The gray lines are the 95% confidence interval for the trend line (*black*). (From Fujiwara et al. [42])

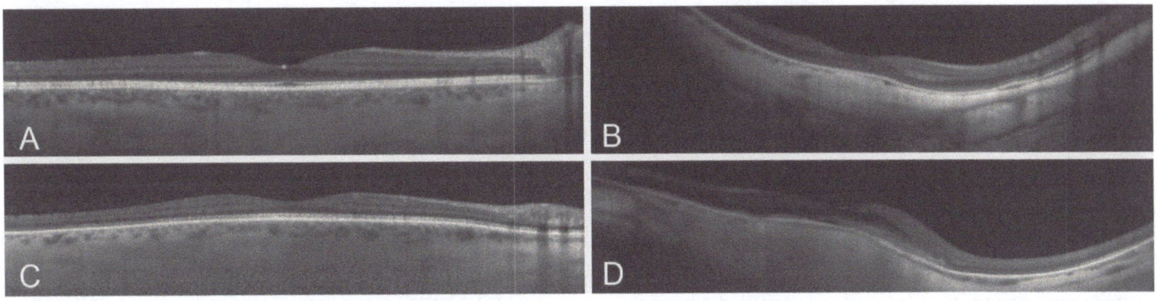

Fig. 15.14 Cross-sectional imaging of the choroid using EDI OCT. Subfoveal choroidal thickness was measured vertically from the outer border of the RPE to the inner border of the sclera. (**a**) The choroidal thickness measured 233 μm in a normal eye (55-year-old), and (**b**) 23 μm (−20-dipoter in 27-year-old), (**c**) 223 μm (−6.75 diopter, 61-year-old), and (**d**) 37 μm (−15.75 diopter, the same patient as (**c**)) in three representative eyes with high myopia. (From Fujiwara et al. [42])

The age-dependent decrease in choroidal thickness suggests that in addition to undergoing choroidal thinning due to progressive stretching from increasing axial elongation, highly myopic eyes also experience the same age-related choroidal attenuation that affect normal eyes. Since both the choroid and the retina are stretched in highly myopic eyes, the choroid - although thinner than normal - may still be able to supply the proportionally thin retina with necessary oxygen and nutrients. This is consistent with the fairly normal visual function in adolescents and young adults with high myopia. The relatively thin choroids seen in younger myopes may be physiologically sufficient even if the same thickness of choroid found in an eye without myopia may be considered pathologic. As such, these patients have what could be termed myopic choroidal thinning. However, as the choroid undergoes age-related attenuation, the available supply may not be sufficient to support the outer retina, the RPE, and even the choroid itself. At some point, the thickness of the choroid seems to make a transition from myopic choroidal thinning to frank myopic choroidal atrophy. The transition point has not been defined at present, but it is possible that functional features such as threshold sensitivities or visual acuity may be part of the definition rather than just choroidal thickness alone. Patients with the loss of the choroid from myopia and age, who have decreased visual function as a consequence, are observed to have what could be termed myopic choroidal atrophy [42].

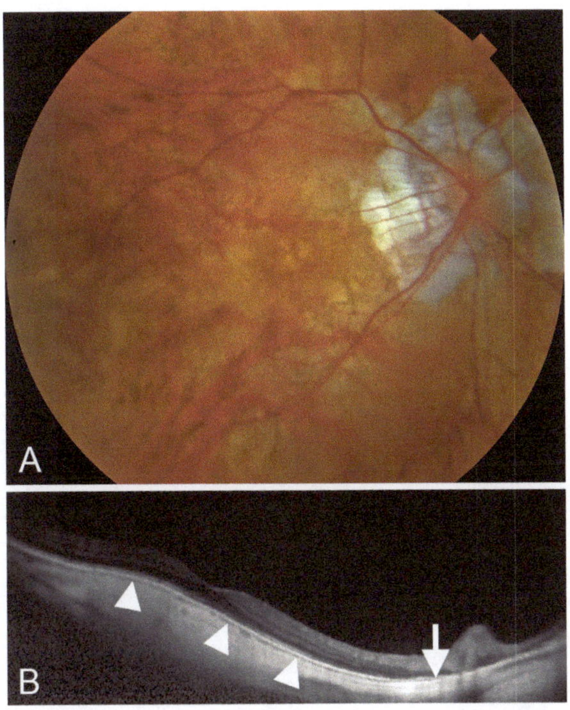

Fig. 15.15 Peripapillary atrophy as compared with the choroidal thickness in high myopia. (**a**) Note that this patient with high myopia has the so-called peripapillary atrophy. (**b**) The EDI OCT image shows the choroid to be very thin (*arrowheads*) with no sharp transition to where the clinically observed "peripapillary" atrophy starts (which is shown by the *arrow*)

Summary for Clinicians

- The choroidal thickness in high myopia is inversely proportional to the diopters of myopia and age
- The choroid in the peripapillary region was exceptionally thin, possibly explaining peripapillary atrophy in myopes
- Myopic choroidal thinning occurs with increasing amounts of myopia, and myopic choroidal atrophy occurs when age-related processes cause the choroid to decrease in thickness sufficient to cause visual dysfunction

15.6 Pigment Epithelial Detachment in Age-Related Macular Degeneration

Although detachment of the RPE associated with AMD is common, theories about the formation of pigment epithelial detachments (PEDs) are remarkably divergent. RPE detachment was described first by Gass and coworkers [43] in 1966, and in 1972, Gass [44] further hypothesized that PEDs occurred in AMD secondary to either serous exudation from choriocapillaris hyperpermeability through an intact Bruch's membrane or by neovascular ingrowth with subsequent exudation from the new vessels directly into the sub-RPE space. Gass thought exudation from neovascularization spread laterally, lifting the surrounding RPE monolayer by hydrostatic dissection up around the leaking vessels. Bird and Marshall [45] proposed that instead of choriocapillaris hyperpermeability or neovascularization, there is increasing deposition of lipid materials into Bruch's membrane with age that rendered it progressively more hydrophobic and impermeable [46]. Pumping of fluid by the RPE toward the hydrophobic Bruch's membrane would cause this fluid to accumulate under the RPE above Bruch's membrane to create a PED, instead of passing through Bruch's membrane. Bird proposed that CNV, if it occurred at all, was an event that occurred secondary to the PED [47]. Kuhn and associates[48] and Slakter and coworkers [49] identified a peculiar vascular configuration, the anastomosis of retinal vessels with underlying CNV, as a risk factor for the development for PED. Hartnett and coworkers, in two publications[50, 51], demonstrated that retinal vessels could grow down to the deep retina and lead to a PED, and they called the vascular change a "deep retinal vascular anomaly". Years later, another group renamed this entity, retinal angiomatous proliferation (RAP), and proposed a staging system [52]. However, Gass and coworkers subsequently disagreed with this hypothesis and staging system [53]. Instead, Gass proposed that patients who appeared to have RAP actually had an early sign of occult chorioretinal anastomosis with occult CNV [53]. The outer retina and the RPE were thought to degenerate, and eventually because of this degeneration, the retinal vessels and the CNV came closer together. Solely on the basis of the proximity, the vessels of the retina were theorized to become anastomotic with those of the CNV. In this new theory, Gass retained his older idea that exudation from occult CNV extended laterally with the development of an adjacent PED.

One of the chief difficulties with PEDs is the difficulty of visualizing their contents [54]. It is difficult to image the contents of PEDs by fluorescein angiography because of light absorption and scattering by the RPE and because fluorescein dye leaks into any potential spaces under the RPE to mask the deeper contents. Conventional OCT has poor ability to image structures under the RPE and consequently, many PEDs look hollow. However, these OCT scans do not image the underlying choroid, so one cannot be certain if deeper portions within the PED are filled with fluid with no reflectivity or just are not imaged in the first place. Using OCT with enhanced imaging of the contents of the PED, as evidenced by imaging of the complete thickness of the choroid in a series of patients, led to interesting findings.

After a series of anti-VEGF injections, some patients can appear to retain PEDs that appear to be "hollow" by conventional OCT. A small series examined with EDI OCT showed that these PEDs were filled with lamellar hyperreflective material (Fig. 15.16). Histologic examination of excised CNV following anti-VEGF treatment showed paucicellular fibrotic scarring [53] with a cross-sectional appearance similar to what was seen by EDI OCT examination. Other patients, those with serous detachment of the RPE, appeared to have collections of material along the back surface of the RPE (Figs. 15.17 and 15.18). Areas of hotspots seen during angiography, suggestive of RAP vs. occult retinal choroidal anastomosis, had spider-like projections extending into the contents of the PED. Anti-VEGF injections were associated with contraction of this material, such that the material could form sheets across the inner chord diameter of the PED. The contracture of the material has been associated with tears of the RPE (Figs. 15.19–15.21).

Angiographic correlation of the material showed that areas of collection of the sub-RPE material was associated with increased fluorescence and late staining, suggesting that the material is composed, at least in part, of fibrovascular proliferation. Hotspots in PEDs colocalized with what appeared to be retinal choroidal anastomosis. However, the appearance of the retina was different from what Gass and coworkers proposed. Gass thought the anastomosis occurred because there was degeneration of the RPE as well as the outer retina such that the retinal vessels came into close contact with the vessels of the CNV [53]. Because of their physical proximity, the vessels were supposed to have become anastomotic. In EDI OCT scans, the outer retina does not appear to be degenerated and autofluorescence shows an intact RPE. This implies that there must be some other mechanism leading to anastomotic connections between the retina and CNV. CNV has been proposed to grow because of increased VEGF levels under the RPE; and by extension, retinal vessel growth from the inner to the outer retina was proposed

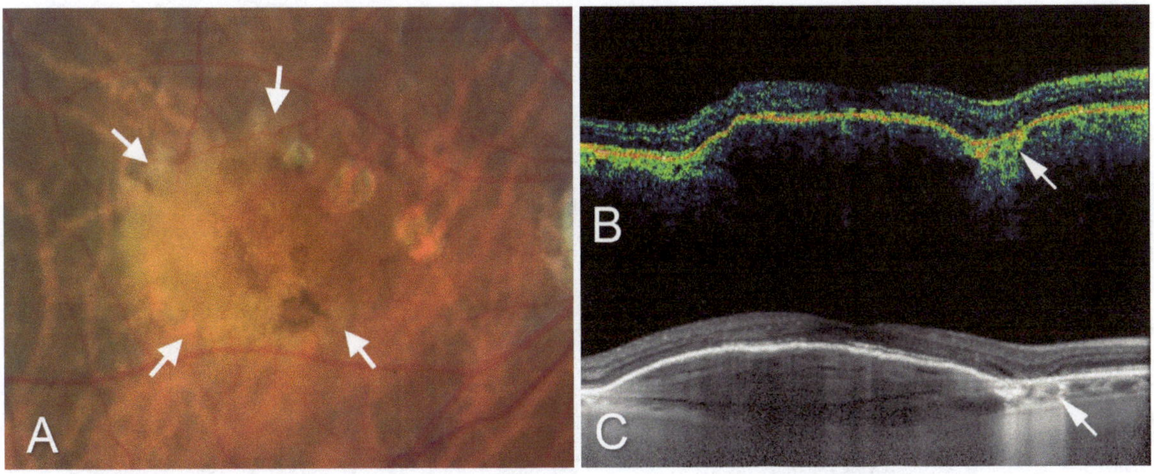

Fig. 15.16 (**a**) This patient received photodynamic therapy with triamcinolone and then more than 18 intravitreal injections directed against vascular endothelial growth factor, without a change in the size of his fibrovascular pigment epithelial detachment (PED) (**a**) which is delimited by the *arrows*. (**b**) Note that the Stratus OCT shows the PED to have no solid internal contents, suggesting it was filled with fluid. The choroid seen through an area of atrophy shows little details, while the choroid not visible under the PED. (**c**) An EDI OCT image shows a multilamellar material filling the contents of the PED. Note that the choroid is visible under the PED. The area of atrophy in the choroid shows the choroidal details as expected (*arrow*)

to arise from increased VEGF levels in the outer retina [55]. VEGF is released in response to a number of stimuli, so the growth of the vessels with eventual anastomotic connection could occur by an active process rather than the passive one, as described by Gass. The EDI OCT findings in PEDs so far has not supported the pathophysiologic processes and stages, as proposed to occur in RAP.

Summary for Clinicians

- There are numerous opposing theories concerning the formation of PEDs in AMD
- Each theory is limited by incomplete information concerning the contents of PEDs
- Untreated PEDs appear to have evidence of fibrovascular proliferation, oftentimes coursing up the back surface of the detached RPE
- Contracture of the fibrovascular material may lead to tears of the RPE
- Treated cases appear to contain material consistent with multilamellar scar-containing vessels

15.7 Additional Diseases such as Choroidal Tumors and Glaucoma

EDI OCT has the ability to image the choroid, but still suffers the problems of decreased signal secondary to absorption and scattering from blood and pigment. For example, it is not particularly helpful in examining pigmented tumors. On the other hand, it is possible to visualize the choroidal infiltration caused by nonpigmented tumors. For example, it is possible to see and measure lymphomatous collections and amelanotic melanomas. EDI OCT imaging can be helpful in ruling out the possibility of choroidal thickening. Glaucoma may involve both vascular and structural abnormalities. The choroidal contribution from the choroid was mentioned previously. The optic nerve can be imaged using the EDI technique to gain information about the lamina cribosa, the pores of which can easily be visualized.

15.8 Volume Rendering

OCT pictures are generally shown as 2D b-scan images acquired through the thickness of the retina. Some older time-domain OCT instruments created *en face* images that allowed inspection of lateral relationships among various retinal structures. The problem with simple en face imaging is that the eye is a curved structure and so an en face image cut across multiple retinal planes. This made image interpretation exceedingly difficult. In addition, small changes in position or scan depth from one image to the next produced vastly different representation of the eye. However, it is simple to obtain a large number of adjacent b-scan images with any typical SD OCT. After the successive images are aligned, a 3D

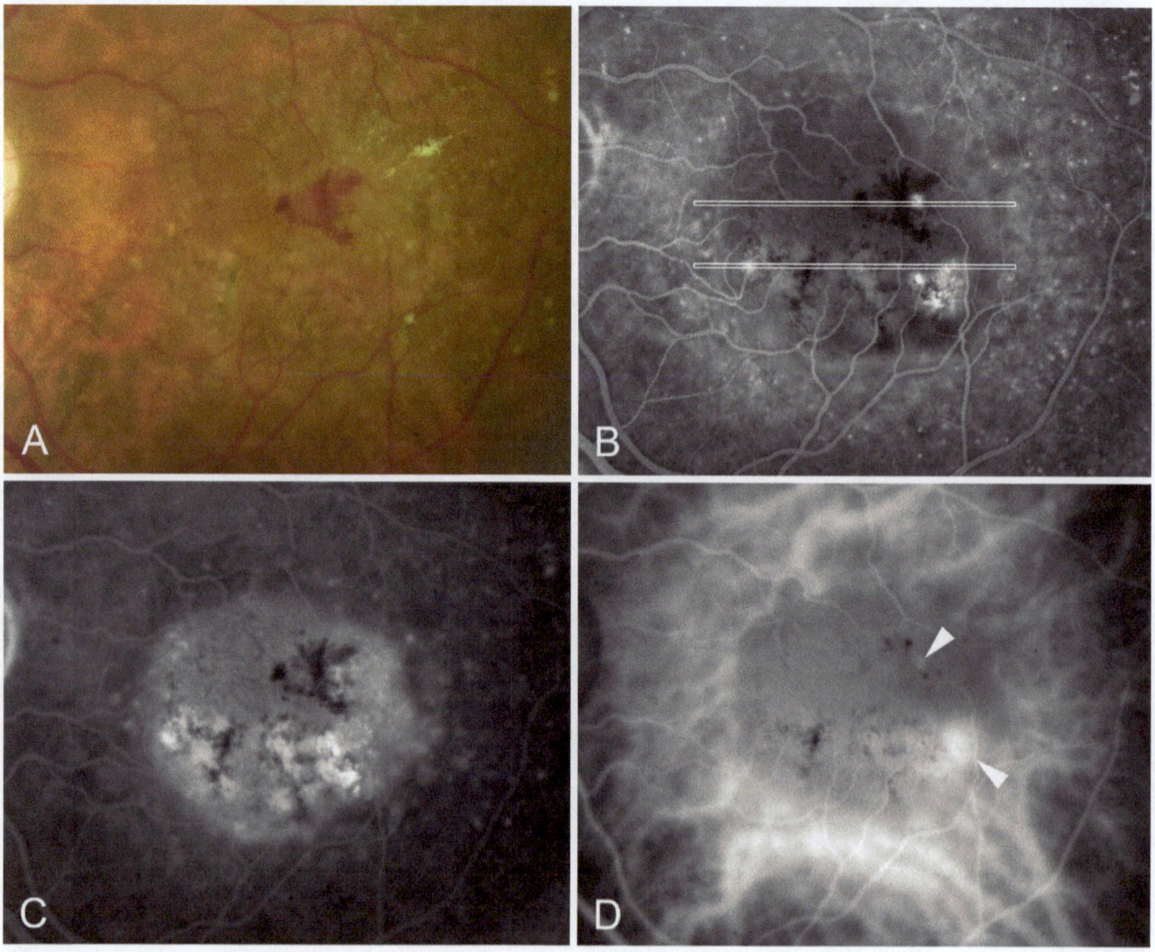

Fig. 15.17 Intra- and subretinal hemorrhage overlying a PED (**a**). Early during fluorescein angiography, the PED (**b**) showed generalized decreased fluorescence with two areas of increased fluorescence, one contiguous with the retinal hemorrhage and a second area inferiorly. This patient was seen emergently because of a 3-day history of visual acuity change. The two lines correspond to sections examined with the EDI OCT. (**c**) Later, in the fluorescein angiogram, there was a generalized increase in fluorescence within the PED. (**d**) Early during the indocyanine green (ICG) angiographic sequence, there were two areas of increased fluorescence that corresponded to what was seen in the fluorescein angiogram. Since the pigmentation in the RPE is thought not to represent a major impediment to the passage of near-infrared light used in ICG angiography, the hyperfluorescent areas were considered to represent actual neovascularization and not transmission defects through the RPE. (From Spaide [54]; used with permission)

volume can be reconstructed. The noise reduction through averaging can be done to each component of b-scan prior to creating the 3D volume.

Volume rendering in this instance takes the advantage of the regular rectangular size of the successive 2D images, which were acquired at a fixed interval by the OCT instrument. Many SD OCT instruments rely on their inherently fast scan rate to assemble a series of b-scans with the assumption that the patient did not make any significant saccades during the scan interval. A projection image of the successive b-scans can be made, and this projection image looks similar to a monochromatic image of the fundus, such as one acquired by a fundus camera or scanning laser ophthalmoscope. Usually, a series of b-scans obtained without eye tracking will show artifacts in the projection image showing that eye movement occurred during the scan interval. With mathematical techniques such as cross-correlation between b-scans, it is possible to partially compensate for eye saccades. However, image averaging is very difficult because there is little in the way of any feedback to know where in the eye the scan is taking

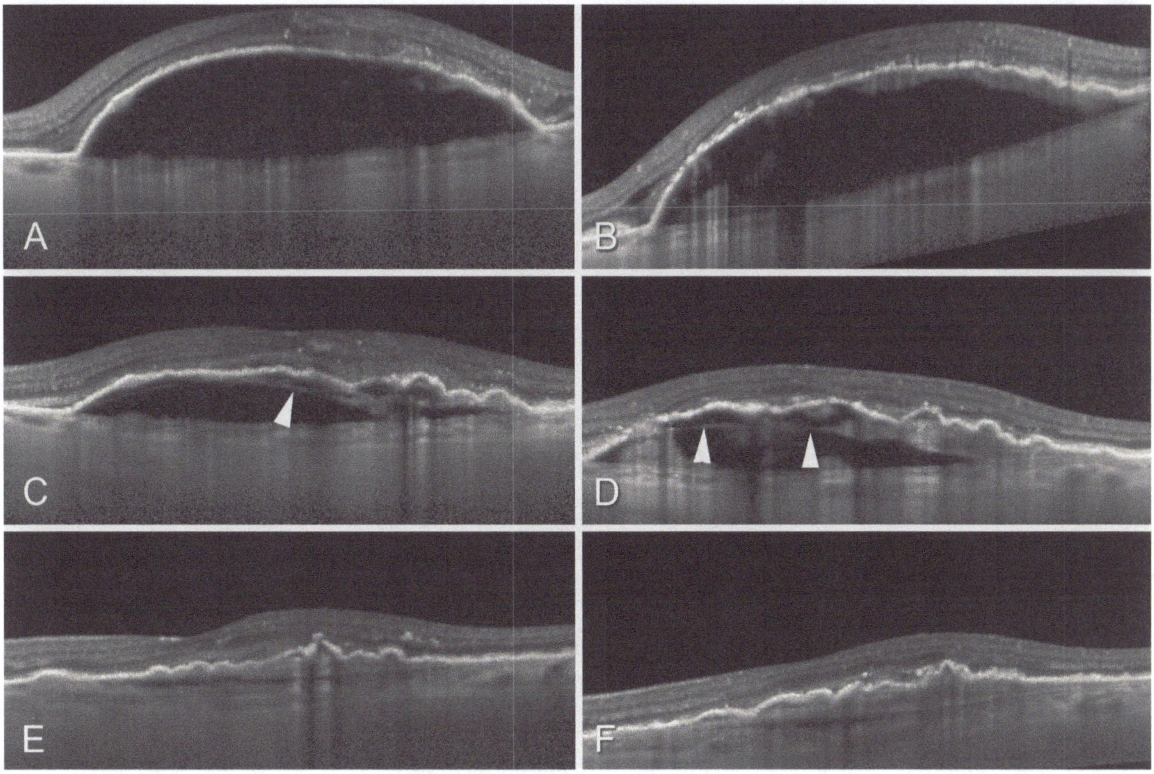

Fig. 15.18 EDI OCT of a fibrovascular PED and its response to intravitreal ranibizumab treatment. The sections on the left correspond to the upper line in the early phase fluorescein angiogram and the sections on the right correspond to the second line. (**a**) Prior to treatment, the section through the "hotspot" on both the fluorescein and ICG angiograms shows a small collection of material posterior to the RPE within the PED. Note that the hyperreflective line corresponding to the RPE has variable thickness throughout the extent of the PED. (**b**) A section taken inferiorly shows a more extensive accumulation of material along the back surface of the PED. There was an accumulation near the edge of the PED of similar material, but the extent of hyperfluorescence in the fluorescein and ICG angiograms cannot be attributed solely to this accumulation, implicating the material on the back surface of the PED as being fibrovascular in nature. (**c**) One week after intravitreal ranibizumab injection, there was a partial collapse of the PED. Note the separation of the hyperreflective line (*arrowhead*) from the back surface of the PED. (**d**) The correspondence in shape between the pretreatment and 1 week post treatment accumulation within the PED is more evident inferiorly. Note the separation and straightening of the sub-RPE material after the ranibizumab injection, even though the PED is collapsing. This implies there was tensile traction within the detached material. (**e, f**) One month after injection, there was flattening of the PED over a hyperreflective material containing several subtle lamellae. (From Spaide [54]; used with permission)

place during any particular b-scan. Eye-tracking techniques can assure that the successive b-scans are repeatedly acquired from the same location. A common method to render volume images uses a technique called ray casting. Uniform resampling of nonuniform sampled information when the sampling intervals are known (such as the information derived from conventional OCT instruments) is often best done with polynomial techniques or the use of band-limited sinc functions. The resultant ray is assigned gradients of shading based on the density and location of the resampled points which are composited to create a planar set of data representing the 3D attributes as seen from the viewing point. This planar data is used to make the display image shown, for example, on a computer monitor. An example of 3D volume rendering of the choroid is shown in Fig. 15.22. With faster OCT scanning and different scanning strategies, it will be possible to easily generate choroidal volume scans in the future.

15.9 Summary

The choroid, although difficult to image, accounts for the majority of blood flow in the eye, and is central to several major diseases affecting visual function. A simple method

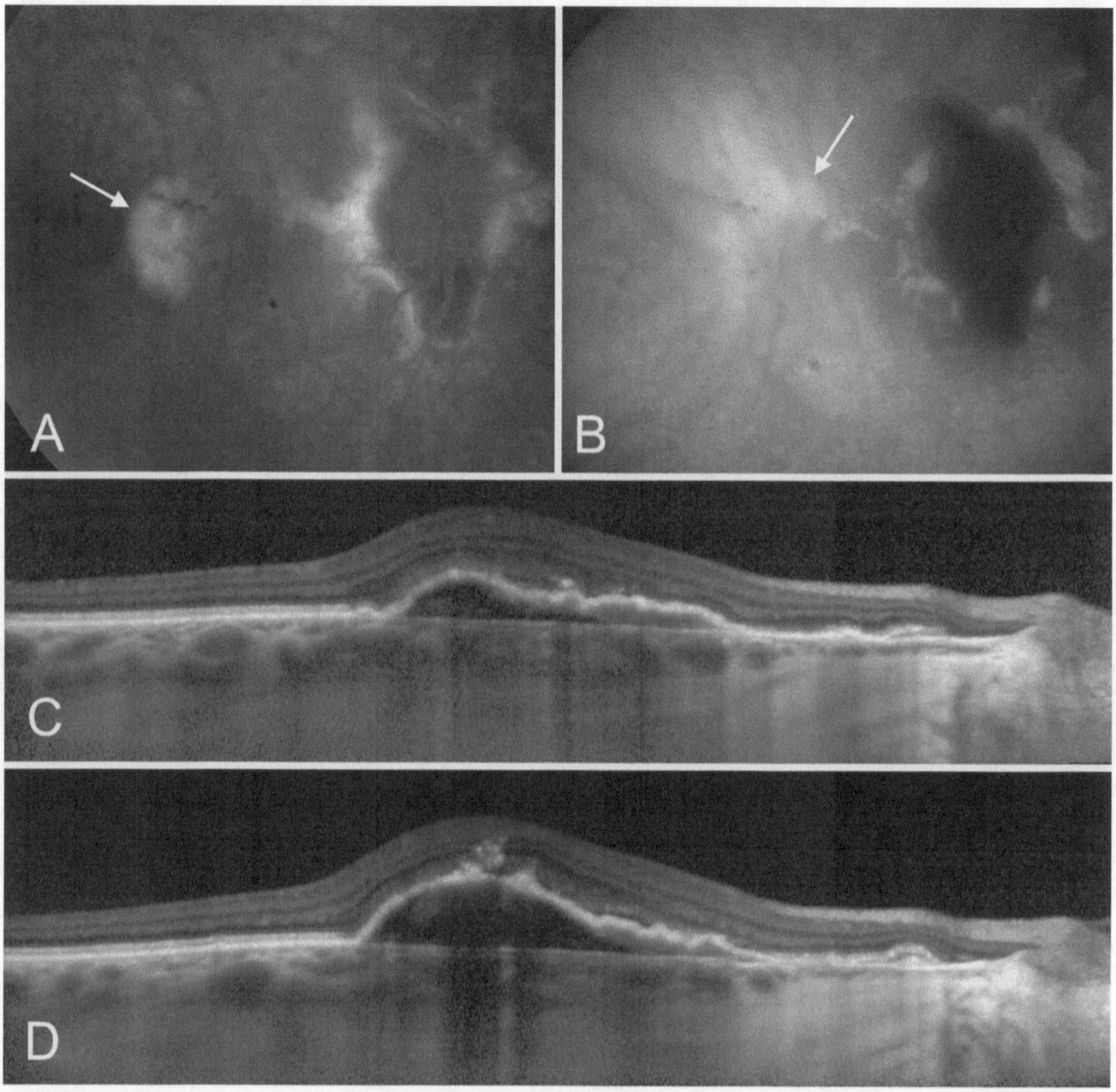

Fig. 15.19 Pretreatment characteristics of an eye that developed a tear in the RPE. (**a**) Note the heterogeneously filled PED (*arrow*) as seen during the midphase of a fluorescein angiogram. (**b**) The ICG angiogram showed a plaque of hyperfluorescence located to the nasal side of the PED (*arrow*). (**c, d**) EDI OCTs taken through the PED shows material on the back surface of the nasal side of the PED

to visualize the choroid was presented, and this technique allows visualization in nearly every patient. The choroidal thickness in normal eyes can be measured and used as a comparison to that found in various disease states. Primary atrophy of the choroid occurs with age and produces a condition differentiable from typical AMD. Myopic degeneration may have a significant contribution from choroidal thinning induced by both the degree of myopia as well as age. Volume-rendering techniques allow visualization and evaluation of the volume of the choroid. The same imaging techniques can be applied to the optic nerve to investigate glaucoma.

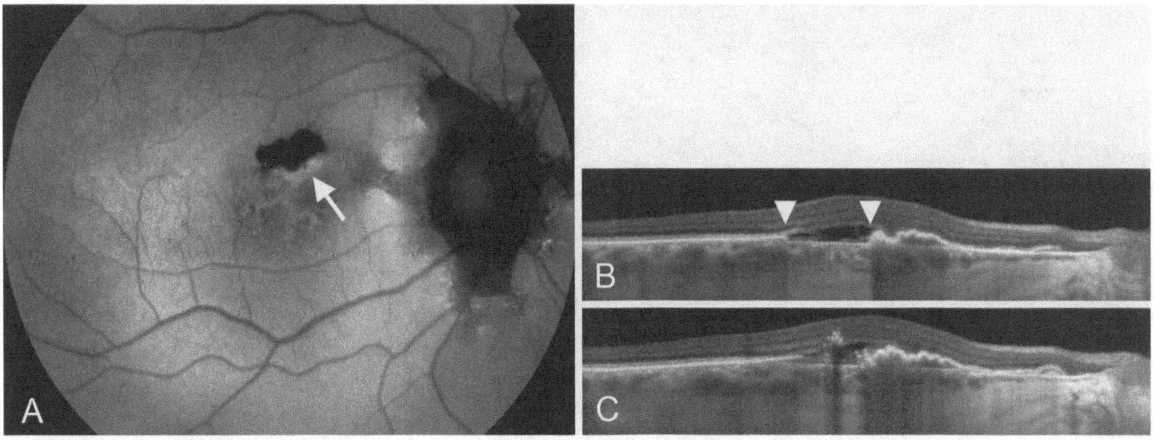

Fig. 15.20 After formation of the tear. (**a**) One month after intravitreal ranibizumab, the autofluorescence photograph shows a hypoautofluorescent defect with an area of increased autofluorescence from the scrolled RPE (*arrow*). (**b**, **c**) Corresponding EDI OCTs taken through the same areas as in Fig. 15.19c, d. Note the gap in the RPE (*arrowheads*) with increased light penetration to the choroid. The corrugated retinal pigment epithelial monolayer sits on the reflective material seen in the pre-rip EDI OCTs

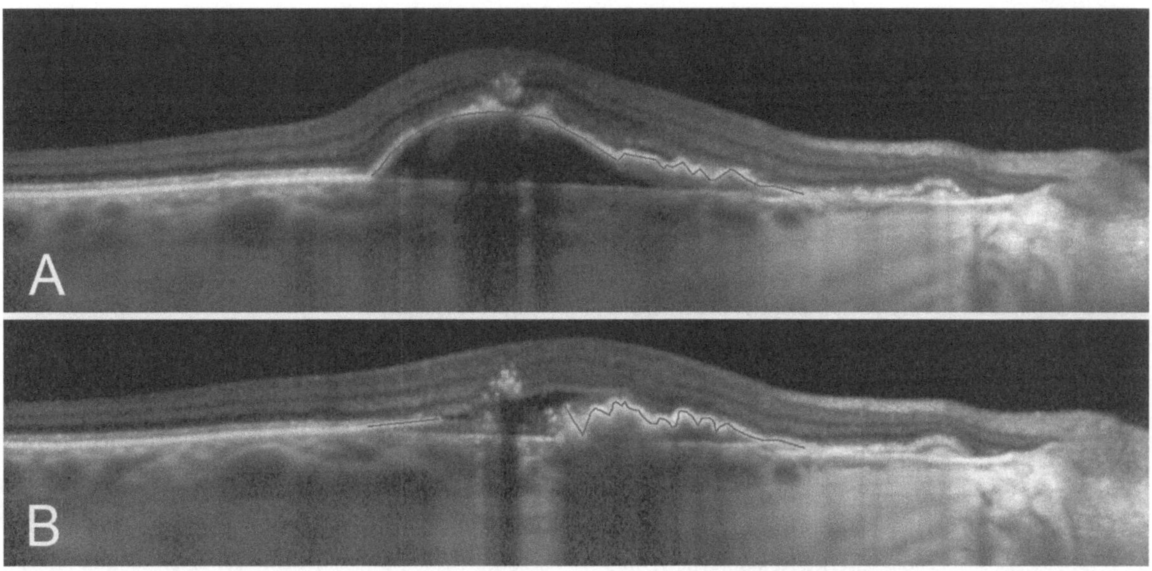

Fig. 15.21 Pre- and post-rip comparison. (**a**) The pre-rip EDI OCT with a *red line* drawn through the center of the RPE monolayer shows the portion that filled with fluorescein to be the ballooned region to the left. The area corresponding to the hyperfluorescent plaque is seen on the right with the overlying RPE showing corrugations. (**b**) After the rip, which appeared to occur in the ballooned area of the detachment, the RPE was thrown into more obvious folds. This suggests contraction of the underlying CNV. Even though anti-VEGF agents are associated with decreased signs of exudation, it is possible that they may contribute to contracture of fibrovascular tissue; much the same has been seen in preretinal proliferation in diabetics

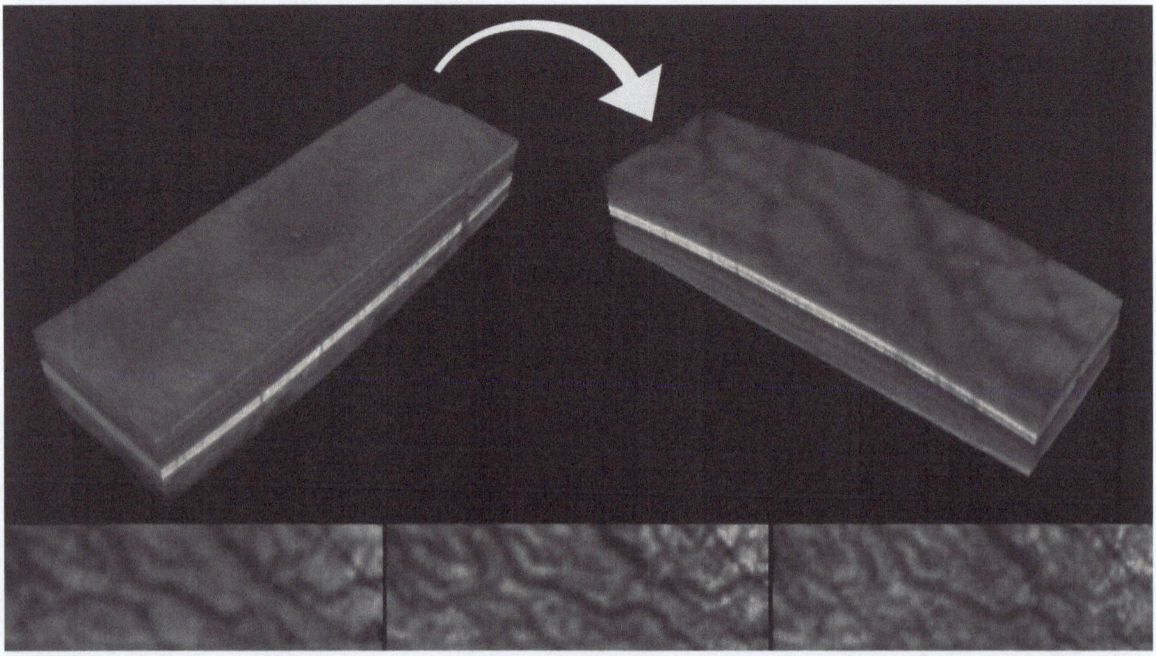

Fig. 15.22 Volume rendering of the same eye as in Fig. 15.4. The block of images was obtained in a 5 by 30° area and volume rendered using a raycasting technique. The block could be freely rotated in space and successive sections could be removed from the sclerad surface of the choroid (*bottom row*)

References

1. Cioffi GA, Granstam E, Alm A (2003) Ocular circulation. In: Kaufman PL, Alm A (eds) Adler's physiology of the eye. Clinical application, 10th edn. Mosby, St. Louis, pp 747–784
2. Seo JH, Yu YS, Kim JH et al (2007) Correlation of visual acuity with foveal hypoplasia grading by optical coherence tomography in albinism. Ophthalmology 114:1547–1551
3. Povazay B, Hermann B, Unterhuber A et al (2007) Three-dimensional optical coherence tomography at 1050 nm versus 800 nm in retinal pathologies: enhanced performance and choroidal penetration in cataract patients. J Biomed Opt 12:041211
4. Brezinski M (2006) Optical coherence tomography theory. In: Brezinski M (ed) Optical coherence tomography. Principles and applications. Elsevier, New York, pp 97–145
5. Fujimoto J, Drexler W (2009) Introduction to optical coherence tomography. In: Fujimoto J, Drexler W (eds) Optical coherence tomography. Technology and application. Springer, Heidelberg, pp 1–45
6. Izatt JA, Choma MA (2009) Theory of optical coherence tomography. In: Fujimoto J, Drexler W (eds) Optical coherence tomography. Technology and application. Springer, Heidelberg, pp 47–72
7. Chui TY, Song H, Burns SA (2008) Individual variations in human cone photoreceptor packing density: variations with refractive error. Invest Ophthalmol Vis Sci 49:4679–4687
8. Spaide RF, Koizumi H, Pozonni MC (2008) Enhanced depth imaging spectral-domain optical coherence tomography. Am J Ophthalmol 146:496–500
9. Chui TY, Yap MK, Chan HH, Thibos LN (2005) Retinal stretching limits peripheral visual acuity in myopia. Vision Res 45:593–605
10. Margolis R, Spaide RF (2009) A pilot study of enhanced depth imaging optical coherence tomography of the choroid in normal eyes. Am J Ophthalmol 147:811–815
11. Kiel JW, van Heuven WA (1995) Ocular perfusion pressure and choroidal blood flow in the rabbit. Invest Ophthalmol Vis Sci 36:579–585
12. Polak K, Luksch A, Berisha F et al (2007) Altered nitric oxide system in patients with open-angle glaucoma. Arch Ophthalmol 125:494–498
13. Lütjen-Drecoll E (2006) Choroidal innervation in primate eyes. Exp Eye Res 82:357–361
14. Chou PI, Lu DW, Chen JT (2001) Adrenergic supersensitivity of rabbit choroidal blood vessels after sympathetic denervation. Curr Eye Res 23:352–356
15. Reitsamer HA, Zawinka C, Branka M (2004) Dopaminergic vasodilation in the choroidal circulation by d1/d5 receptor activation. Invest Ophthalmol Vis Sci 45:900–905
16. Shimura M, Uchida S, Suzuki A, Nakajima K, Aikawa Y (2002) Reflex choroidal blood flow responses of the eyeball following somatic sensory stimulation in rats. Auton Neurosci 97:35–41

17. Delgado E, Marques-Neves C, Rocha I et al (2009) Intrinsic vasomotricity and adrenergic effects in a model of isolated rabbit eye. Acta Ophthalmol 87:443–449
18. Ramrattan RS, van der Schaft TL, Mooy CM et al (1994) Morphometric analysis of Bruch's membrane, the choriocapillaris, and the choroid in aging. Invest Ophthalmol Vis Sci 35:2857–2864
19. Feeney-Burns L, Burns RP, Gao CL (1990) Age-related macular changes in humans over 90 years old. Am J Ophthalmol 109:265–278
20. Sarks SH (1976) Ageing and degeneration in the macular region: a clinico-pathological study. Br J Ophthalmol 60: 324–341
21. Spaide RF (2009) Age-related choroidal atrophy. Am J Ophthalmol 147:801–810
22. Sarks SH (1973) Senile choroidal sclerosis. Br J Ophthalmol 57:98–109
23. Grossniklaus HE, Green WR (1992) Pathologic findings in pathologic myopia. Retina 12:127–133
24. Coletta NJ, Watson T (2006) Effect of myopia on visual acuity measured with laser interference fringes. Vision Res 46: 636–651
25. Curtin BJ (1977) The posterior staphyloma of pathologic myopia. Trans Am Ophthalmol Soc 75:67–86
26. Hirata A, Negi A (1998) Morphological changes of choriocapillaris in experimentally induced chick myopia. Graefes Arch Clin Exp Ophthalmol 236:132–137
27. Hotchkiss ML, Fine SL (1981) Pathologic myopia and choroidal neovascularization. Am J Ophthalmol 91:177–183
28. Kitaguchi Y, Bessho K, Yamaguchi T, Nakazawa N, Mihashi T, Fujikado T (2007) In vivo measurements of cone photoreceptor spacing in myopic eyes from images obtained by an adaptive optics fundus camera. Jpn J Ophthalmol 51:456–461
29. Klein RM, Curtin BJ (1975) Lacquer crack lesions in pathologic myopia. Am J Ophthalmol 79:386–392
30. Lai TY, Fan DS, Lai WW, Lam DS (2008) Peripheral and posterior pole retinal lesions in association with high myopia: a cross-sectional community-based study in Hong Kong. Eye 22:209–213
31. Luu CD, Lau AM, Lee SY (2006) Multifocal electroretinogram in adults and children with myopia. Arch Ophthalmol 124:328–334
32. Morgan IG (2003) The biological basis of myopic refractive error. Clin Exp Optom 86:276–288
33. Okabe S, Matsuo N, Okamoto S, Kataoka H (1982) Electron microscopic studies on retinochoroidal atrophy in the human eye. Acta Med Okayama 36:11–21
34. Saw SM, Gazzard G, Shih-Yen EC, Chua WH (2005) Myopia and associated pathological complications. Ophthalmic Physiol Opt 25:381–391
35. Vongphanit J, Mitchell P, Wang JJ (2002) Prevalence and progression of myopic retinopathy in an older population. Ophthalmology 109:704–711
36. Atchison DA, Schmid KL, Pritchard N (2006) Neural and optical limits to visual performance in myopia. Vision Res 46:3707–3722
37. Moriyama M, Ohno-Matsui K, Futagami S et al (2007) Morphology and long-term changes of choroidal vascular structure in highly myopic eyes with and without posterior staphyloma. Ophthalmology 114:1755–1762
38. Quaranta M, Arnold J, Coscas G et al (1996) Indocyanine green angiographic features of pathologic myopia. Am J Ophthalmol 122:663–671
39. Akyol N, Kükner AS, Ozdemir T, Esmerligil S (1996) Choroidal and retinal flow changes in degenerative myopia. Can J Ophthalmol 31:113–119
40. To'mey KF, Faris BM, Jalkh AE, Nasr AM (1981) Ocular pulse in high myopia: a study of 40 eyes. Ann Ophthalmol 13:569–571
41. Geijssen HC, Greve EL (1987) The spectrum of primary open angle glaucoma. I: senile sclerotic glaucoma versus high tension glaucoma. Ophthalmic Surg 18:207–213
42. Fujiwara T, Imamura Y, Margolis R, Slakter JS, Spaide RF (2009) Enhanced depth imaging optical coherence tomography of the choroid in highly myopic eyes. Am J Ophthalmol 148:445–450
43. Gass JD, Norton EW, Justice J Jr (1966) Serous detachment of the retinal pigment epithelium. Trans Am Acad Ophthalmol Otolaryngol 70:990–1015
44. Gass JD (1972) Drusen and disciform macular detachment and degeneration. Trans Am Ophthalmol Soc 70:409–436
45. Bird AC, Marshall J (1986) Retinal pigment epithelial detachments in the elderly. Trans Ophthalmol Soc U K 105:674–682
46. Morre DJ, Hussain AA, Marshall J (1995) Age-related variation in the hydraulic conductivity of Bruch's membrane. Invest Ophthalmol Vis Sci 36:1290–1297
47. Casswell AG, Kohen D, Bird AC (1985) Retinal pigment epithelial detachments in the elderly: classification and outcome. Br J Ophthalmol 69:397–403
48. Kuhn D, Meunier I, Soubrane G, Coscas G (1995) Imaging of chorioretinal anastomoses in vascularized retinal pigment epithelium detachments. Arch Ophthalmol 113:1392–1398
49. Slakter JS, Yannuzzi LA, Schneider U et al (2000) Retinal choroidal anastomoses and occult choroidal neovascularization in age-related macular degeneration. Ophthalmology 107:742–753
50. Hartnett ME, Weiter JJ, Garsd A, Jalkh AE (1992) Classification of retinal pigment epithelial detachments associated with drusen. Graefes Arch Clin Exp Ophthalmol 230:11–19
51. Hartnett ME, Weiter JJ, Staurenghi G, Elsner AE (1996) Deep retinal vascular anomalous complexes in advanced age-related macular degeneration. Ophthalmology 103:2042–2053
52. Yannuzzi LA, Negrão S, Iida T et al (2001) Retinal angiomatous proliferation in age-related macular degeneration. Retina 21:416–434

53. Gass JD, Agarwal A, Lavina AM, Tawansy KA (2003) Focal inner retinal hemorrhages in patients with drusen: an early sign of occult choroidal neovascularization and chorioretinal anastomosis. Retina 23:741–751
54. Spaide RF (2009) Enhanced depth imaging optical coherence tomography of retinal pigment epithelial detachment in age-related macular degeneration. Am J Ophthalmol 147:644–652
55. Linsenmeier RA, Padnick-Silver L (2000) Metabolic dependence of photoreceptors on the choroid in the normal and detached retina. Invest Ophthalmol Vis Sci 41:3117–3123

Chapter 16

Spectral-Domain Optical Coherence Tomography in Central Serous Chorioretinopathy

16

Sandeep Saxena, Carsten H. Meyer, Hans-Martin Helb, and Frank G. Holz

Core Messages

- Central serous chorioretinopathy (CSC) typically affects young and middle-aged males and is characterized by serous retinal detachment at the macula secondary to increased permeability of choroidal vessels and a barrier defect in the retinal pigment epithelium (RPE)
- Spectral-domain optical coherence tomography (OCT) offers a new approach to diagnose, prognosticate, and monitor the clinical course of the disease and its response to therapy
- Morphologic alterations in the RPE, detached retina, and subretinal space around the fluorescein leakage sites can be observed in acute CSC
- Three-dimensional (3D) OCT imaging delineates the microstructural changes that occur within the photoreceptor layers and demonstrates the spatial relationship between the laterally spreading or scattering microstructures and the fovea in the eyes with CSC.
- Primarily, the outer segment layer is altered in CSC
- Visual prognosis in patients with CSC can be linked to retinal morphological changes by OCT
- Presence of correlation between foveal thickness and visual acuity has been observed
- Topographic changes in CSC can be very elegantly visualized and documented with 3D-reconstruction.

16.1 Introduction

Central serous chorioretinopathy (CSC) [1–4] that typically affects middle-aged males is characterized by serous retinal detachment at the macula secondary to increased permeability of the choroidal vessels and a barrier defect in the retinal pigment epithelium (RPE) [5, 6]. Ultrastructural studies in animal models of CSC have shown defects in RPE, which might favor a breakdown in the outer blood-retinal barrier [7].

Presenting symptoms include central visual loss, a sudden decrease in vision that can be corrected with an increased hyperopic correction, metamorphopsia, central scotoma, and decreased color saturation. The symptoms are usually self-limiting, but can recur in the same or the opposite eye. The association of the disease with type A personality, systemic hypertension, and corticosteroid intake is well known.

Although eyes with CSC usually have a good visual prognosis, prolonged and recurrent macular detachment may lead to degenerative changes and poor visual outcome [8, 9].

Acute CSC: The acute form is classically unilateral and characterized by one or more focal leaks at the level of RPE on fluorescein angiography. The neurosensory detachment contains clear subretinal fluid, but may be cloudy or have subretinal fibrin in some cases. This form is self-limiting and does not lead to gross visual deficit after resolution.

Chronic CSC: The chronic form is believed to be due to diffuse RPE disease and is usually bilateral. It presents with diffuse RPE atrophic changes, varying degrees of subretinal fluid, RPE alterations, and RPE tracks. It is characterized by diffuse areas of RPE leakage on fluorescein angiography. It has a relatively poorer visual prognosis.

Management options for CSC include observation, focal laser photocoagulation, and low-fluence photodynamic therapy [10–13].

> **Summary for the Clinician**
>
> - CSC affects young and middle-aged males in their third to fifth decades, and is secondary to increased permeability of choroidal vessels and a barrier defect in the RPE
> - Although eyes with CSC usually have a good visual prognosis, prolonged and recurrent macular detachment may lead to degenerative changes and poor visual outcome

16.2 Optical Coherence Tomography

Optical coherence tomography (OCT) functions as a type of optical biopsy, providing information on retinal pathology in situ and in real time, with resolutions approaching that of excisional biopsy and histopathology. OCT is potentially useful as a non invasive diagnostic technique for quantitative examination. It offers a new approach to diagnose, prognosticate, and monitor the clinical course of the disease and its response to therapy.

OCT features of CSC are [14]:

Acute CSC

(i) Thickening of the neurosensory retina with detachment.
(ii) Retinal pigment epithelial detachment.
(iii) Combination of both.
(iv) Presence of moderately high reflective mass bridging the detached neurosensory retina and RPE with subretinal fibrin.

Chronic CSC

(i) Foveal atrophy and thinning.
(ii) Cystoid changes at the fovea.

Associated Complications

(i) RPE tear (rip).
(ii) Choroidal neovascularization.

16.3 Role of Optical Coherence Tomography

OCT plays a significant role in:

(i) Diagnosis of the disease,
(ii) Progression of the disease,
(iii) Prediction of visual acuity recovery, and
(iv) Explanation of poor visual acuity recovery.

16.4 Spectral-Domain Optical Coherence Tomography

The development of high-speed spectral detection technique has enabled a significant improvement in ophthalmic OCT imaging performance. Three-dimensional, high-resolution OCT can provide information on intraretinal morphology that is not available from any other noninvasive diagnostic modality. High-speed imaging facilitates the acquisition of 3D data sets, thus enabling volumetric rendering and the generation of OCT fundus images that precisely and reproducibly register OCT images to fundus features [15]. High-speed ultrahigh-resolution OCT generates images of retinal pathologies with improved quality, more comprehensive retinal coverage, and more precise registration than time-domain OCT. The speed preserves the retinal topography, thus enabling the visualization of subtle changes associated with the disease. High-definition high-transverse pixel density OCT images improve visualization of photoreceptor and pigment epithelial morphology as well as thin intra retinal structures. Three-dimensional (3D) OCT enables comprehensive retinal coverage, reduces sampling errors, and enables assessment of 3D pathology. This new technology has become a useful tool for elucidating disease pathogenesis and improving disease management [16].

High-resolution OCT has been used to identify typical changes in CSC. Topographic changes in CSC can be visualized with 3D reconstructions in all locations. Retinal thickness can be measured and quantified precisely. The results may be presented in 2D and 3D maps. High-resolution OCT is able to provide essential additional information about CSC when combined with appropriate analyzing programmes. Apart from precise volumetric measurements, exact localization of the pathological deviations can be achieved (Fig. 16.1) [17].

> **Summary for the Clinician**
>
> - 3D, high-resolution OCT can provide information on intraretinal morphology that is not available from any other noninvasive diagnostic modality.
> - 3D OCT enables comprehensive retinal coverage, reduces sampling errors, and enables assessment of 3D patholoxgy.

Morphologic alterations in the RPE, detached retina, and subretinal space around the fluorescein leakage sites can be observed in acute CSC [18]. Among the leakage sites, spectral-domain OCT shows RPE abnormalities in the majority of the cases. Pigment epithelial detachment and protruding or irregular RPE layer can also be observed. However, higher resolution of the leakage site reveals

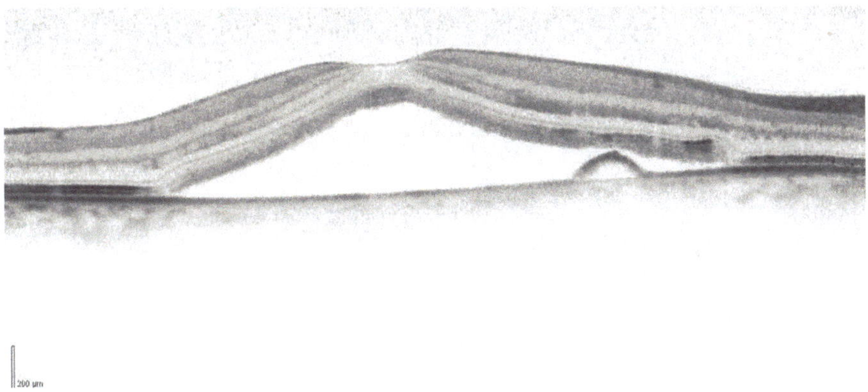

Fig. 16.1 Central serous chorioretinopathy (CSC): Spectral-domain OCT shows serous detachment of the retina associated with a retinal pigment epithelial detachment. Also, thickening of the layer associated with outer segments of the photoreceptors is evident

proliferating RPE cells at the leakage site (Figs. 16.2a, b and 16.3). Fibrinous exudates in the subretinal space and sagging/dipping of the posterior layer of the neurosensory retina above the leakage sites may also be noted (Fig. 16.4). An RPE defect at the edge of or within the PED may be evident through which fluid might pass from the sub-RPE to the subretinal area. The posterior surface of the detached retina is smooth or granulated. The smooth posterior detached retina becomes granulated in the presence of residual subretinal fluid (Figs. 16.5 and 16.6). Persistent PED may also be observed despite SRF resolution.

> **Summary for the Clinician**
>
> - Among the leakage sites, spectral-domain OCT shows RPE abnormalities in the majority of cases. Pigment epithelial detachment and protruding or irregular RPE layer can also be observed.
> - Fibrinous exudates in the subretinal space and sagging/dipping of the posterior layer of the neurosensory retina above the leakage sites may also be noted.
> - The posterior surface of the detached retina may be smooth or granulated.
> - Persistent PED may also be observed despite SRF resolution.

En face OCT has been found to detect alterations of RPE in the form of PED or a small bulge of RPE in the eyes with CSC. Most alterations of RPE are associated with choroidal abnormalities [19]. OCT-ophthalmoscope has also been found to detect morphologic changes easily and noninvasively at the point of dye leakage in the eyes with CSC. Transverse images (C-scan) clearly showed serous retinal detachment and irregular lesions in RPE. These findings agree with the location of lesions in areas of fluorescein dye leakage on fluorescein angiography. Longitudinal images (B-scan) of irregular RPE lesions in transverse images show PED and small protrusion of the RPE layer and rough RPE layer [20]. 3D single-layer RPE map has been found to reveal abnormal pattern in the asymptomatic eyes of patients with unilateral CSC [21].

3D OCT imaging delineates the microstructural changes that occur within the photoreceptor layers and demonstrates the spatial relationship between the laterally spreading or scattering microstructures and the fovea in the eyes with CSC. Visualization of the 3D relationship between the external limiting membrane and each photoreceptor layer before and after macular reattachment facilitates understanding of the anatomic and vision changes that result from CSC [22].

Visual prognosis in patients with CSC can be linked to retinal morphological changes by OCT [23–25]. Pathologic changes in the foveal photoreceptor layer show a line corresponding to back reflection from the external limiting membrane visible in images from eyes with all stages of CSC. Back reflection from the photoreceptor inner and outer segment junction (IS/OS) is absent before, but is present after reattachment. Primarily, the outer segment layer is altered in CSC. Punctate areas of intense reflectivity are observed more frequently in the outer segment layer of the detached retinas in cases of chronic or recurrent versus acute CSC. Eyes with large defects in the subfoveal IS/OS have poor visual acuity when compared with eyes with small or no defects which have good visual acuity [22].

Photoreceptor-segment morphologic changes at the detached retina show elongation of the photoreceptor outer segments and decreased thickness of the outer nuclear layer [26]. The outer nuclear layer thickness is positively correlated with the best-corrected visual acuity (BCVA) in resolved CSC. Discontinuity of the IS/OS line

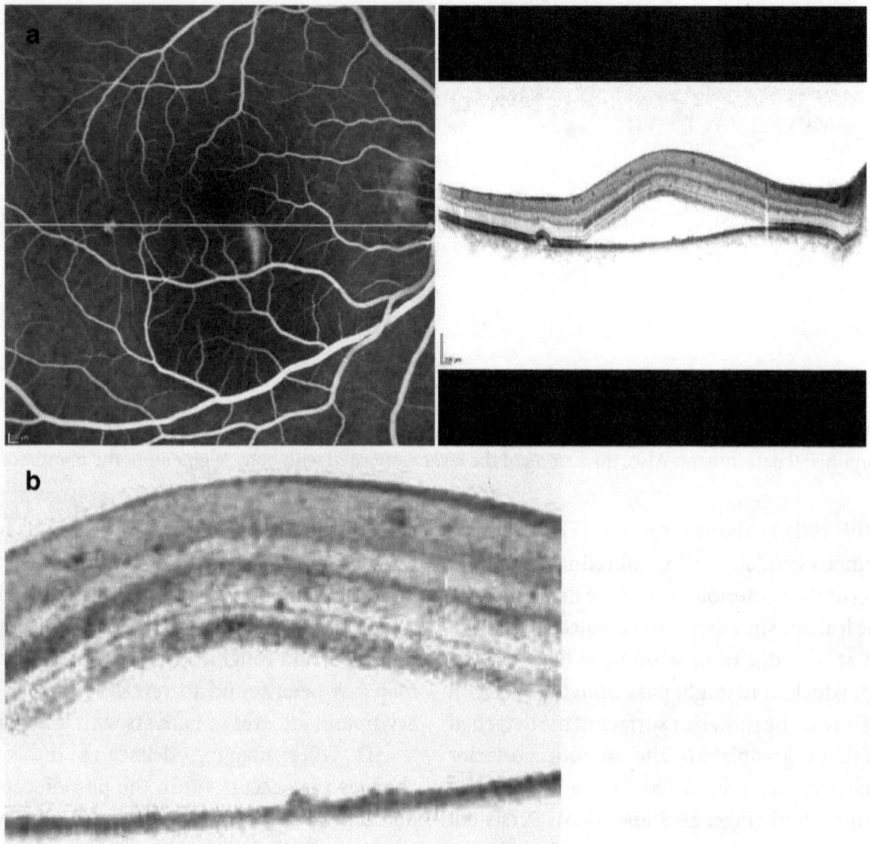

Fig. 16.2 (**a**) CSC: Fluorescein angiography shows a pigment epithelial detachment and a leakage site. Spectral-domain OCT shows corresponding retinal pigment epithelial detachment associated with serous detachment of the retina and proliferating RPE cells corresponding to the leakage site. (**b**) CSC: Spectral-domain OCT (high magnification) shows serous detachment of the retina associated with proliferating RPE cells

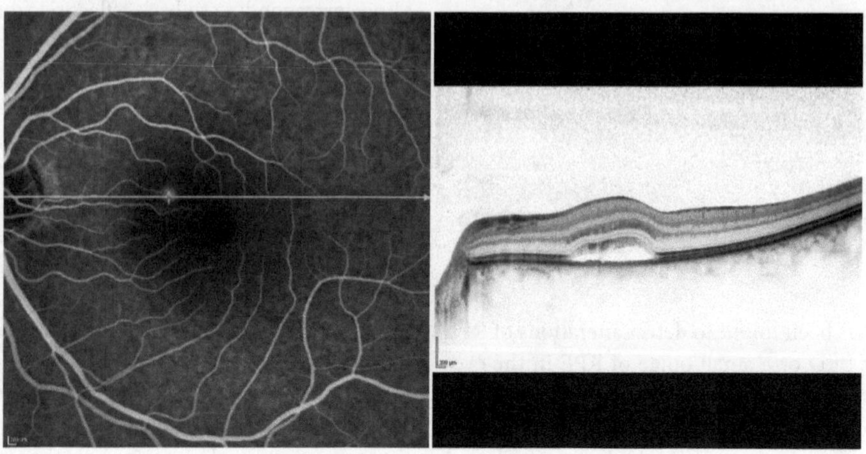

Fig. 16.3 CSC: Fluorescein angiography shows an ink blot appearance. Spectral-domain OCT shows serous detachment of the retina associated with proliferating RPE cells corresponding to the leakage site

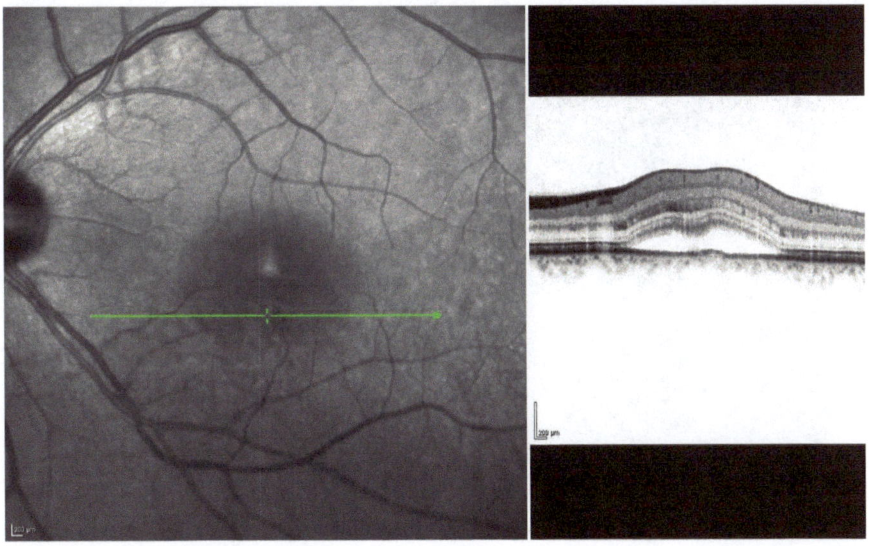

Fig. 16.4 CSC: Infrared photograph shows a serous detachment of the macula. Spectral-domain OCT shows serous detachment of the retina, retinal pigment epithelial detachment, and sagging/dipping of the posterior layer of the neurosensory retina

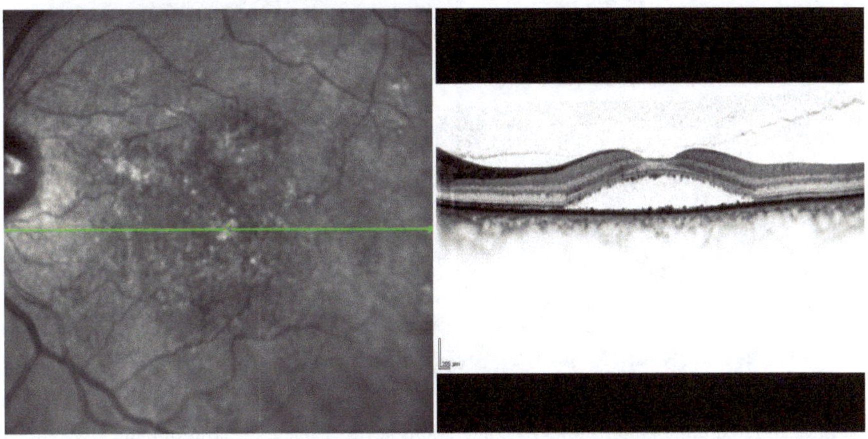

Fig. 16.5 Chronic CSC: Infrared photograph shows a serous detachment of the macula along the retinal pigment epithelium (RPE) alterations. Spectral-domain OCT shows serous detachment of the retina and granulated posterior detached retina in the presence of residual subretinal fluid. Irregular, granulated retinal pigment epithelial layer is also observed

is prevalent in eyes with thinner outer nuclear layer and lower BCVA [27].

In patients with acute phase of CSC, the detached neurosensory retina is thickened and visual acuity is kept well before and after resolution of subretinal fluid [28]. However, in cases with chronic CSC prolonged for several years, the persistent macular detachment may cause degenerative changes in RPE and the neurosensory retina, which results in a poor visual outcome (Fig. 16.7) [23, 29]. Foveal thickness can be a factor predictive of visual outcome in patients with persistent CSC. Presence of correlation between foveal thickness and visual acuity has been observed [23]. Even simple measurements of foveal thickness on OCT images can provide objective information for the management of CSC. Final visual acuity correlates with initial and final foveal thickness. Damage of the neurosensory retina may reflect in foveal thickness at final examination and visual outcome [30]. Both foveal thickness and visual acuity have been observed to be proportional to the duration of symptoms, which lead to foveal attenuation and atrophy, which may result from prolonged absence of contact between photoreceptors and retinal pigment epithelial cells [31].Visual recovery after macular reattachment may be predicted by

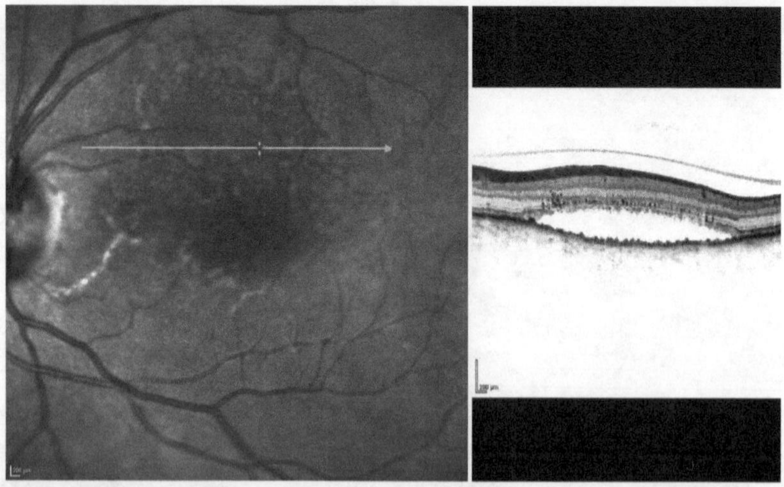

Fig. 16.6 Chronic CSC: Infrared photograph shows a serous detachment of the macula along the RPE alterations. Spectral-domain OCT shows serous detachment of the retina, granulated posterior detached retina, and granulated irregular retinal pigment epithelial layer

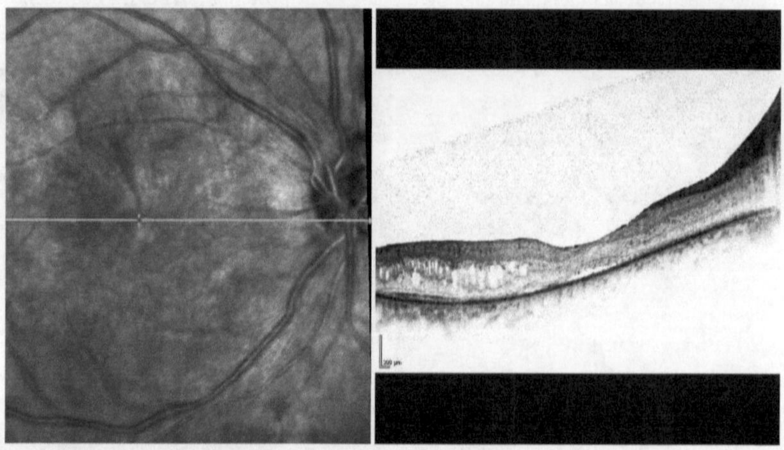

Fig. 16.7 Chronic CSC: Infrared photograph shows RPE alterations at the macula. Spectral-domain OCT shows residual serous detachment of the retina along with cystic changes

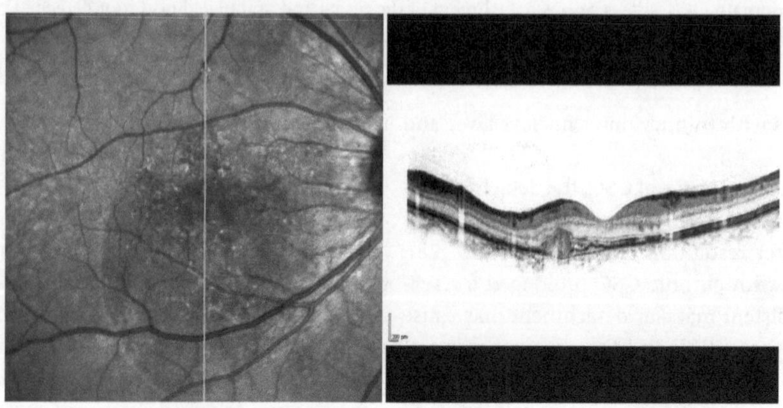

Fig. 16.8 Chronic CSC: Infrared photograph shows serous retinal detachment with RPE alterations and choroidal neovascularization. Spectral-domain OCT shows a choroidal neovasular membrane

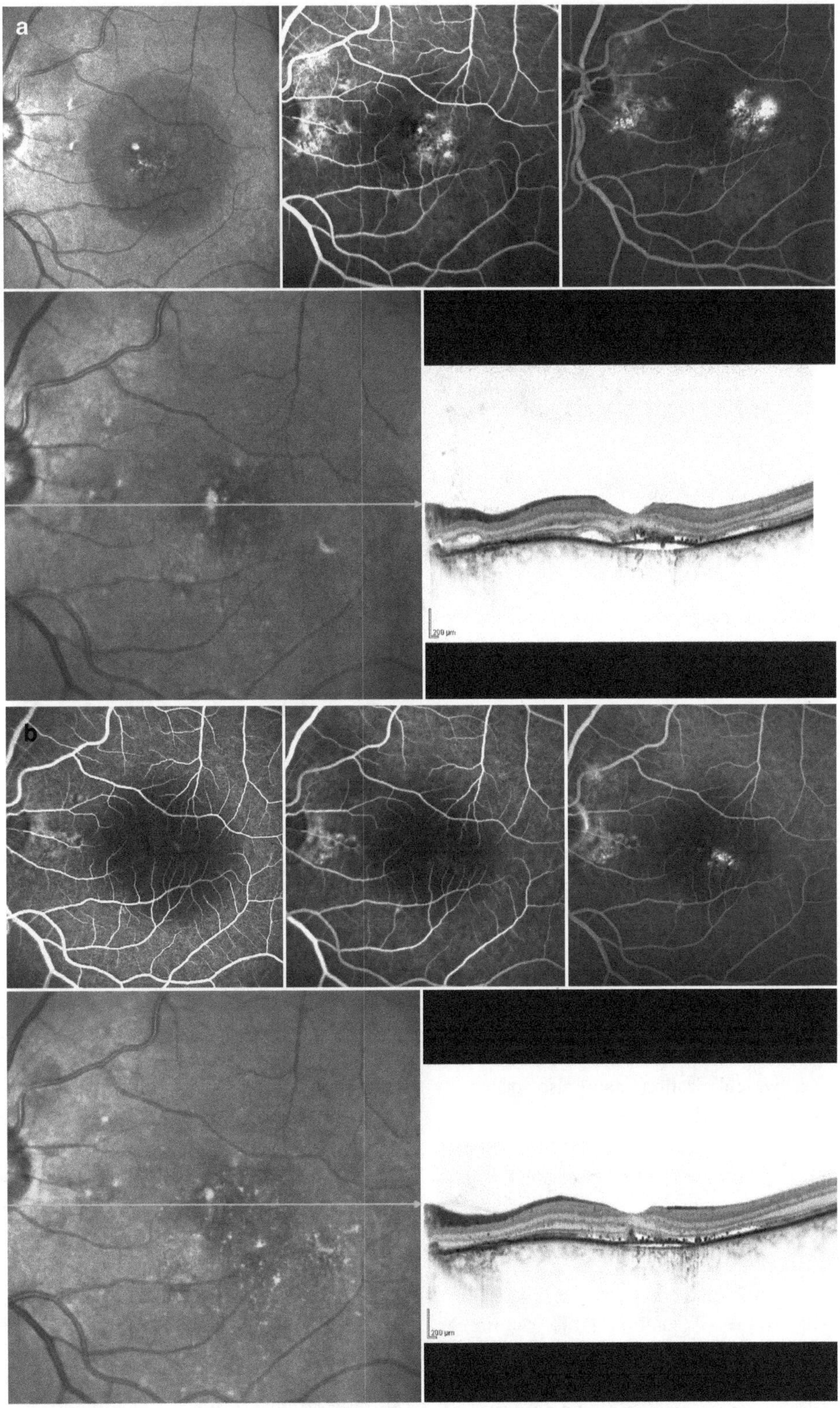

Fig. 16.9 (**a**) Photodynamic therapy in CSC: pre treatment. (**b**) Photodynamic therapy in CSC: post treatment [13]

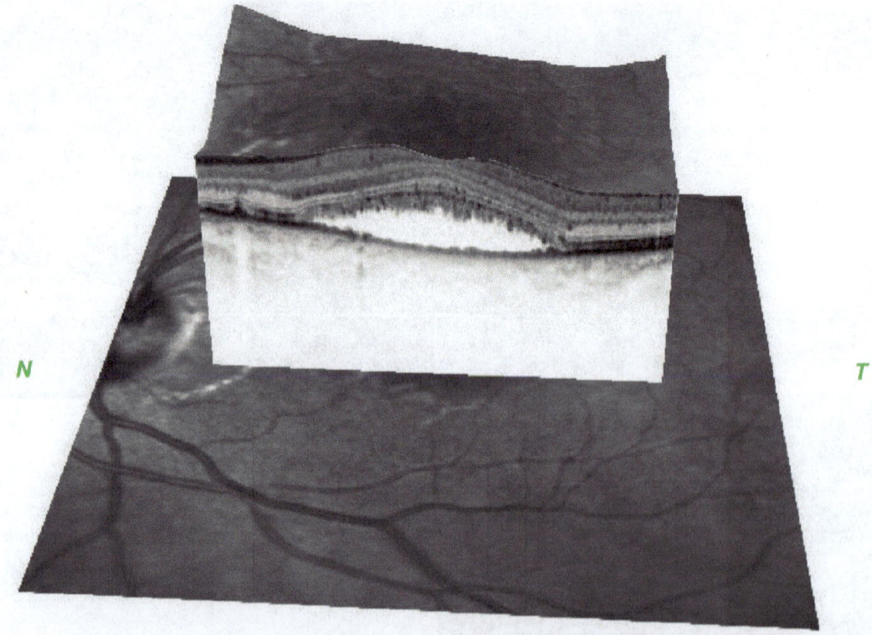

Fig. 16.10 Topographic changes in CSC can be visualized and documented very well with 3D reconstruction

preserved undamaged outer photoreceptor layer and higher visual acuity at presentation [25]. Prolonged and recurrent retinal detachment at the macula causes an apoptotic mechanism which is involved in the process of degeneration of photoreceptor death [32, 33]. This process may cause thinning of foveal thickness after the resolution of subretinal fluid.

Accumulation of abnormal production of outer segment of the neurosensory retina is related to clinical manifestations in OCT as a granulated profile on the outer surface of the detached retina, and in fundus camera or scanning laser ophthalmoscope as an autofluorescence in the eyes with CSC [34–37].

Choroidal neovascularization may also occur in patients with CSC (Fig. 16.8).

Summary for the Clinician

- 3D OCT imaging delineates the microstructural changes that occur within the photoreceptor layers in the eyes with CSC.
- Visualization of the 3D relationship between the external limiting membrane and each photoreceptor layer before and after macular reattachment facilitates understanding of the anatomic and vision changes that result from CSC.

Effect of therapy can also be observed on spectral-domain OCT [38]. Furthermore, resolution of serous retinal detachment and quantitative macular thickness can be documented very well (Figs. 16.9a, b).

The spectral-domain OCT can create 3D area scans by combining B-scans. As it is possible to acquire high-density volumetric data of the macula, the OCT data can be processed to provide comprehensive structural information. With 3D image reconstruction, the 3D area scans can be manipulated and viewed from multiple angles. The unprecedented visualization provided by this technology enables determination of specific alterations in the retinal anatomy characteristics. Topographic changes in CSC can be very elegantly visualized and documented with 3D reconstruction (Fig. 16.10).

The *X*, *Y*, and *Z* planes for slicing are defined as follows:

X plane is the horizontal B-scan as it is acquired. The anatomical features shown in the X plane are real, as the eye movement is negligible.

Y plane is the vertical reconstructed B-scan. The eye movement in the reconstructed B-scan is quite noticeable.

Z plane is a reconstructed en face image. It is also called the coronal scan.

The relationship among the *X*, *Y*, and *Z* planes can be observed exquisitely [39].

References

1. Gass JDM (1960) Pathogenesis of disciform detachment of the neuroepithelium, II: idiopathic central serous choroidopathy. Am J Ophthalmol 63:578–615
2. Gass JDM (1997) Specific diseases causing disciform macular detachment. In: Stereoscopic atlas of macular diseases: diagnosis and treatment. Mosby, St Louis, pp 49–70
3. Kitaya N, Nagaoka T, Hikichi T et al (2003) Features of abnormal choroidal circulation in central serous chorioretinopathy. Br J Ophthalmol 87:709–712
4. Spaide RF, Campeas L, Haas A et al (1996) Central serous chorioretinopathy in younger and older adults. Ophthalmology 103:2070–2079
5. Guyer DR, Yannuzzi LA, Slakter JS et al (1994) Digital indocyanine green videoangiography of central serous chorioretinopathy. Arch Ophthalmol 112:1057–1062
6. Iida T, Kishi S, Hagimura N, Shimizu K (1999) Persistent and bilateral choroidal vascular abnormalities in central serous chorioretinopathy. Retina 19:508–512
7. Yoshioka H, Katsume Y, Akune H (1982) Experimental central serous chorioretinopathy in monkey eyes: fluorescein angiographic findings. Ophthalmologica 185:168–178
8. Jalkh AE, Jabbour N, Avila MP et al (1984) Retinal pigment epithelium decompensation. I. Clinical features and natural course. Ophthalmology 91:1544–1548
9. Yannuzzi LA, Shakin JL, Fisher YL, Altomonte MA (1984) Peripheral retinal detachments and retinal pigment epithelial atrophic tracts secondary to central serous pigment epitheliopathy. Ophthalmology 91:1554–1572
10. Helb HM, Charbel Issa P, Fleckenstein M et al (2009) Clinical evaluation of simultaneous confocal scanning laser ophthalmoscopy imaging combined with high-resolution, spectral domain optical coherence tomography. Acta Ophthalmol. Aug 25. [Epub ahead of print]
11. Hassenstein A, Meyer CH (2009). Clinical use and research applications of Heidelberg retinal angiography and spectral-domain optical coherence tomography - a review. Clin Experiment Ophthalmol. Jan;37(1):130–43
12. Mennel S, Barbazetto I, Meyer CH et al (2007) Ocular photodynamic therapy – standard applications and new indications (Part II). Ophthalmologica 221:282–291
13. Meyer CH, Mennel S (2007) Therapie der idiopathischen Chorioretinopathia centralis serosa mit der Photodynamischen Therapie. In: Lang GE (ed) Die PDT in der Augenheilkunde. Springer, Verlag pp 57–62
14. Bhende M, Nair BK (2006) Central serous chorioretinopathy. In: Saxena S, Meredith TA (eds) Optical coherence tomography in retinal diseases. Jaypee, New Delhi, pp137–144
15. Drexler W, Fujimoto JG (2008) State-of-the-art retinal optical coherence tomography. Prog Retin Eye Res 27:45–88
16. Srinivasan VJ, Wojtkowski M, Witkin AJ et al (2006) High-definition and 3-dimensional imaging of macular pathologies with high-speed ultrahigh-resolution optical coherence tomography. Ophthalmology 113:2054–2059
17. Stock G, Ahlers C, Sayegh R et al (2008) Three-dimensional imaging in central serous chorioretinopathy. Ophthalmologe 105:1127–1134
18. Fujimoto H, Gomi F, Wakabayashi T et al (2008) Morphologic changes in acute central serous chorioretinopathy evaluated by fourier-domain optical coherence tomography. Ophthalmology 115:1494–1500
19. Hirami Y, Tsujikawa A, Sasahara M et al (2007) Alterations of retinal pigment epithelium in central serous chorioretinopathy. Clin Experiment Ophthalmol 35:225–230
20. Mitarai K, Gomi F, Tano Y (2006) Three-dimensional optical coherence tomographic findings in central serous chorioretinopathy. Graefes Arch Clin Exp Ophthalmol 244: 1415–1420
21. Gupta P, Gupta V, Dogra MR et al (2009) Morphological changes in the retinal pigment epithelium on spectral-domain OCT in the unaffected eyes with idiopathic central serous chorioretinopathy. Int Ophthalmol. Jan 30. [Epub ahead of print]
22. Matsumoto H, Kishi S, Otani T, Sato T (2008) Elongation of photoreceptor outer segment in central serous chorioretinopathy. Am J Ophthalmol 145:162–168
23. Eandi CM, Chung JE, Piccolino FC, Spaide RF (2005) Optical coherence tomography in unilateral resolved central serous chorioretinopathy. Retina 25:417–421
24. Matsumoto H, Sato T, Kishi S (2009) Outer nuclear layer thickness at the fovea determines visual outcomes in resolved central serous chorioretinopathy. Am J Ophthalmol 148: 105–110
25. Ojima Y, Hangai M, Sasahara M et al (2007) Three-dimensional imaging of the foveal photoreceptor layer in central serous chorioretinopathy using high-speed optical coherence tomography. Ophthalmology 114:2197–2207
26. Hee MR, Puliafito CA, Wong C et al (1995) Optical coherence tomography of central serous chorioretinopathy. Am J Ophthalmol 120:65–74
27. Piccolino FC, de la Longrais RR, Ravera G et al (2005) The foveal photoreceptor layer and visual acuity loss in central serous chorioretinopathy. Am J Ophthalmol 139:87–99
28. Iida T, Hagimura N, Sato T, Kishi S (2000) Evaluation of central serous chorioretinopathy with optical coherence tomography. Am J Ophthalmol 129:16–20
29. Iida T, Yannuzzi LA, Spaide RF et al (2003) Cystoid macular degeneration in chronic central serous chorioretinopathy. Retina 23:1–7
30. Furuta M, Iida T, Kishi S (2009) Foveal thickness can predict visual outcome in patients with persistent central serous chorioretinopathy. Ophthalmologica 223:28–31

31. Wang M, Sander B, Larsen M (2002) Retinal atrophy in idiopathic central serous chorioretinopathy. Am J Ophthalmol 133:787–793
32. Berglin L, Algvere PV, Seregard S (1997) Photoreceptor decay over time and apoptosis in experimental retinal detachment. Graefes Arch Clin Exp Ophthalmol 235: 306–312
33. Hisatomi T, Sakamoto T, Goto Y et al (2002) Critical role of photoreceptor apoptosis in functional damage after retinal detachment. Curr Eye Res 24:161–172
34. Spaide RF, Klancnik JM Jr (2005) Fundus autofluorescence and central serous chorioretinopathy. Ophthalmology 112: 825–833
35. Framme C, Walter A, Gabler B et al (2005) Fundus autofluorescence in acute and chronic-recurrent central serous chorioretinopathy. Acta Ophthalmol Scand 81: 161–167
36. Kon Y, Iida T, Maruko I, Saito M (2008) Optical coherence tomography – ophthalmoscope of central serous chorioretinopathy with precipitates. Retina 28:864–869
37. von Ruckmann A, Fitzke FW, Fan J et al (2002) Abnormalities of fundus autofluorescence in central serous retinopathy. Am J Ophthalmol 133:780–786
38. Lang GE, Mennel S, Spital G et al (2009) Verschiedene Indikationen der photodynamischen Therapie in der Augenheilkunde. Klin Monatsbl Augenheilkd. 2009 Sep; 226(9):725–39
39. Saxena S, Singh K (2009) Three dimensional retinal imaging in spectral domain optical coherence tomography. In: Saxena S, Sadda S (eds) Emerging technologies in retinal diseases. Jaypee, New Delhi, pp 67–121

Chapter 17

New Developments in Optical Coherence Tomography Technology

17

Wolfgang Drexler, Rainer Leitgeb, and Christoph K. Hitzenberger

Core Messages

- Optical coherence tomography (OCT) represents the fasted adopted retinal imaging modality in the history of ophthalmology.
- Three-dimensional (3D) retinal OCT at 1,060 nm (as opposed to 800 nm) enables wide-field 3D visualization of the entire choroid, fairly irrespective of the patient's fundus pigmentation.
- 3D OCT at 1,060 nm (as opposed to 800 nm) promises improved clinical feasibility for retinal imaging in patients with opaque ocular media in the anterior eye segment (e.g., cataract or corneal haze).
- Combining adaptive optics and OCT technology might pave the way for in vivo cellular resolution retinal imaging for routine diagnosis in the eye clinic.
- Extensions of OCT are recently developed that enable noninvasive depth resolved functional imaging of the retina, providing blood flow or physiologic tissue information. These extensions of OCT should not only improve image contrast, but should also enable the differentiation of retinal pathologies via localized metabolic properties or functional state.
- Polarization sensitive (PS)-OCT provides intrinsic, tissue-specific contrast of birefringent and depolarizing tissue.
- PS-OCT can be used to identify and segment the retinal pigment epithelium (RPE) based on its depolarizing property, and to analyze the retinal nerve fiber layer (RNFL) based on its birefringence
- Doppler OCT (D-OCT) provides quantitative information about retinal perfusion, in addition to standard OCT structure tomograms.
- D-OCT promises to improve early diagnosis by detecting microcirculation abnormalities as precursors of retinal diseases, and in general, vascular diseases.

17.1 Background and Motivation

Optical coherence tomography (OCT) is a rapidly emerging noninvasive, optical diagnostic imaging modality enabling in vivo cross-sectional or volumetric tomographic visualization of internal microstructure in the biological systems at resolution levels of a few micrometers [1]. Advances in the photonics technology including high-speed detectors, ultrabroad bandwidth, and tunable light sources as well as novel contrast mechanisms have recently revolutionized imaging performance and clinical feasibility of retinal OCT. In this view, OCT is now not only considered as an optical counterpart of ultrasound imaging, but also as an optical analog to computed tomography and magnetic resonance imaging, not enabling full body imaging, but noninvasive optical biopsy, i.e., micron/cellular resolution 3D visualization of superficial (up to 1–2 mm) tissue morphology [2, 3].

The eye provides easy optical access to the anterior segment and the retina due to its essentially transparent nature. Hence, ophthalmic and especially retinal imaging has so far not only been the first, but also the most successful clinical application for OCT since its initiation in the late-1980s and early 1990s. Objectively, this is evidenced by the fact that about 50% of all OCT publications so far have been published in ophthalmic journals. In addition, eight companies offer this technology in its recent generation for 3D retinal OCT - all of them working in the 800 nm wavelength region. Consequently, retinal OCT represents the fastest adopted imaging technology in the history of ophthalmology.

While commercial retinal OCT systems (Stratus OCT) were based on the so-called time-domain OCT, enabling up to 400 A-scans (one-dimensional measurements) per second, the fourth generation (spectral or Fourier domain based) commercial retinal OCT systems, nowadays, can perform up to 100 times more measurements per second, enabling either highly sampled (high definition) 2D tomograms or 3D (volumetric) imaging of the retina [4, 5]. The clinical benefit of these instruments is demonstrated in highly sampled 3D visualization of the retina during a reasonable short data acquisition time, resulting in more reliable and reproducible 2D thickness maps of (intra)retinal layers. From a clinical perspective, segmentation of retinal tomograms is extremely important. Reliable, reproducible algorithms that automatically detect interfaces between all major intraretinal layers in healthy as well as pathologic retinas in a short amount of time are still a challenge for software engineers. Nevertheless, segmentation is essential not only to provide normative databases that might contribute to improved diagnosis of retinal pathologies, but also for improved understanding of retinal pathogenesis as well as enhanced (objective) monitoring of various novel therapy approaches. Furthermore, the clinically most feasible and at the same time least time-intensive representation of the large amount of data acquired by these commercial fourth-generation retinal OCT systems is still a matter of discussion. However, reducing the wealth of information about intraretinal microstructure simply to two-dimensional (2D) thickness maps is definitely an underutilization of the state-of-the-art high-speed, high-resolution retinal OCT. It is also noteworthy that in addition to clinical cross-sectional or longitudinal patient trials, the tremendous potential of 3D retinal OCT is also to noninvasively monitor the development of retinal-disease progression or efficacy of novel therapy approaches in various animal models of retinal diseases.

Recent scientific efforts focus on the development of OCT not only to provide morphologic tissue information at cellular resolution, but also to enable either contrast enhancement or extraction of *depth-resolved* functional tissue properties. The contrast of presently available commercial OCT systems - time domain as well as spectral domain - is based on the intensity of backscattered light. However, as it is well known from microscopy, intensity-based imaging is frequently unable to directly differentiate between different tissues. Polarization sensitive (PS)-OCT has the advantage of additional information carried in the polarization state of the backscattered light. By measuring this polarization state, PS-OCT generates an intrinsic, tissue-specific contrast that can be used for tissue identification, segmentation, and for quantitative measurements. Being an interferometric technique, OCT can trace small structural changes, such as flowing red blood cells even within small retinal vessels with absolute precision. This unique capability of Doppler OCT (D-OCT) to quantitatively contrast depth-resolved retinal and sub-retinal microcirculation promises new perspectives beyond standard angiography for early diagnosis of retinal diseases as well as for pharmacological research.

Summary for the Clinician

- Fourth-generation commercial retinal OCT based on Fourier or spectral domain (as opposed to time-domain (e.g., Stratus OCT) OCT significantly enable improved data acquisition speed for 3D retinal OCT.
- Clinically relevant (2D or 3D) representation of retinal OCT data and automated, time-effective, robust, and reliable quantification of all major intraretinal layers still remain a challenge.
- Despite an increase in data acquisition speed by two orders of magnitude - from 400 A-scans/s to 40,000 A-scans/s - sufficient isotropic sampling, i.e., equidistant spacing between voxels in all three dimensions is still not possible, unless using additional technological efforts, e.g., an eye tracker or significantly faster detector technology.
- Spectral- or Fourier-domain OCT technology, despite its significantly higher data-acquisition efficacy - resulting in higher data-acquisition speed - has transferred motion artifacts from a one-dimensional problem (between adjacent A-scans) to a 3D one (between adjacent B-scans).
- In contrast to time-domain OCT (e.g., Stratus OCT), spectral- or Fourier-domain OCT suffers from a scanning depth dependent system sensitivity as well as axial resolution decay, resulting in reduced detection sensitivity and axial resolution due to involuntary axial eye motions.

17.2 Three-Dimensional Imaging of the Choroid

At the moment, all commercially available retinal OCT instruments work in the 800 nm wavelength region. This is mainly due to the availability of cost-effective, compact light sources and detectors in this wavelength range. Although these commercial 3D retinal OCT systems at 800 nm can resolve all major intraretinal layers, they only enable limited penetration beyond the retina strongly depending on the patient's fundus pigmentation, thus resulting in limited visualization of the choroid. In contrast to the common 800 nm region, scattering is reduced in the 1,060 nm water absorption window [6], which was demonstrated with time-domain OCT based systems in ex vivo porcine retinas [7] and in vivo in healthy human subjects [6]. Moreover, in clinical OCT, turbid ocular media (e.g., cataract or corneal haze) represent a significant challenge when imaging the retina [8]. These studies triggered ongoing interest at this wavelength region for 3D visualization of the vascular structure of the retina and the choroid, and to investigate the involvement of individual parts of the blood supply with the development and progress of retinal diseases like age-related macular degeneration [9–14].

Ophthalmic spectrometer based OCT relies on the availability of high-speed camera technology as well as suitable broadband light sources (>70 nm). While silicon-based cameras use the 400–920 nm wavelength region, high-speed linear arrays (≥20,000 spectra/s) with sufficient (>1,024) pixels of 1 μm and beyond were not readily available. To circumvent this problem, alternative high-speed tunable sources have been developed [14, 15], which are currently rather challenging to operate, quite expensive, need complicated detection electronics, and offer only limited optical bandwidth usually centered at the shorter portion of the 1,060 nm wavelength band, where melanin absorption is up to 2.5 times higher, restricting high axial resolution OCT imaging and penetration. Several groups recently demonstrated 3D OCT at 1,060 nm with enhanced visualization of the choroid up to the sclera. A cost-effective, easy-to-implement system was used based on a high-speed InGaAs linear 1,024 pixel array (SUI-Goodrich), enabling 47,000 A-scans/s, 5–8 μm of axial resolution, and 2.6 mm of scanning depth in tissue. The high-speed 3D retinal OCT system for 1,060 nm was interfaced to a preliminary patient module, modified for operation at 1,060 nm to enable clinical retinal imaging at this wavelength and compared with an OCT system operating at 800 nm. Figure 17.1 depicts the comparison of 3D OCT at 800 vs. 1,060 nm in a normal (cf. Fig. 17.1a–d) and pathologic (cf. Fig. 17.1e–h) eye, i.e., of a patient with retinitis pigmentosa [16, 17]. Three-dimensional rendering resulting in *en face* scans of the choroid for 800 nm (cf. Fig. 17.1a, e) and 1,060 nm

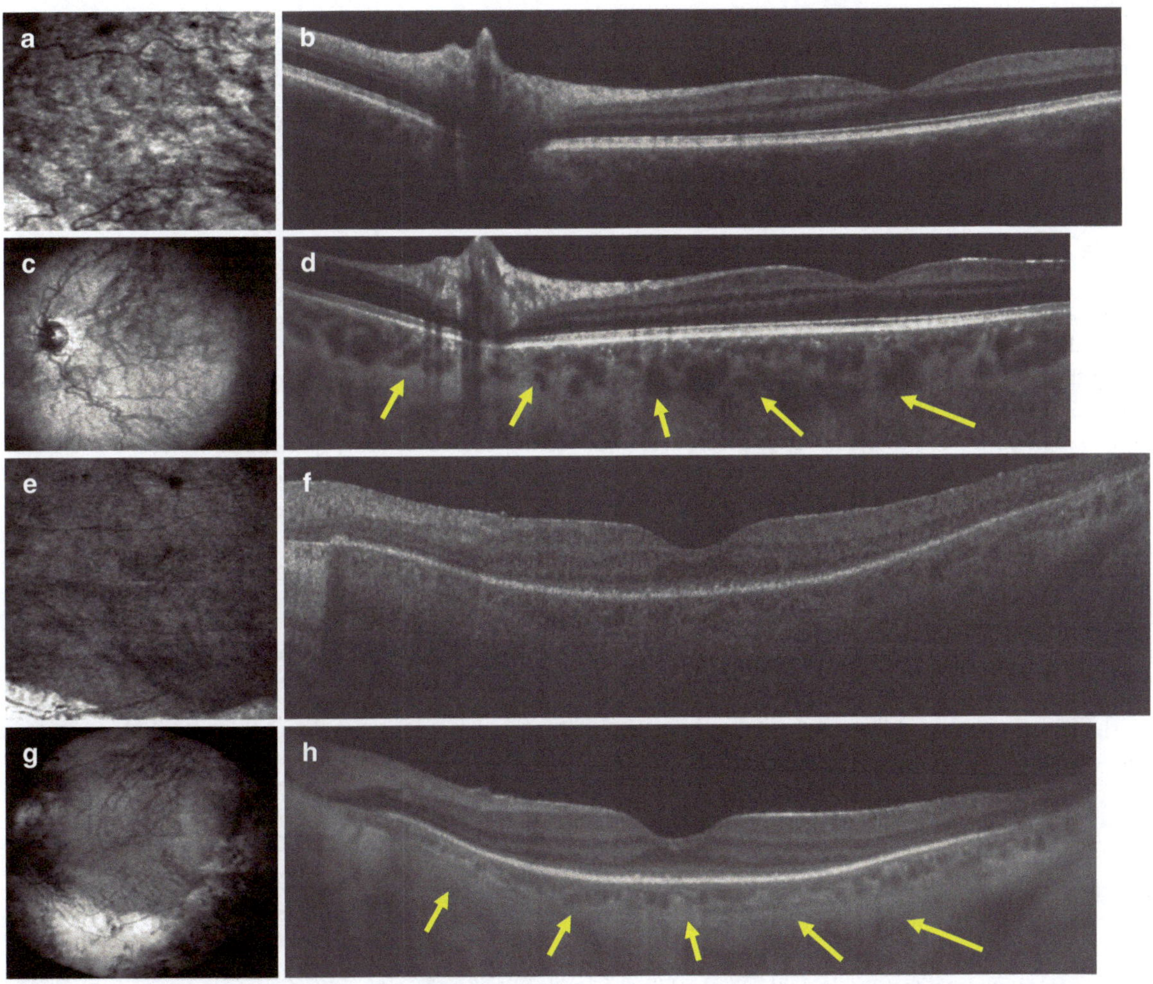

Fig. 17.1 OCT at 800 and 1,060 nm of a normal retina (**a–d**) and a patient with retinitis pigmentosa (**e–h**): high definition (4,096 depth scans) 800 nm 3D OCT scan over 35° (**b, f**); high-definition (2,048 pixel) 1,060 nm 3D OCT scan over 35° (**d, h**); *en face* widefield (35° × 35°, **c, g**); *en face* zoom in fundus image of the choroid using 1,060 nm 3D-OCT (**a, e**); *arrows* indicate enhanced choroidal visualization (*yellow arrows* in Figure **d, h** indicate the choroidal–scleral interface) (adapted from ref. [17])

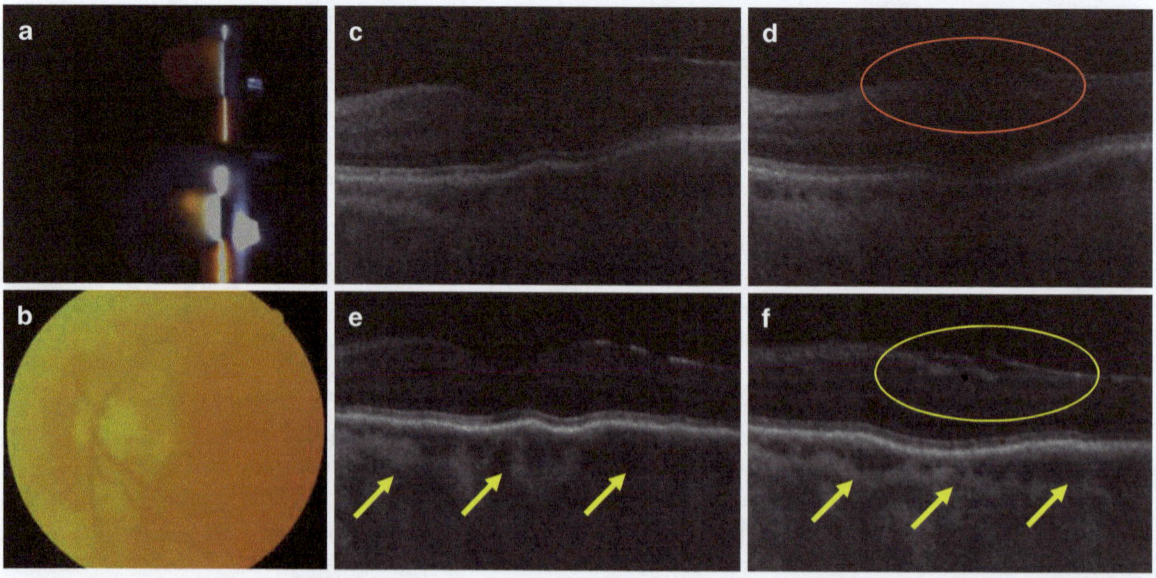

Fig. 17.2 Three-dimensional retinal 1,060 nm OCT in a patient with a cataract grade of N04 NC5 C4 P5 according to LOCS III. Digital slit lamp biomicroscopy of the cataract lens with two different magnifications (**a**), color fundus photography with standard illumination (**b**). Two representative cross-sections from a 3D stack of the same patient for 800 nm OCT (**c**, **d**) and approximately at the same retinal location for 1,060 nm OCT (**e**, **f**). Severe central signal attenuation in 800 nm OCT (*red circle* **d**) due to significantly increased scattering caused by lens opacification. Clear image of the retina despite the cataract using 1,060 nm OCT (*yellow circle* in **f**) and the choroidal-scleral interface (*yellow arrows* **e**, **f**)

(cf. Fig. 17.1c, g), and high definition B-scans for 800 nm (cf. Fig. 17.1b, f) as well as 1,060 nm (cf. Fig. 17.1d, h) demonstrated improved penetration, and hence visualization of the choroid (cf. yellow arrows in Fig. 17.1d, h indicating the choroidal–scleral interface). Thus, high-speed 3D 1,060-nm retinal OCT now enables unprecedented visualization of all three choroidal layers giving access to the entire choroidal vasculature and thickness. In addition to unprecedented visualization of choroidal vasculature without the use of any contrast agent, 2D choroidal thickness maps might have significant impact on the early diagnosis of retinal pathologies like glaucoma and age-related macular degeneration and might therefore contribute to a better understanding of retinal pathogenesis.

Another advantage of 3D retinal OCT at 1,060 nm is its significantly improved clinical feasibility in patients with turbid ocular media in the anterior eye segment, e.g., cataract or corneal haze. Figure 17.2 shows a patient with a cataract grade of N04 NC5 C4 P5 according to LOCS III (lens opacification classification system III), indicating a progressed cataract grade. Figure 17.2a depicts the digital slit lamp biomicroscopy of the cataract lens with two different magnifications, while Fig. 17.2b shows a color fundus photography with standard illumination, both indicating a particularly centrally localized obscuration due to progressed cataract. Figures 17.2c–f indicate two representative cross-sections from a 3D stack of the same patient for 800 nm OCT (cf. Fig. 17.2c, d), and approximately at the same retinal location for 1,060 nm OCT (cf. Fig. 17.2e, f). While cataract causes a severe central signal attenuation in 800 nm OCT (cf. red ellipse in Fig. 17.2d) due to significantly increased scattering caused by lens opacification, 1,060 nm OCT is found to clearly visualize the retina despite the cataract delineating the epiretinal membrane (cf. yellow circle in Fig. 17.2f) as well as the choroidal–scleral interface (cf. yellow arrows in Fig. 17.2e, f).

Summary for the Clinician

- All fourth-generation commercial retinal OCT systems working on the principle of Fourier or spectral domain are based on light source technology operating in the 800 nm wavelength region.
- 3D retinal OCT at 1,060 nm (a similar wavelength region as that of lasers used for YAG-capsulotomy) enables deeper penetration and hence better visualization of the choroid, which is significantly less dependent on the patient's fundus pigmentation when compared with the 800 nm retinal OCT systems.

- In addition to visualizing all intraretinal layers, 3D retinal OCT at 1,060 nm enables visualization and quantification of all choroidal layers as well as the entire choroid itself.
- In patients with opaque ocular media in the anterior eye segment (e.g., corneal haze or cataract), 3D retinal OCT at 1,060 nm enables improved clinical feasibility to visualize retinal morphology, despite scattering and hence OCT signal attenuating, and turbid ocular media of the anterior eye segment.
- Despite several proof-of-principle demonstrations of significantly improved OCT imaging performance (especially of the choroid), sound clinical studies on larger, properly selected patient cohorts are necessary to demonstrate the improved clinical impact and therefore verify the increased technological effort of 3D retinal OCT at 1,060 nm.

17.3 In Vivo Cellular Resolution Retinal Imaging

For ophthalmic retinal OCT imaging, the cornea and the lens act as the "imaging objective," thereby determining the numerical aperture and hence the beam diameter in the retina. The highest transverse resolution for OCT imaging is determined by the smallest achievable spot size on the retina. This diameter specifies the transverse OCT resolution that is of the order of ~20 µm for a beam of ~1 mm diameter (at 800 nm) - approximately a factor 4–5 worse than common axial OCT resolutions. This can be improved by dilating the pupil and increasing the measurement beam diameter. Studies have shown that the largest pupil size still yields diffraction limited focusing of ~3 mm, enabling theoretical retinal spot sizes of about 5–7 µm [18]. In practice, however, for large incident beam diameters, ocular aberrations limit this minimum focused spot site on the retina, even for monochromatic illumination. Adaptive optics (AO) is a promising approach to correct ocular aberrations in order to decrease the spot size on the retina and improve transverse resolution in OCT [19]. AO has been successfully interfaced to ophthalmic imaging techniques, such as conventional, flood illuminated [20], or scanning fundus imaging systems [21] used to provide higher contrast and transverse resolution, achieving in vivo, *en face* visualization of photoreceptors as well as ganglion and retinal pigment epithelium (RPE) cells in animal models [22]. Integrating AO with ultrahigh resolution 3D OCT promises to enable retinal visualization with isotropic resolution of a few micrometers [23–27].

AO has recently been interfaced to ultrahigh resolution 3D OCT for in vivo cellular resolution retinal imaging. In the present approach, a deformable mirror (Mirao52, Imagine Eyes, France) with a unique performance in terms of amplitude (±50 µm stroke) and linearity was used, allowing for correcting highly aberrated normal or pathologic eyes [28]. Furthermore, a 140–160 nm Ti:sapphire laser (Femtolasers Integral, Femtolaser, Vienna, Austria) in combination with a CMOS Basler sprint spL4096–140k camera (Basler AG Germany) was used, enabling 160,000 A-scans/s with 1,536 pixels, resulting in ultrahigh speed (625 frames of 256 × 768 pixels) cellular resolution retinal imaging with isotropic resolution of 2–3 µm. At this data acquisition speed, only minimal motion artifacts are encountered and no eye tracker is needed, and hence, volumetric cellular resolution imaging of the living human retina is accomplished.

Figures 17.3 and 17.4 demonstrate a possible concept for clinical cellular resolution AO OCT in a patient with Type 2 Macular Telangiectasia. In addition to standard clinical examination (color fundus photography (cf. Fig. 17.3a), fundus autofluorescence (cf. Fig. 17.3b), and fluorescein angiography in early (cf. Fig. 17.3c) and late phase (cf. Fig. 17.3d)), a commercial 3D OCT is used to prescreen a larger volume (cf. representative B-scans in Fig. 17.3e–g as well as 3D rendering of the entire scanned volume in Fig. 17.3h) to indentify suspicious locations. These areas are then investigated (at the moment, still with a separate system) with AO OCT (cf. Fig. 17.3i–l as well as Fig. 17.4). In this case, the central foveal region was significantly impaired (cf. Fig. 17.3e–g as well as i and j), whereas AO OCT revealed reasonable cellular morphology at 6° parafoveal at the photoreceptor level (cf. Fig. 17.3k, l). Figure 17.4 depicts the cross-sectional and *en face* tomograms for the OCT volumes depicted in Fig. 17.3i–l. Figure 17.4a shows a slightly peripheral region that seems to cover three different stages with normal (green arrow), affected (yellow arrows), and impaired (red arrows) appearance. While the green portion seems to be comparable to the normal, increased signal in the inner nuclear layer is detected (cf. Fig. 17.4a green arrow). In the yellow region that is free of any cyst, a signal increase in the outer nuclear layer and a slight signal loss in the inner plexiform layer is observed. Furthermore, the increase in the signal reflected from the external limiting membrane (cf. Fig. 17.4a, second yellow arrow from the

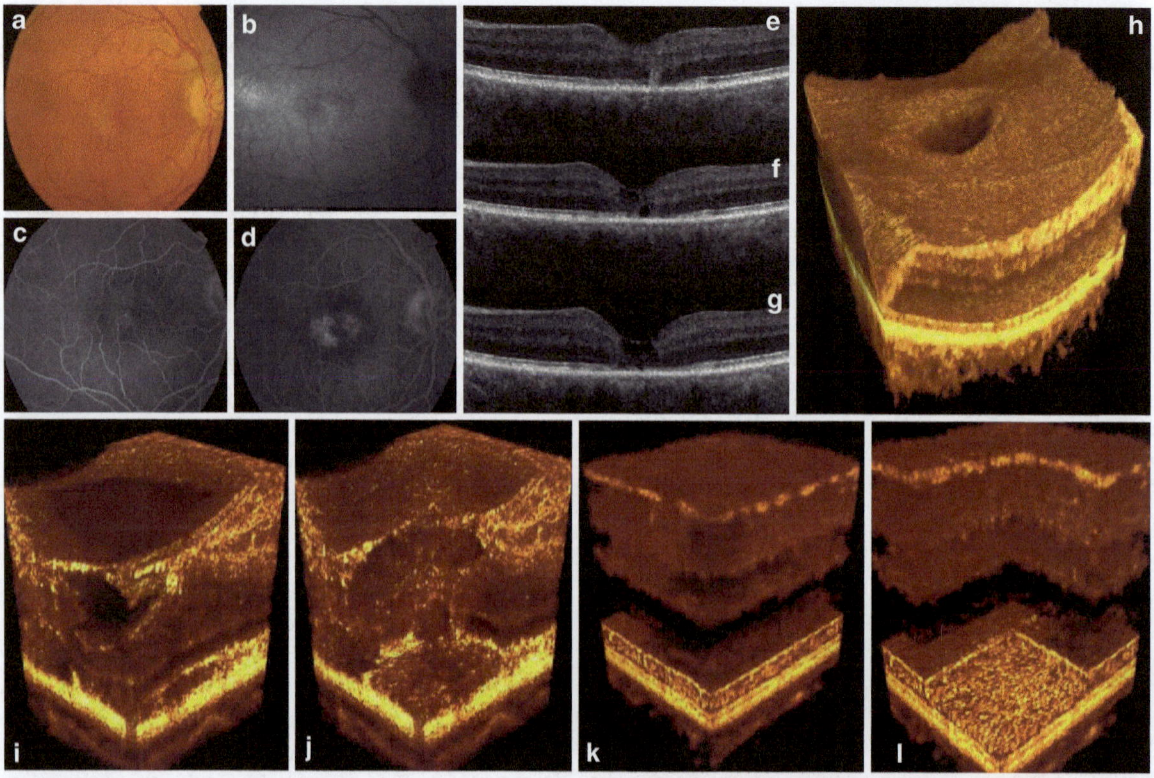

Fig. 17.3 Possible strategy for clinical cellular resolution OCT in a patient with Type 2 Macular Telangiectasia: color fundus photography (**a**), fundus autofluorescence (**b**), and fluorescein angiography in early (**c**) and late phase (**d**); Commercially available OCT is used to pre-screen a larger volume representative B-scans (**e–g**) and 3D rendering of the entire scanned volume (**h**) using a commercial 3D OCT to indentify suspicious locations; these areas are then investigated with AO OCT at cellular resolution level at 0° (**i, j**) and 6° (**k, l**) (adapted from ref. [17])

top) might indicate changes in the tight junctions. The region that is associated with the photoreceptor outer segment (cf. Fig. 17.4a 3rd + 4th yellow arrow from top) has a significant signal decrease, which might indicate photoreceptor outer segment atrophy, or retraction of the RPE. In the red region, the cyst (cf. Fig. 17.4 A 1st red arrow from top) separates the inner plexiform layer from the underlying layers. The photoreceptor inner segment seems to be shorter than normal (cf. Fig. 17.4b), and the junction between the inner and outer photoreceptor segment is almost invisible. Visualization of the microstructural morphology of the central outer nuclear layer (cf. Fig. 17.4c) as well as the central RPE (cf. Fig. 17.4d) has also been accomplished. Cellular resolution AO OCT in the same eye at 6° nasal reveals reasonable appearance of the nerve fiber bundles (cf. Fig 17.4e), capillaries at the level of the inner nuclear layer (cf. Fig. 17.4f), as well as photoreceptor density of 9,260 cones/mm^2 at the level of the inner/outer segment junction (cf. Fig. 17.4g) and of 8,870 cones/mm^2 at the tips of the outer photoreceptor segments (cf. Fig. 17.4h).

Summary for the Clinician

- State-of-the-art commercially available 3D retinal OCT systems accomplish "only" high axial resolution. Transverse resolution determined by the measurement beam diameter and the optical quality of the human eye (mainly that of the cornea and the lens) are generally one order of magnitude worse than the axial OCT resolution.
- By using a wavefront sensor in combination with a deformable mirror (adaptive optics), individual optical aberrations of the investigated eyes can be measured and compensated to enable a significantly smaller focus in the retina, and hence, improved transverse resolution in addition to the high axial resolution accomplished by OCT. In this way, cellular features of the living human retina can be visualized (pending on sufficient optical contrast, despite high isotropic resolution of AO OCT).

- Owing to limited numerical aperture and optical contrast, tightly packed photoreceptors in the foveal center cannot be directly visualized at the moment. In parafoveal regions (larger than ~1–2°), this becomes less challenging due to increased photoreceptor diameters and less tight packaging.
- In eyes with good optical quality (reduced lower and higher order aberrations), photoreceptors can also be visualized in the parafoveal regions without the use of adaptive optics.
- Despite several proof-of-principle demonstrations of significantly improved OCT imaging performance, sound clinical studies on larger, properly selected patient cohorts are necessary to demonstrate improved clinical impact, and therefore, verify the increased technological effort combining adaptive optics with high resolution, ultrahigh speed OCT for in vivo cellular resolution retinal imaging.

17.4 Polarization Sensitive Retinal OCT

Currently available commercial OCT instruments record images based on backscattered intensity. While intensity-based OCT provides cross-sectional and 3D images of the retina with high resolution, it cannot directly differentiate the tissues. However, light has additional properties that can be measured and used to generate tissue-specific contrast. The polarization state of light is such a property that can be changed by various light-tissue interactions and thus can be used to generate tissue-specific contrast. These effects are used by PS-OCT. PS-OCT requires a more complex instrumental setup than intensity-based OCT. The sample is typically illuminated either with circularly polarized light or with different polarization states successively. Furthermore, the light has to be detected in two orthogonal polarization channels to provide the necessary polarization information. In addition to the usual intensity-based images, PS-OCT acquires images of retardation, birefringent axis orientation, and images containing information on depolarization. Initially implemented as time-domain OCT [29, 30], PS-OCT techniques were

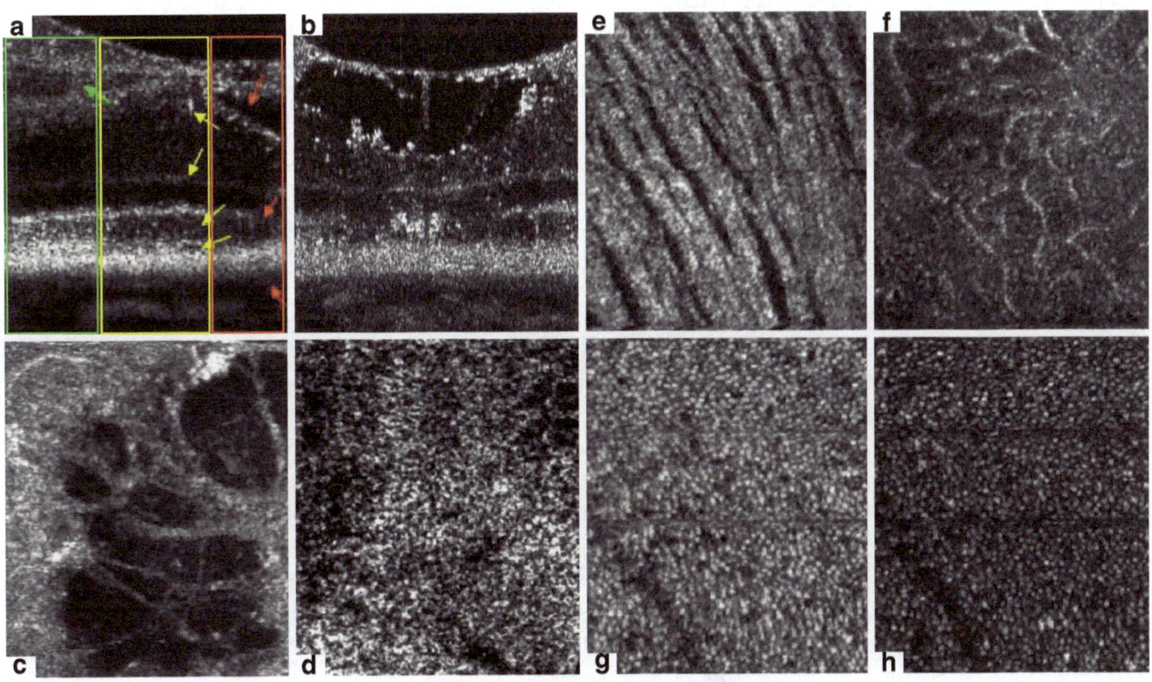

Fig. 17.4 Possible strategy for clinical cellular resolution OCT in a patient with Type 2 Macular Telangiectasia: *en face* AO OCT images from volumes depicted in Fig. 173i–l; cross-sections (**a**, **b**) and *en face* images at the level of the outer nuclear layer (**c**) and retinal pigment epithelium (**d**) at 0°; *arrows* in (**a**) indicate areas of little (*green*), medium (*yellow*), and significant (*red*) impairment; *en face* images at the level of the nerve fiber bundles at 6° (**e**); capillaries in the inner nuclear layer at 6° (**f**); inner/outer photoreceptor junction at 6° (**g**) and at the level of the tips of the outer photoreceptors at 6°(**h**) (adapted from ref. [17])

later adapted to spectral-domain OCT, finally providing ocular imaging with similar speed and sensitivity as intensity-based spectral-domain OCT [31–33]. Two polarization changing light-tissue interaction mechanisms are of special interest for retinal imaging: birefringence and depolarization. Birefringence is found in fibrous tissues consisting of long, parallel fibrils that are surrounded by material of different refractive index (form birefringence). Depolarization can be caused by multiple light-scattering at large particles or scattering at nonspherical particles.

PS-OCT was demonstrated in the anterior and posterior segments of the human eye in vivo. Detailed PS-OCT studies of the ocular fundus led to a classification of tissues into polarization preserving (e.g., photoreceptor layer), birefringent (e.g., retinal nerve fiber layer (RNFL), Henle's fiber layer, sclera, scar tissue) [31, 34–37], and polarization scrambling or depolarizing (e.g., RPE, choroidal nevus) [31, 35–38]. Furthermore, PS-OCT was recently used to identify the reasons for atypical scanning laser polarimetry patterns [39] (increased penetration of probing light into the birefringent sclera). The results of these studies indicate two possible future applications of PS-OCT for the diagnosis of retinal diseases:

(i) A recent animal study has shown that a damage of the optic nerve leads to a reduced RNFL birefringence, before RNFL thickness changes are detectable by intensity-based OCT [40]. As depth-resolved retardation measurements by PS-OCT directly provide quantitative information on RNFL birefringence [33, 34, 41], glaucoma-induced RNFL damage might be detected at an early stage, possibly improving glaucoma diagnosis.

(ii) The depolarization (or polarization scrambling) caused by RPE can directly be used to identify, visualize [36, 37, 42], and segment [43] this layer whose integrity is decisive for photoreceptor metabolism, and therefore, for visual function. As RPE segmentation by PS-OCT exploits an intrinsic, tissue-specific contrast mechanism, it is likely to be less affected by factors like illumination conditions, presence of vessels, or irregular RPE shape in the vicinity of lesions like drusen, detachments, atrophies, or neovascularizations. Therefore, PS-OCT is an interesting tool for diagnosis and follow-up studies of diseases associated with RPE alterations like AMD.

Figure 17.5 shows an example of B-scans obtained by a spectral-domain PS-OCT instrument (center wavelength of 840 nm) in a healthy human fovea. The images are extracted from a 3D data set that was recorded in ~ 3 s. Figure 17.5a shows the conventional intensity image derived from the data set, where the three strongly reflecting boundaries of the posterior retina are marked (IS/OS,

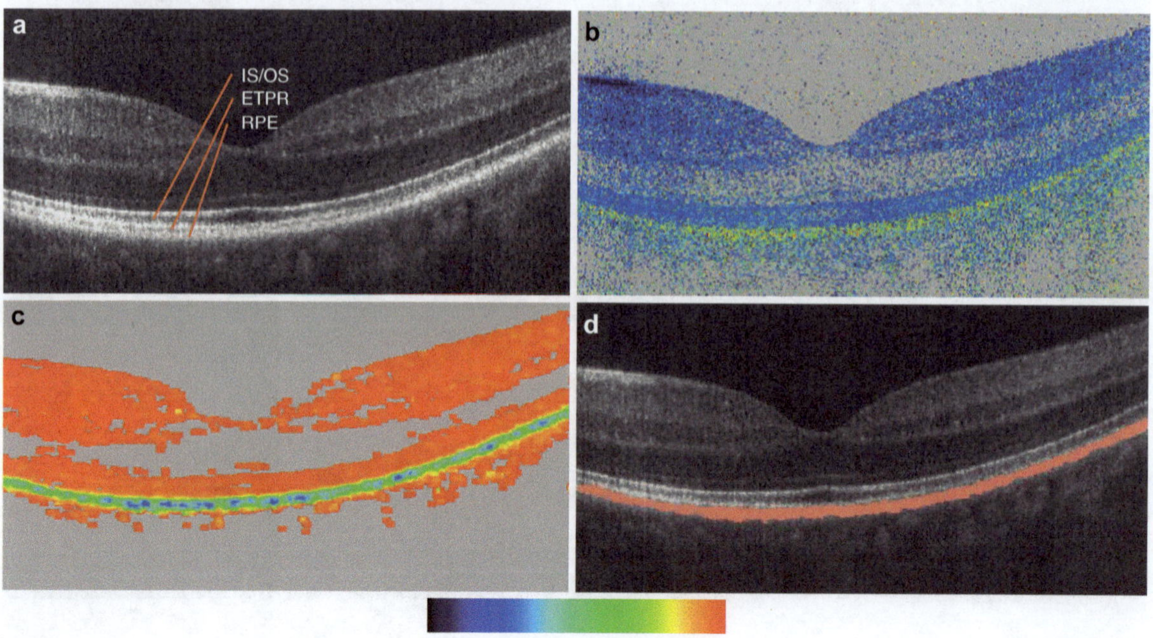

Fig. 17.5 PS-OCT B-scan images of healthy human fovea in vivo. (**a**) Intensity (log scale); (**b**) retardation (*color bar*: 0°–90°); (**c**) degree of polarization uniformity DOPU (*color bar*: 0–1). (**d**) Overlay of intensity image with RPE segmented by DOPU data (*red*). Image size: 15° (horizontal) × 0.75 mm (vertical, optical distance). (From Götzinger et al. [43] by permission of the Optical Society of America)

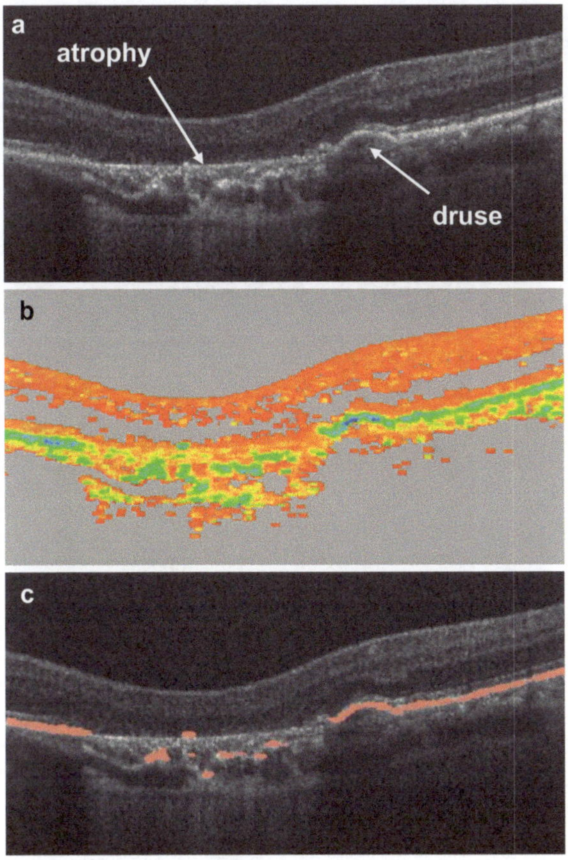

Fig. 17.6 PS-OCT images of retina with AMD. (**a**) Intensity; (**b**) DOPU (*color bar*: see fig. 17.1c); (**c**) intensity overlaid with segmented RPE. Image size: 15° (horizontal) × 1 mm (vertical). (From Götzinger et al. [43] by permission of the Optical Society of America)

boundary between inner and outer photoreceptor segments; ETPR, end tips of photoreceptors; RPE). The retardation image (Fig. 17.5b) shows the different polarizing properties of retinal tissue in this region: most tissues preserve the polarization state, i.e., do not introduce or change retardation (blue colors), only the RPE scrambles the polarization state, generating random retardation values (the mix of all color values appears green in this presentation). Figure 17.5c shows the degree of polarization uniformity (DOPU) [43], a quantity closely related to the degree of polarization known from classical polarization optics. DOPU is high (orange to red colors) in all layers except the RPE, indicating the depolarization caused by the RPE. The DOPU image was used to segment the RPE and to generate an overlay image showing intensity (gray scale) and the segmented RPE in red (Fig. 17.5d).

Similar PS-OCT imaging was performed in numerous patients. Figure 17.6 shows an example of a PS-OCT B-scan obtained in the retina of a patient with AMD. A large atrophy is visible on the left-hand side of the image, discernible by the increased light penetration into the deeper layers in the intensity image (Fig. 17.6a). Figures 17.6b, c show the DOPU and the overlay image (segmented RPE in red), clearly showing the atrophy. An evaluation of the entire 3D data set allows determination of the lesion area, a quantity important for follow-up studies, therapy monitoring, and control.

Figure 17.7 shows an area of advanced AMD with a scar. It can be noted that a thickened hyperreflective band has replaced the RPE, and no polarization scrambling is observed. Instead, enhanced birefringence caused by the fibrotic scar tissue is observed in the retardation image (Fig. 17.7b) with areas of varying fibril orientation (axis orientation image Fig. 17.7c). The fundus image (Fig. 17.7d) shows the trace of the B-scan (white line).

Summary for the Clinician

- PS-OCT provides, in addition to the usual intensity-based images, images of retardation, birefringent axis orientation, and depolarization.
- PS-OCT provides intrinsic, tissue-specific contrast of birefringent (e.g., RNFL) and depolarizing (e.g., RPE) tissue.
- Spectral-domain PS-OCT achieves the same imaging speed, sensitivity, and resolution as commercial intensity-based spectral-domain OCT instruments.
- PS-OCT can possibly be used for glaucoma diagnosis (by RNFL birefringence measurements) and for the diagnosis of RPE disturbances associated with diseases like AMD and others (by measuring depolarization).
- Several hundred patients have been imaged by PS-OCT, with encouraging results. Additional studies are necessary to demonstrate the benefit of the additional technical effort.

17.5 Doppler (Blood Flow) Retinal OCT

Assessment of blood flow and microcirculation is certainly the most direct window to tissue, organ, and general health status. There are different modalities in biomedicine that allow measuring perfusion including ultrasound or CT. In contrast, optical methods such as Laser Doppler flowmetry (LDF) or D-OCT have the advantage of being noncontact, label-free, employing nonhazardous radiation. Like ultrasound flow imaging, they make use of the Doppler effect, named after the

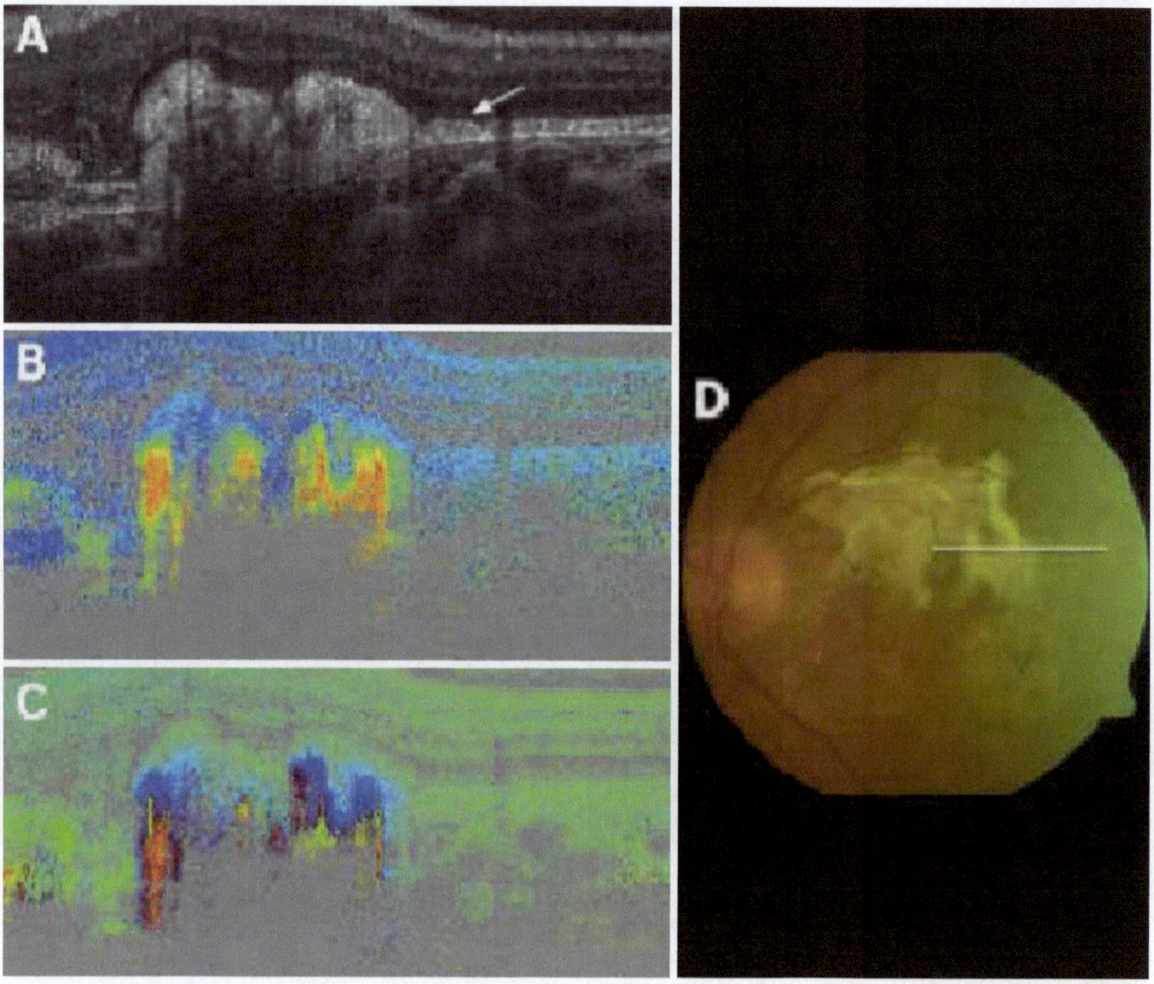

Fig. 17.7 PS-OCT images of retina with advanced AMD and fibrosis. (**a**) Intensity; (**b**) retardation; (**c**) axis orientation; (**d**) fundus image (*white line*: B-scan trace). (From Michels et al. [37] by permission of the British Journal of Ophthalmology)

Austrian scientist, Christian Doppler, who described the phenomenon that moving sources appear at higher or lower frequency depending on their relative speed toward or away from the observer. Analogously, light scattered at moving red blood cells experiences a shift in optical frequency that is directly proportional to the flow velocity. LDF analyzes the total spectral content of light scattered from perfused tissue volumes illuminated by a laser. Hence, the extraction of defined absolute flow velocities is not possible due to multiple scattering within the irradiated volume at various angles. Also, depth localization is difficult and mainly determined by the penetration depth of the laser light and its coherence properties [44]. Nevertheless, the easy implementation of the technique allowed a number of clinical studies on retinal blood flow. The results stressed the clinical importance of detecting early changes in retinal perfusion as precursor of important diseases such as glaucoma, diabetic retinopathy, and age-related macula degeneration [45–47]. Of equal impact were several pharmacological studies that helped in understanding the role of endothelial cells and its release of vasoactive substances such as nitride oxide (NO) for perfusion regulation. The major drawback of LDF is the limited depth discrimination: it would, e.g., be of clinical importance to clearly separate choroidal perfusion from inner retinal blood flow.

Compared with LDF, D-OCT not only allows for micron depth localized flow imaging and efficient separation of different flow beds, but also allows absolute quantification of flow within retinal vessels down to the size of small metarterioles and venules. Early implementations of D-OCT were based on time-domain OCT [48–50], and further improvements enabled initial in vivo results of retinal perfusion [51, 52]. Nowadays, Fourier (also frequency or spectral) domain (FD) OCT is gradually replacing time-domain OCT in ophthalmic imaging, owing to its intrinsic

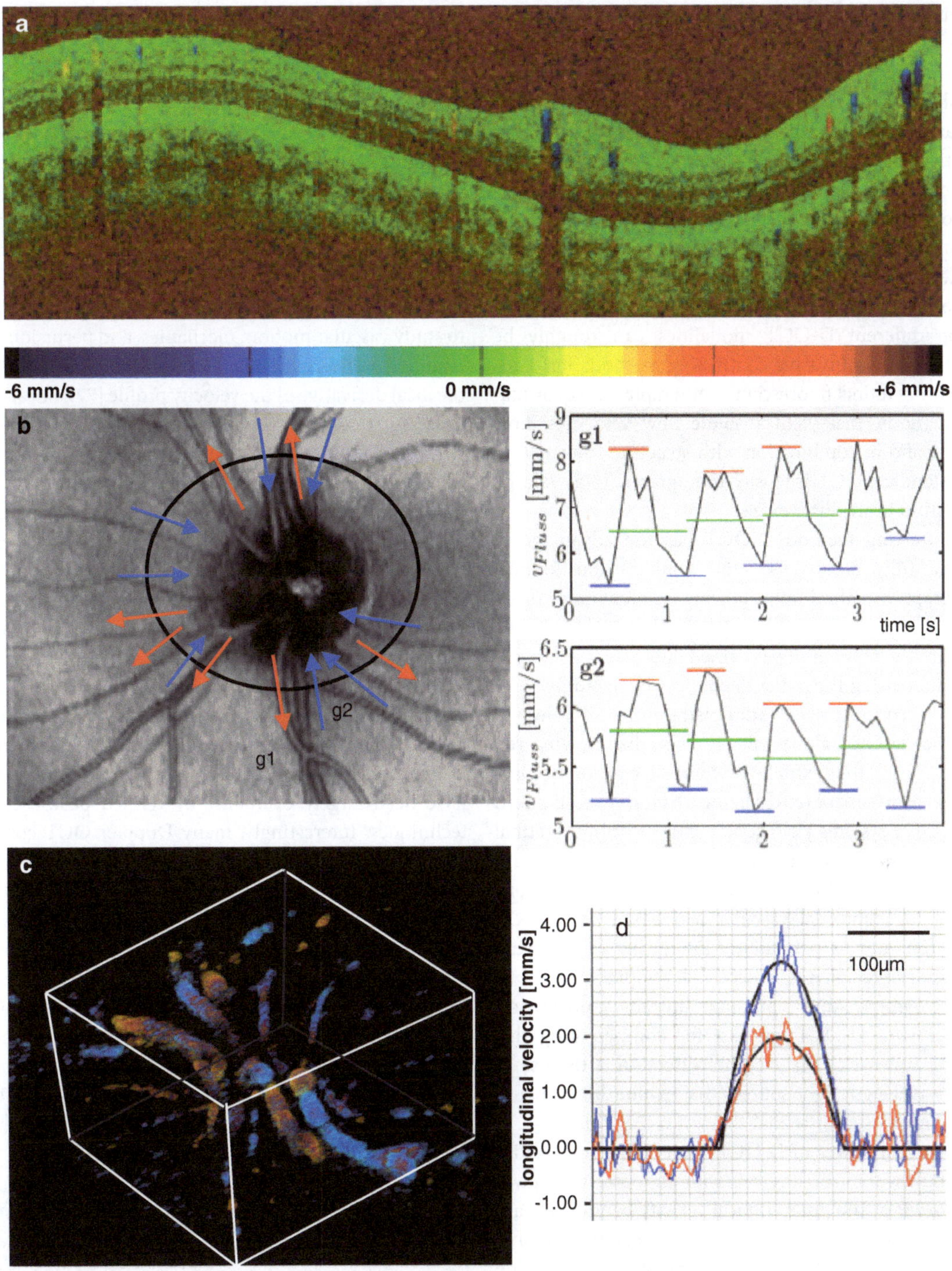

Fig. 17.8 (**a**) Typical D-OCT tomogram displaying color coded axial velocity information of a circum-papillar OCT scan at the position indicated as black circle in (B) (3000 A-scans recorded at 30 kHz); (**b**) (*lhs*) fundus projection of 3D OCT intensity data obtained at the nervus opticus. Arrows indicate flow directions as seen from 3D plots an allow associating veins and arteries (*blue* and *red*). (*rhs*) For vessels denoted g1 and g2 a time series consisting of 60 circular scans yields pulsatile characteristics of vessels (*red*: systolic flow velocites, *blue*: diastolic velocities, *green*: pulse averaged velocities). The pulsatility index ($PI = (v_{max} - v_{min})/v_{avg}$) of g1 is calculated as 0.36 with a relative error of 17.16% and of g2 0.16 with 19.64% relative error. Although average velocities are similar in both vessels arterial (g1) and venous (g2) flow are easily distinguished by assessment of their pulsatile dynamics. (**c**) Quantitative volumetric angiography map of perfusion at the nervus opticus. (**d**) High velocity sensitivity together with gated reconstruction allows measuring systolic (*blue line*) and diastolic (*red line*) profiles within individual vessels. (reproduced from [60])

sensitivity and speed advantage [53, 54] as well as its ability for in vivo 3D imaging [5, 55–59]. The advantages can be effectively exploited by functional extensions such as Doppler (FD) OCT resulting in higher velocity sensitivity and large bandwidth [60–63]. Today, D-OCT has become an active field of research, and recent developments such as resonant Doppler imaging [64], optical microangiography [65], joint frequency and time-domain D-OCT [66], and other different flow filtering methods [67, 68] provide a wide spectrum of exciting possibilities to characterize and contrast perfusion of full retinal volumes.

The different D-OCT modalities can roughly be divided into noninvasive contrasting methods for complementing retinal fluorescent angiography and quantitative methods, that yield absolute flow velocities, flow profiles, and in combination with structure information from standard OCT intensity tomograms, total volume flow within individual vessels.

Contrasting method D-OCT has the advantage of being a fully noninvasive and nonhazardous optical angiographic method [69], allowing frequent monitoring of disease and treatment progression. This might help one to reduce the number of performed fluorescent angiographies, increasing the patient's comfort by avoiding side-effects of contrast agent administration. It is however clear that D-OCT alone will only visualize moving red blood cells and thus exhibits no contrast, e.g., for the clinically relevant case of retinal hemorrhages. Also, standard retinal OCT systems yield good contrast for inner retinal structures, but choroidal structures suffer from lower signal and scattering losses, limiting the potential for contrasting the choroidal vascular bed based on D-OCT alone. The latter is particularly interesting for studying the pathogenesis of AMD. Recent developments of optical angiography thus combine intensity information together with D-OCT contrast for compensating this original drawback [70]. Another direction is the use of larger wavelength light sources that exhibit better penetration into posterior retinal structures [71, 72].

The actual power of D-OCT is its ability to quantify blood flow within small vessels with high precision down to the order of 100 μm/s. Typical velocity bandwidths are in the range of 10 mm/s, which covers most of the retinal perfusion. It should however be mentioned that only the velocity component parallel to the observation direction can be quantified. For determination of the true flow speed, the angle between flow vector or vessel and the illumination direction needs to be known. Different methods have been explored for absolute retinal blood velocity values, either in postprocessing by extracting the angle from 3D tomograms [73, 74] or by optical means, using two defined illumination directions for angle independent flow measurement [75]. Another possibility is to acquire data from two concentric circum-papillar scans of different radii, by measuring the local vessel gradient between both the scans [76]. Patient's movement however limits the reproducibility of the angle reconstruction, and retinal tracking may be highly beneficial. The angular dependence may be avoided by using angle-independent parameters to characterize flow such as resistance index or pulsatility index, known from ultrasound Doppler imaging.

Fast imaging sequences of vessel dynamics together with blood flow quantification offers unique capabilities to study vascular motion, mechanics, and perfusion regulation. The shearing stress can be readily obtained from the local derivative of the velocity profile [77]. Shear stress causes small deformations of the endothelial cells, which triggers a variety of biochemical and vasomotor functional reactions [78] such as the production of NO. Vascular stiffness is another parameter that can be assessed via the pulsatile properties of retinal vessels. Current studies evoking flicker-stimulated vasomotion investigate the relation of retinal vascular stiffness and predisposition to general vascular diseases based on fast fundus imaging technology [79].

In summary, currently, we have a manifold of D-OCT techniques, yielding qualitative as well as quantitative information with high precision. Initial problems of D-OCT such as phase wrapping or bulk motion artifacts have been largely overcome by refined postprocessing techniques. Interestingly, many Doppler OCT concepts might be easily integrated into commercial OCT platforms, as they mainly involve software adaptations, although retinal tracking would be of advantage. However, the clinical importance still needs to be fully exploited and demonstrated, despite initial promising attempts [80]. Being a fast-evolving field in the last years, D-OCT has the potential to not only become a standard ophthalmology research tool, but also an indispensable diagnosis instrument for enhancing current angiographic techniques far beyond today's capabilities.

Summary for the Clinician

- D-OCT provides, in addition to standard OCT, intensity contrast information about retinal perfusion.
- Quantitative D-OCT uniquely allows extracting true velocity information of retinal blood flow that can be used in combination with the measured vessel geometry from intensity tomograms to determine total volume flow, dynamic pulsatile flow profiles, vessel compliance, or shear stress.

- Qualitative D-OCT methods yield vascular contrast similar to fluorescent angiography, but with the important difference that only blood in motion can be visualized.
- Novel D-OCT instruments with enhanced penetration promise assessing both inner retinal and choroidal perfusion dynamics with high contrast and sensitivity.
- Quantitative D-OCT gives insight into vascular dynamics and mechanics. The assessment of vascular stiffness is an important factor for determining vascular-disease predisposition.
- Patient studies are currently underway with the hope to exploit the full potential of modern D-OCT concepts for early diagnosis of perfusion disorders, such as precursors of retinal disease (AMD, diabetic retinopathy, glaucoma) as well as for pharmacological research.

Acknowledgements The authors acknowledge all the members of the Biomedical Imaging Group at the School of Optometry and Vision Sciences, Cardiff University, Alan C. Bird and Catherine A. Egan, Medical Retina Service, Moorfields, London, United Kingdom; B. Baumann, E. Götzinger, M. Pircher, T. Schmoll, C. Kolbitsch, L. Schmetterer and H. Sattmann, Center for Biomedical Engineering and Physics, Medical University of Vienna; C. Ahlers, W. Geitzenauer, S. Michels, and U. Schmidt-Erfurth, Department of Ophthalmology, Medical University of Vienna, T. Lasser, A. Bachmann, R. Michaely, and M. Villiger, Ecole Polytechnique Federale de Lausanne, Switzerland. Financial and equipment support by the following institutions is also acknowledged: Cardiff University, FP6-IST-NMP-2 STREPT (017128), Action Medical Research (AP1110), DTI (1544C), European Union project FUN OCT (FP7 HEALTH, contract no. 201880); FEMTOLASERS GmbH, Carl Zeiss Meditec Inc., Exalos Inc, Maxon Computer GmbH, Multiwave Photonics and The Lowy Foundation, Sydney, Australia; Austrian Science Fund (P19624).

References

1. Huang D, Swanson EA, Lin CP, Schuman JS, Stinson WG, Chang W, Hee MR, Flotte T, Gregory K, Puliafito CA, Fujimoto JG (1991) Optical coherence tomography. Science 254:1178–1181
2. Drexler W, Fujimoto JG (2008) Optical coherence tomography: technology and applications. Springer, Verlag
3. Drexler W, Fujimoto JG (2008) State-of-the-art retinal optical coherence tomography. Prog Retin Eye Res 27:45–88
4. Fercher AF, Hitzenberger CK, Kamp G, El-Zaiat SY (1995) Measurement of intraocular distances by backscattering spectral interferometry. Opt Commun 117:43–48
5. Leitgeb R, Hitzenberger CK, Fercher AF (2003) Performance of fourier domain vs. time domain optical coherence tomography. Opt Express 11:889–894
6. Unterhuber A, Považay B, Hermann B, Sattmann H, Chavez-Pirson A, Drexler W (2005) In vivo retinal optical coherence tomography at 1040 nm-enhanced penetration into the choroid. Opt Express 13:3252–3258
7. Považay B, Bizheva K, Hermann B, Unterhuber A, Sattmann H, Fercher AF, Drexler W, Schubert C, Ahnelt PK, Mei M, Holzwarth R, Wadsworth WJ, Knight JC, Russel PS (2003) Enhanced visualization of choroidal vessels using ultrahigh resolution ophthalmic OCT at 1050 nm. Opt Express 11:1980–1986
8. Považay B, Hermann B, Unterhuber A, Hofer B, Sattmann H, Zeiler F, Morgan JE, Falkner-Radler C, Glittenberg C, Binder S, Drexler W (2007) Three-dimensional optical coherence tomography at 1050 nm versus 800 nm in retinal pathologies: enhanced performance and choroidal penetration in cataract patients. J Biomed Opt 12:041211
9. Makita S, Hong Y, Yamanari M, Yatagai T, Yasuno Y (2006) Optical coherence angiography. Opt Express 14: 7821–7840
10. Lee EC, de Boer JF, Mujat M, Lim H, Yun SH (2006) In vivo optical frequency domain imaging of human retina and choroid. Opt Express 14:4403–4411
11. Yasuno Y, Hong YJ, Makita S, Yamanari M, Akiba M, Miura M, Yatagai T (2007) In vivo high-contrast imaging of deep posterior eye by 1-μm swept source optical coherence tomography and scattering optical coherence angiography. Opt Express 15:6121–6139
12. Hong Y, Makita S, Yamanari M, Miura M, Kim S, Yatagai T, Yasuno Y (2007) Three-dimensional visualization of choroidal vessels by using standard and ultra-high resolution scattering optical coherence angiography. Opt Express 15: 7538–7550
13. Makita S, Fabritius T, Yasuno Y (2008) Full-range, high-speed, high-resolution 1-μm spectral-domain optical coherence tomography using BM-scan for volumetric imaging of the human posterior eye. Opt Express 16: 8406–8420
14. Huber R, Adler DC, Srinivasan VJ, Fujimoto JG (2007) Fourier domain mode locking at 1050 nm for ultra-high-speed optical coherence tomography of the human retina at 236,000 axial scans per second. Opt Lett 32:2049–2051
15. Srinivasan VJ, Adler DC, Chen Y, Gorczynska I, Huber R, Duker J, Schuman JS, Fujimoto JG (2008) Ultrahigh-speed optical coherence tomography for three-dimensional and en face imaging of the retina and optic nerve head. Invest Ophthalmol Vis Sci iovs.08–2127%U http://www.iovs.org/cgi/content/abstract/iovs.2108–2127v2121
16. Povazay B, Hermann B, Hofer B, Kajic V, Simpson E, Bridgford T, Drexler W (2009) Wide field optical coherence

17

tomography of the choroid in vivo. Invest Ophthalmol Vis Sci 50:1856–1863

17. Považay B, Hofer B, Torti C, Hermann B, Tumlinson AR, Esmaeelpour M, Egan CA, Bird AC, Drexler W (2009) Impact of enhanced resolution, speed and penetration on three-dimensional retinal optical coherence tomography. Opt Express 17:4134–4150
18. Howland HC, Howland B (1977) A subjective method for the measurement of monochromatic aberrations of the eye. J Opt Soc Am 67:1508–1518
19. Liang JZ, Williams DR, Miller DT (1997) Supernormal vision and high-resolution retinal imaging through adaptive optics. J Opt Soc Am A Opt Image Sci Vis 14:2884–2892
20. Roorda A, Williams DR (1999) The arrangement of the three cone classes in the living human eye. Nature 397:520–522
21. Roorda A, Romero-Borja F, Donnelly WJ, Queener H, Hebert TJ, Campbell MCW (2002) Adaptive optics scanning laser ophthalmoscopy. Opt Express 10:405–412
22. Gray DC, Merigan W, Wolfing JI, Gee BP, Porter J, Dubra A, Twietmeyer TH, Ahmad K, Tumbar R, Reinholz F, Williams DR (2006) In vivo fluorescence imaging of primate retinal ganglion cells and retinal pigment epithelial cells. Opt Express 14:7144–7158
23. Hermann B, Fernandez EJ, Unterhuber A, Sattmann H, Fercher AF, Drexler W, Prieto PM, Artal P (2004) Adaptive-optics ultrahigh-resolution optical coherence tomography. Opt Lett 29:2142–2144
24. Zhang Y, Rha JT, Jonnal RS, Miller DT (2005) Adaptive optics parallel spectral domain optical coherence tomography for imaging the living retina. Opt Express 13:4792–4811
25. Zhang Y, Cense B, Rha J, Jonnal RS, Gao W, Zawadzki RJ, Werner JS, Jones S, Olivier S, Miller DT (2006) High-speed volumetric imaging of cone photoreceptors with adaptive optics spectral-domain optical coherence tomography. Opt Express 14:4380–4394
26. Zawadzki RJ, Jones SM, Olivier SS, Zhao MT, Bower BA, Izatt JA, Choi S, Laut S, Werner JS (2005) Adaptive-optics optical coherence tomography for high-resolution and high-speed 3D retinal in vivo imaging. Opt Express 13:8532–8546
27. Fernandez EJ, Hermann B, Povazay B, Unterhuber A, Sattmann H, Hofer B, Ahnelt PK, Drexler W (2008) Ultrahigh resolution optical coherence tomography and pancorrection for cellular imaging of the living human retina. Opt Express 16:11083–11094
28. Fernandez EJ, Vabre L, Hermann B, Unterhuber A, Povazay B, Drexler W (2006) Adaptive optics with a magnetic deformable mirror: applications in the human eye. Opt Express 14:8900–8917
29. Hee MR, Huang D, Swanson EA, Fujimoto JG (1992) Polarization-sensitive low-coherence reflectometer for birefringence characterization and ranging. J Opt Soc Am B Opt Phys 9:903–908
30. deBoer JF, Milner TE, vanGemert MJC, Nelson JS (1997) Two-dimensional birefringence imaging in biological tissue by polarization-sensitive optical coherence tomography. Opt Lett 22:934–936
31. Götzinger E, Pircher M, Hitzenberger CK (2005) High speed spectral domain polarization sensitive optical coherence tomography of the human retina. Opt Express 13: 10217–10229
32. Cense B, Mujat M, Chen TC, Park BH, de Boer JF (2007) Polarization-sensitive spectral-domain optical coherence tomography using a single line scan camera. Opt Express 15:2421–2431
33. Yamanari M, Miura M, Makita S, Yatagai T, Yasuno Y (2008) Phase retardation measurement of retinal nerve fiber layer by polarization-sensitive spectral-domain optical coherence tomography and scanning laser polarimetry. J Biomed Opt 13:10
34. Cense B, Chen TC, Park BH, Pierce MC, de Boer JF (2004) Thickness and birefringence of healthy retinal nerve fiber layer tissue measured with polarization-sensitive optical coherence tomography. Invest Ophthalmol Vis Sci 45:2606–2612
35. Pircher M, Götzinger E, Leitgeb R, Sattmann H, Findl O, Hitzenberger CK (2004) Imaging of polarization properties of human retina in vivo with phase resolved transversal PS-OCT. Opt Express 12:5940–5951
36. Pircher M, Götzinger E, Findl O, Michels S, Geitzenauer W, Leydolt C, Schmidt-Erfurth U, Hitzenberger CK (2006) Human macula investigated in vivo with polarization-sensitive optical coherence tomography. Invest Ophthalmol Vis Sci 47:5487–5494
37. Michels S, Pircher M, Geitzenauer W, Simader C, Gotzinger E, Findl O, Schmidt-Erfurth U, Hitzenberger CK (2008) Value of polarisation-sensitive optical coherence tomography in diseases affecting the retinal pigment epithelium. Br J Ophthalmol 92:204–209
38. Götzinger E, Pircher M, Baumann B, Ahlers C, Geitzenauer W, Schmidt-Erfurt U, Hitzenberger CK (2009) Three-dimensional polarization sensitive OCT imaging and interactive display of the human retina. Opt Express 17: 4151–4165
39. Götzinger E, Pircher M, Baumann B, Hirn C, Vass C, Hitzenberger CK (2008) Analysis of the origin of atypical scanning laser polarimetry patterns by polarization sensitive optical coherence tomography. Invest Ophthalmol Vis Sci 49:5366–5372
40. Fortune B, Cull GA, Burgoyne CF (2008) Relative course of retinal nerve fiber layer birefringence and thickness and

retinal function changes after optic nerve transection. Invest Ophthalmol Vis Sci 49:4444–4452

41. Mujat M, Park BH, Cense B, Chen TC, de Boer JF (2007) Autocalibration of spectral-domain optical coherence tomography spectrometers for in vivo quantitative retinal nerve fiber layer birefringence determination. J Biomed Opt 12:6
42. Miura M, Yamanari M, Iwasaki T, Elsner AE, Makita S, Yatagai T, Yasuno Y (2008) Imaging polarimetry in age-related macular degeneration. Invest Ophthalmol Vis Sci 49:2661–2667
43. Götzinger E, Pircher M, Geitzenauer W, Ahlers C, Baumann B, Michels S, Schmidt-Erfurt U, Hitzenberger CK (2008) Retinal pigment epithelium segmentation by polarization sensitive optical coherence tomography. Opt Express 16: 16410–16422
44. Logean E, Schmetterer LF, Riva CE (2000) Optical doppler velocimetry at various retinal vessel depths by variation of the source coherence length. Appl Opt 39:2858–2862
45. Flammer J, Orgul S, Costa VP, Orzalesi N, Krieglstein GK, Serra LM, Renard VX, Stefansson E (2002) The impact of ocular blood flow in glaucoma. Prog Retin Eye Res 21:359–393
46. Friedman E (1997) A hemodynamic model of the pathogenesis of age-related macular degeneration. Am J Ophthalmol 124:677–682
47. Schmetterer L, Wolzt M (1999) Ocular blood flow and associated functional deviations in diabetic retinopathy. Diabetologia 42:387–405
48. Wang XJ, Milner TE, Nelson JS (1995) Characterization of fluid flow velocity by optical Doppler tomography. Opt Lett 20:1337–1339
49. Izatt JA, Kulkarni MD, Yazdanfar S, Barton JK, Welch AJ (1997) In vivo bidirectional color Doppler flow imaging of picoliter blood volumes using optical coherence tomography. Opt Lett 22:1439–1441
50. Chen Z, Milner TE, Dave D, Nelson JS (1997) Optical Doppler tomographic imaging of fluid flow velocity in highly scattering media. Opt Lett 22:64–66
51. Yazdanfar S, Rollins AM, Izatt JA (2000) Imaging and velocimetry of the human retinal circulation with color Doppler optical coherence tomography. Opt Lett 25: 1448–1450
52. Yazdanfar S, Rollins AM, Izatt J (2003) In vivo imaging of human retinal flow dynamics by color Doppler optical coherence tomography. Arch Ophthalmol 121:235–239
53. Schmidt-Erfurth U, Leitgeb RA, Michels S, Povazay B, Sacu S, Hermann B, Ahlers C, Sattmann H, Scholda C, Fercher AF, Drexler W (2005) Three-dimensional ultrahigh-resolution optical coherence tomography of macular diseases. Invest Ophthalmol Vis Sci 46:3393–3402
54. Nassif N, Cense B, Park BH, Yun SH, Chen TC, Bouma BE, Tearney GJ, de Boer JF (2004) In vivo human retinal imaging by ultrahigh-speed spectral domain optical coherence tomography. Opt Lett 29:480–482
55. Fercher AF, Hitzenberger CK, Kamp G, Elzaiat SY (1995) Measurement of intraocular distances by backscattering spectral interferometry. Opt Commun 117:43–48
56. de Boer JF, Cense B, Park BH, Pierce MC, Tearney GJ, Bouma BE (2003) Improved signal-to-noise ratio in spectral-domain compared with time-domain optical coherence tomography. Opt Lett 28:2067–2069
57. Choma MA, Sarunic MV, Yang C, Izatt J (2003) Sensitivity advantage of swept source and Fourier domain optical coherence tomography. Opt Express 11:2183–2189
58. Wojtkowski M, Leitgeb R, Kowalczyk A, Bajraszewski T, Fercher AF (2002) In vivo human retinal imaging by Fourier domain optical coherence tomography. J Biomed Opt 7:457–463
59. Wojtkowski M, Srinivasan V, Fujimoto JG, Ko T, Schuman JS, Kowalczyk A, Duker JS (2005) Three-dimensional retinal imaging with high-speed ultrahigh-resolution optical coherence tomography. Ophthalmology 112:1734–1746
60. Leitgeb RA, Schmetterer L, Drexler W, Fercher AF, Zawadzki RJ, Bajraszewski T (2003) Real-time assessment of retinal blood flow with ultrafast acquisition by color Doppler Fourier domain optical coherence tomography. Optics Express 11:3116–3121
61. Leitgeb RA, Schmetterer L, Hitzenberger CK, Fercher AF, Berisha F, Wojtkowski M, Bajraszewski T (2004) Real-time measurement of in vitro flow by Fourier-domain color Doppler optical coherence tomography. Opt Lett 29:171–173
62. White BR, Pierce MC, Nassif N, Cense B, Park BH, Tearney GJ, Bouma BE, Chen TC, de Boer JF (2003) In vivo dynamic human retinal blood flow imaging using ultra-high-speed spectral domain optical Doppler tomography. Opt Express 11:3490–3497
63. Schmoll T, Kolbitsch C, Leitgeb RA (2009) Ultra-high-speed volumetric tomography of human retinal blood flow. Opt Express 17:4166–4176
64. Bachmann AH, Villiger ML, Blatter C, Lasser T, Leitgeb RA (2007) Resonant Doppler flow imaging and optical vivisection of retinal blood vessels. Opt Express 15:408–422
65. An L, Wang RK (2008) In vivo volumetric imaging of vascular perfusion within human retina and choroids with optical micro-angiography. Opt Express 16:11438–11452
66. Szkulmowski M, Szkulmowska A, Bajraszewski T, Kowalczyk A, Wojtkowski M (2008) Flow velocity estimation using joint spectral and time domain optical coherence tomography. Opt Express 16:6008–6025
67. Tao YK, Davis AM, Izatt JA (2008) Single-pass volumetric bidirectional blood flow imaging spectral domain optical coherence tomography using a modified Hilbert transform. Optics Express 16:12350–12361

17

68. Kolbitsch C, Schmoll T, Leitgeb RA (2009) Histogram-based filtering for quantitative 3D retinal angiography. J Biophotonics 2:416–425
69. Makita S, Hong Y, Yamanari M, Yatagai T, Yasuno Y (2006) Optical coherence angiography. Opt Express 14:7821–7840
70. Hong Y, Makita S, Yamanari M, Miura M, Kim S, Yatagai T, Yasuno Y (2007) Three-dimensional visualization of choroidal vessels by using standard and ultra-high resolution scattering optical coherence angiography. Opt Express 15: 7538–7550
71. Unterhuber A, Pova?ay B, Hermann B, Sattmann H, Chavez-Pirson A, Drexler W (2005) In vivo retinal optical coherence tomography at 1040 nm - enhanced penetration into the choroid. Opt Express 13:3252–3258
72. Yasuno Y, Hong Y, Makita S, Yamanari M, Akiba M, Miura M, Yatagai T (2007) In vivo high-contrast imaging of deep posterior eye by 1-um swept source optical coherence tomography andscattering optical coherence angiography. Opt Express 15:6121–6139
73. Michaely R, Bachmann AH, Villiger ML, Blatter C, Lasser T, Leitgeb RA (2007) Vectorial reconstruction of retinal blood flow in three dimensions measured with high resolution resonant Doppler Fourier domain optical coherence tomography. J Biomed Opt 12:041213–041217
74. Makita S, Fabritius T, Yasuno Y (2008) Quantitative retinal-blood flow measurement with three-dimensional vessel geometry determination using ultrahigh-resolution Doppler optical coherence angiography. Opt Lett 33: 836–838
75. Werkmeister RM, Dragostinoff N, Pircher M, G^tzinger E, Hitzenberger CK, Leitgeb RA, Schmetterer L (2008) Bidirectional Doppler Fourier-domain optical coherence tomography for measurement of absolute flow velocities in human retinal vessels. Opt Lett 33:2967–2969
76. Wang YM, Bower BA, Izatt JA, Tan O, Huang D (2008) Retinal blood flow measurement by circumpapillary Fourier domain Doppler optical coherence tomography. J Biomed Opt 13:064003
77. van Leeuwen TG, Kulkarni MD, Yazdanfar S, Rollins AM, Izatt JA (1999) High-flow-velocity and shear-rate imaging by use of color Doppler optical coherence tomography. Opt Lett 24:1584–1586
78. Davies PF, Tripathi SC (1993) Mechanical stress mechanisms and the cell. An endothelial paradigm. Circ Res 72:239–245
79. Vilser W, Nagel E, Lanzl I (2002) Retinal vessel analysis-new possibilities. Biomed Tech 47(Suppl 1):682–685
80. Wang Y, Fawzi A, Tan O, Gil-Flamer J, Huang D (2009) Retinal blood flow detection in diabetic patients by Doppler Fourier domain optical coherence tomography. Opt Express 17:4061–4073

Chapter 18

Toward Molecular Imaging

18

Steffen Schmitz-Valckenberg, M. Francesca Cordeiro,
Fred W. Fitzke, and Frank G. Holz

Core Messages

- Molecular imaging is a relatively new field that aims at the visualization and follow-up of cellular dysfunction of molecular disease mechanisms in living organisms.
- Early recognition of malfunction and direct visualization of pharmacodynamics may result in optimization of therapeutic strategies and better treatment success. Furthermore, enhanced diagnosis may also have a major economic impact.
- The key element of molecular imaging is the use of biomarkers. These reporting molecules are used as probes to help image and detect particular targets or pathways.
- In ophthalmology, molecular imaging has already been successfully applied in several animal models, using both exogenous and endogenous fluorescent probes.

New diagnostic tools provide increasingly more accurate insights into disease development and pathophysiological dysfunctions, at the cellular and biochemical level. "Molecular imaging" aims at the *in vivo* identification of organic and cellular malfunction even before the occurrence of anatomical changes. Thus, it is expected that in addition to better knowledge of pathological mechanisms, molecular imaging will allow for earlier diagnosis, optimization of therapeutic strategies, and early assessment of success or failure of therapy (monitoring). Medicines of the future will see a major paradigm shift by molecular imaging and the introduction of molecular medicine (Fig. 18.1).

Well-established therapeutic approaches are based on the diagnosis and treatment of diseases, when symptoms or clinical signs of the disease are already present. Late recognition and delayed initiation of therapeutic measures means costly treatment and possibly a lower chance of successful treatment. For example, one great challenge of glaucoma is the fact that the definitive diagnosis can only be made when major damage has already occurred. It is estimated that visual field defects cannot be detected until there is 20–40% retinal ganglion cells loss [1]. Current diagnostic tools do not allow for in vivo visualization of damage to these key cells in glaucoma. With regard to another major cause of visual disability: although anti-vascular endothelial growth factor (VEGF)-therapy represents a breakthrough in the treatment of age-related macular degeneration, some patients still do not benefit from the treatment or may not achieve satisfactory functional outcomes. Recent data further indicate that another group of patients with exudative AMD with initial treatment response fails to favorably respond to anti-VEGF treatment after some time [2–4]. One major disadvantage of anti-VEGF therapy as with many other current therapies is indeed the inability to actually visualize the pharmacodynamics of the drug in vivo. Does the agent actually reach its target? Does it have a sufficient treatment effect? Is the dose correct? Does the patient or is he/she developing resistance against the drug? The biological characterization of disease and their treatments in real time by molecular imaging aims to select the best treatment strategy ("theragnostics"), including optimization of dose and detection of drug resistance.

In current clinical practice imaging techniques are designed primarily for the detection of anatomical and morphological structures, while they have very low sensitivity to changes on the biological level. Notably, better insights in diseases and patients are possible by *ex vivo* diagnostics and histopathology based on clinical biopsy

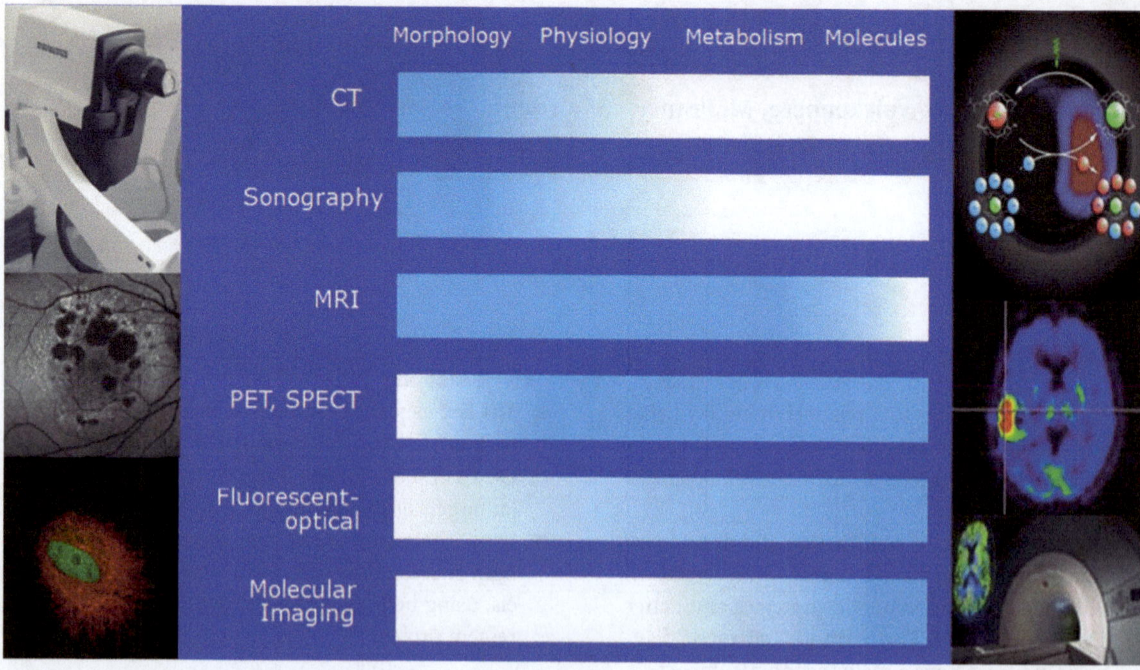

Fig. 18.1 Routine imaging methodologies such as computer tomography or ultrasonography aim to detect anatomical alterations at the macroscopic level; mapping of metabolic changes is today already possible with imaging methods like fundus autofluorescence imaging. The next step, molecular imaging, using biomarkers in the form of fluorescent-labeled markers, may allow for an early diagnosis and better and quicker treatment of disease. This may result in a major paradigm shift of medicine

and tissue collection. However, it is still not known how much alteration of intrinsic activity occurs as a result of tissue fixation and processing ("artifacts"). Furthermore, methods relying on postmortem analysis do not enable the effects to be monitored in real time. This also means that the same organisms or tissue cannot be studied over time.

Looking at in vivo diagnostics in ophthalmology, fluorescein angiography for example allows for functional imaging and visualization of leakage, enabling assessment of the breakdown of the retinal vascular barrier. However, the fluorescent dye Fluorescein Sodium, is a non-specific marker. This "cold" labeling does not allow for direct binding of target substances. In contrast, fundus autofluorescence imaging already represents a technology to image direct target substances by allowing for metabolic mapping of the retinal pigment epithelium [5–7], which has been made possible with the development of confocal scanning laser ophthalmoscopy with its improved sensitivity and increased image contrast [8]. However, no individual reporting molecules are detectable by fundus autofluorescence yet. Outside ophthalmology, molecular imaging technology has already been applied in patients. Using positron emission tomography (PET) and radioactive-labeled annexin A5 as apoptosis marker, programmed cell death has been visualized in vivo in heart insufficiency [9]. Six hours after injection, the biological marker showed binding to ischemic cardiac tissue. This demonstration of molecular imaging directly in patients is impressive, although it was not possible to resolve individual cells binding the marker. Hereby, a major challenge is the investigation of interior organs with no direct optical access. In ophthalmology, the eye with its unique optical properties offers easy access to deep anatomic structures, and, thus, provides a promising organ for in vivo visualization of molecular processes in the interior of the body at high resolution.

The hand tools for molecular imaging of the eye are already present in early stages of development. Innovative technologies such as high-resolution optical coherence tomography and confocal scanning laser ophthalmoscope already allow today for real-time presentation of ocular structures with high sensitivity and high image contrast. On the other hand, growing knowledge has been gained on cellular metabolic pathways in eye diseases in recent years. Furthermore, several developments in the field of biochemistry now allow for better labeling of target substances and reporting molecules. Hereby, fluorescent optical approaches appear to be particularly promising for molecular imaging. When compared with the PET technique, they are not as costly and there are no concerns of radiations. The latter in particular, limits the repeated application of PET technology in the same individual that would be important to monitor molecular processes at different time points in longitudinal studies. One other major advantage of fluorescent optical approaches is the fact that they are not limited to exogenous probes. In animal experiments, transgenic animals can express an endogenous fluorescent target molecule. These endogenous probes would be obviously limited to preclinical evaluations while exogenous probes may represent translational biomarkers, e.g., first used and investigated in animals and then translated to the clinical application. Both these approaches - endogenous and exogenous fluorescent probes - have been already used in animal experiments in ophthalmology.

In 2004, Cordeiro and co-workers were able to image individual retinal ganglion cell apoptosis in vivo in the glaucoma rat model in real time [10]. They also demonstrated the ability to visualize single nerve cell apoptosis over hours, days, and months and showing that the effects depend on the magnitude of the initial apoptotic inducer in several models of neurodegenerative disease in rat and primate. This was succeeded by injecting fluorescent-labeled annexin 5 into the vitreous and using the confocal scanning laser ophthalmoscope for identification of single apoptosing cells. This technology, which has been subsequently given the acronym DARC (detection of apoptosing retinal cells), has been used to assess drug efficacy in glaucoma and has also been shown to be useful to evaluate neuroprotective strategies [11–14]. In experimental glaucoma, amyloid-beta deposition as a hallmark for the devastating neurodegenerative condition of Alzheimer's disease was colocalized with apoptotic retinal ganglion cells and induced significant retinal ganglion cell apoptosis in vivo in a dose- and time-dependent manner. It was further demonstrated that targeting different components of the Abeta formation and aggregation pathway can effectively reduce glaucomatous RGC apoptosis in vivo, and finally, that combining treatments (triple therapy) was more effective than monotherapy. Overall, DARC appears to be a meaningful clinical end point that is based on the direct assessment of the retinal ganglion cell death process, not only being useful in assessing treatment efficacy, but also leading to the early identification of patients with glaucoma. The next step, translation of this technology to glaucoma patients, is underway.

It is well known by numerous postmortem studies that programmed cell death in the eye is not limited to the ganglion cells and glaucoma. The process of apoptosis is implicated in disorders throughout the retina [15]. In two easy accessible models of retinal damage, laser-induced retinal damage and acute light exposure, the DARC technique has also been used to visualize apoptotic processes in the animal model beyond retinal ganglion cell death. Individual hyperfluorescent spots as ongoing retinal cell death were seen after supra-threshold laser exposure inside laser burns in vivo (Fig. 18.2), mainly in the inner nuclear layer [16]. These observations were confirmed by postmortem analysis that showed apoptotic cells in the

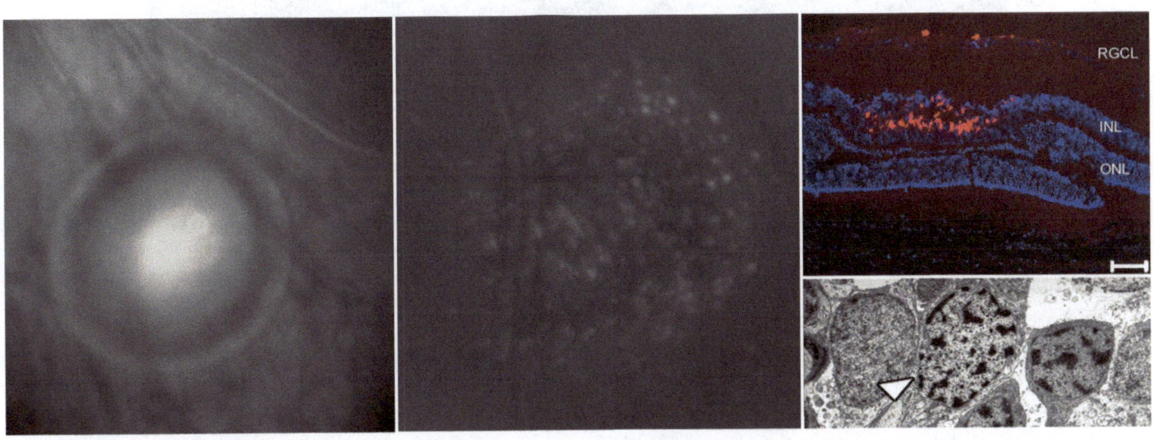

Fig. 18.2 Molecular imaging of real-time individual retinal cell apoptosis after laser exposure in rats after intravitreal injection of fluorescent-labeled annexin 5 as biomarker. Near-infrared confocal scanning laser ophthalmoscopy (*left*) shows a roundish laser lesion. Inside this lesion, single hyperfluorescent spots as single cells undergoing programmed cell death reflectance are visible in the fluorescent mode (*middle*). Cross-sectional postmortem analysis through a laser lesion allows for localization of annexin-5 positive spots mainly at the inner nuclear layer (*upper right RGCL* retinal ganglion cell layer; *INL* inner nuclear layer; *ONL* outer nuclear layer; *blue* DAPI; *red* fluorescence labeled annexin 5). Electron microscopy (*lower right*) shows structural changes consistent with apoptosis, including pyknotic nuclei (*arrowhead*) with abnormal distribution of heterochromatin, local swelling of the cytoplasm, and organelle loss in the inner nuclear layer

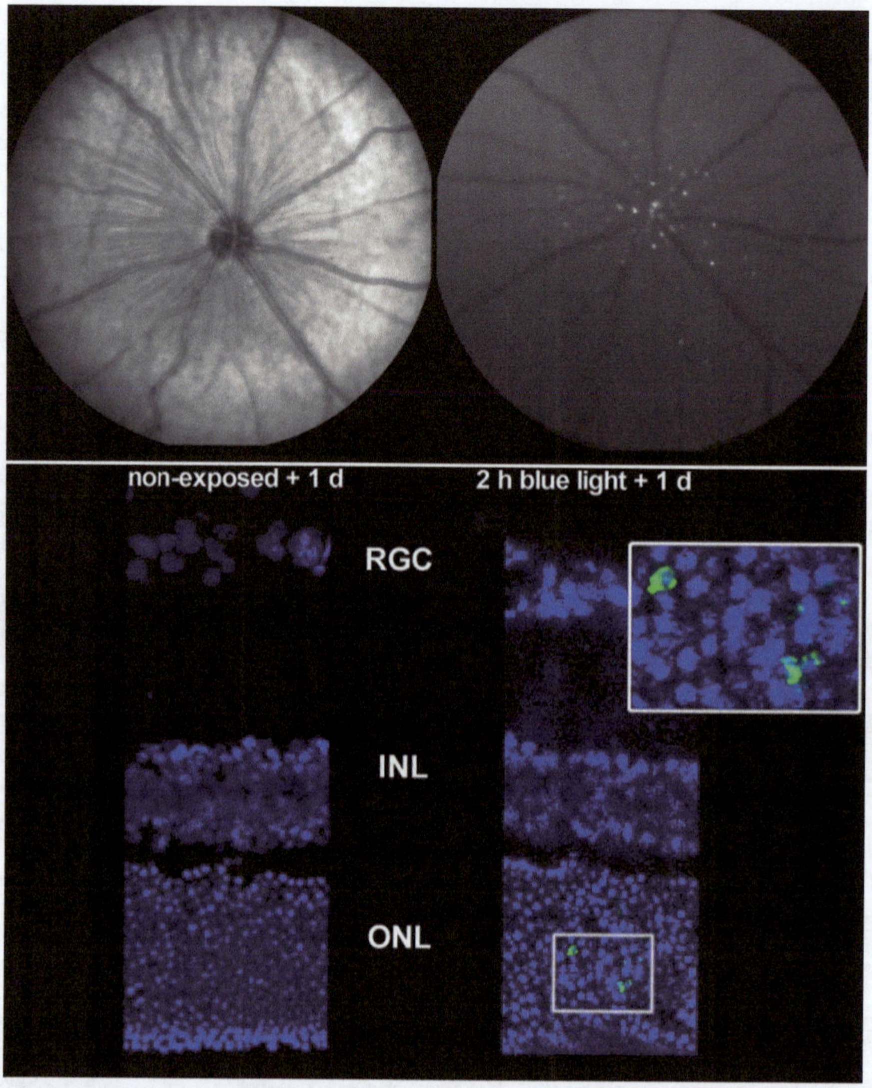

Fig. 18.3 In vivo visualization of photoreceptor apoptosis after acute light exposure over 2 h in rats. By near-infrared confocal reflectance imaging (*upper left*), retinal thinning in the exposed retinal area is visible. Inside this area around the optic nerve head, the fluorescent mode reveals individual hyperfluorescent spots as single cells undergoing apoptosis (*upper right*). Postmortem cross-sectioning confirms damage to and localization of annexin-5 positive cells in the outer nuclear layer (*bottom*). *RGC* retinal ganglion cell layer; *INL* inner nuclear layer; *ONL* outer nuclear layer; *blue* DAPI, *red* fluorescence labeled annexin

inner retina, while severe necrosis was observed at the level of the retinal pigment epithelium and inner choroid. In the model of acute blue light exposure over 2 h in rats, retinal flattening and the development of apoptosis within the irradiated retina occurred one day later and following dark adaptation (Fig. 18.3) [17]. Confocal live scanning through the exposed retina revealed hyperfluorescent apoptotic cells at the level of the outer retina. Histological analysis confirmed the occurrence of photoreceptor cell death and the development of cellular damage at the outer retina. Both these studies using the in vivo DARC technology confirmed previously postmortem reports of retinal cell apoptosis. Overall, the ability to monitor changes as they occur and longitudinally as they progress promises to be a major advancement in the real-time assessment of retinal diseases and treatment effects.

As opposed to the approach with exogenous probes as applied by the DARC technology, Eter and co-workers reported in 2008 about the use of an endogenous probe. In CX(3)CR1(GFP/+) knockin mice, in which dendritic cells, macrophages, and microglia cells are constitutively fluorescent due to genetic modification, they demonstrated in vivo the inflammatory response to laser-induced damage in the fundus of the eye [18]. They revealed that

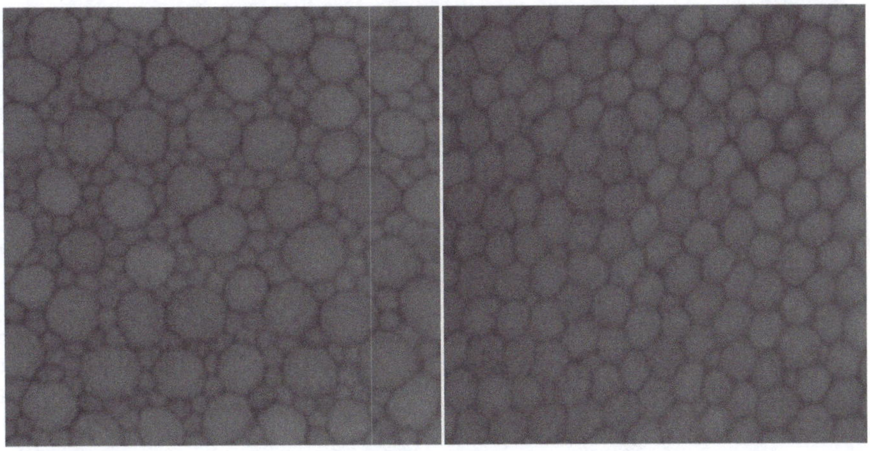

Fig. 18.4 Ex vivo imaging of the photoreceptor mosaic in a human donor eye by two photon-excited fluorescence

the inflammatory response to laser damage was longer than previously thought.

Two major challenges for the further development of molecular imaging in eye disease are the improvement of current imaging methods and the design of reporting biomarkers. The introduction of the confocal scanning laser ophthalmoscope has allowed for recording images of the living retina with enhanced sensitivity and high contrast. It has already been proven to be useful for molecular imaging in ophthalmology in several studies as outlined above. However, as opposed to the reliable analysis of the topographic distribution of the signal over one image, an absolute quantification of fluorescence intensities has not yet been possible in a reliable manner [19]. Several new imaging technologies and new development in the field of optics are available, but must be translated to ophthalmology. For example, the advantages of two-photon excited fluorescence have been already demonstrated on human eye donor tissue ex vivo (Fig. 18.4) [20, 21]. Without any slicing or cutting, the photoreceptor mosaic could be imaged with high resolution through the complete neurosensory retina. This was achieved by using the femtosecond laser. Hereby, the excitation light is effectively concentrated both in space and time, resulting in overall relative low excitation energy and generating a low amount of scattered light. When compared with standard confocal imaging, the result is an improved signal-to-noise ratio and better image contrast, permitting the visualization of more and deeper retinal structures.

Furthermore, promising target molecules for eye disease must be identified and coupled with fluorescent dyes in order to use them as biomarkers for molecular imaging. To be successful, these reporting molecules must be highly sensitive and recordable with available in vivo imaging methods. Not all substances will most likely find the way to the patient. The tolerability, safety profile and – last but not the least – the drug licensure by authorities must not be neglected.

Summaries for the Clinician

- "Molecular imaging" aims at in vivo identification of organic and cellular malfunction before the occurrence of morphological or functional changes.
- Molecular imaging offers great perspectives for earlier diagnoses, monitoring, and individualizing therapies.
- A growing understanding of disease mechanisms and their causes at the molecular level could lead to a transformation in our treatment approach.
- In several animal models, molecular imaging has already been successfully applied in ophthalmology.
- For the sustained development of this new field, multidisciplinary efforts and close cooperation of experts from the field of ocular imaging with specialists in the field of molecular biology and probe development appear to be essential.

References

1. Guo L, Cordeiro MF (2008) Assessment of neuroprotection in the retina with DARC. Prog Brain Res 173:437–450
2. Mitchell P, Korobelnik JF, Lanzetta P et al (2009) Ranibizumab (Lucentis) in neovascular age-related macular degeneration: evidence from clinical trials. Br J Ophthalmol

18

3. Raftery J, Jones J, Clegg A, Lotery A (2007) Ranibizumab (lucentis) versus bevacizumab (avastin): modelling cost effectiveness. Br J Ophthalmol 91:1244–6
4. Rosenfeld PJ, Brown DM, Heier JS et al (2006) Ranibizumab for neovascular age-related macular degeneration. N Engl J Med 355:1419–1431
5. Delori FC, Dorey CK, Staurenghi G et al (1995) In vivo fluorescence of the ocular fundus exhibits retinal pigment epithelium lipofuscin characteristics. Invest Ophthalmol Vis Sci 36:718–729
6. Holz FG, Schmitz-Valckenberg S, Spaide RF, Bird AC (2007) Atlas of fundus autofluorescence imaging. Springer, Berlin
7. von Ruckmann A, Fitzke FW, Bird AC (1995) Distribution of fundus autofluorescence with a scanning laser ophthalmoscope. Br J Ophthalmol 79:407–412
8. Webb RH, Hughes GW, Delori FC (1987) Confocal scanning laser ophthalmoscope. Appl Opt 26:1492–1499
9. Kietselaer BL, Reutelingsperger CP, Boersma HH et al (2007) Noninvasive detection of programmed cell loss with 99mTc-labeled annexin A5 in heart failure. J Nucl Med 48:562–567
10. Cordeiro MF, Guo L, Luong V et al (2004) Real-time imaging of single nerve cell apoptosis in retinal neurodegeneration. Proc Natl Acad Sci U S A 101:13352–13356
11. Guo L, Moss SE, Alexander RA et al (2005) Retinal ganglion cell apoptosis in glaucoma is related to intraocular pressure and IOP-induced effects on extracellular matrix. Invest Ophthalmol Vis Sci 46:175–182
12. Guo L, Salt TE, Maass A et al (2006) Assessment of neuroprotective effects of glutamate modulation on glaucoma-related retinal ganglion cell apoptosis in vivo. Invest Ophthalmol Vis Sci 47:626–633
13. Guo L, Salt TE, Luong V et al (2007) Targeting amyloid-{beta} in glaucoma treatment. Proc Natl Acad Sci U S A. 104:13444–9
14. Maass A, von Leithner PL, Luong V et al (2007) Assessment of rat and mouse RGC apoptosis imaging in vivo with different scanning laser ophthalmoscopes. Curr Eye Res 32:851–861
15. Kermer P, Bahr M (2005) Programmed cell death in the retina. Molecular mechanisms and therapeutic strategies. Ophthalmologe 102:674–678
16. Schmitz-Valckenberg S, Guo L, Maass A et al (2008) Real-time in-vivo imaging of retinal cell apoptosis after laser exposure. Invest Ophthalmol Vis Sci 49:2773–2780
17. Schmitz-Valckenberg S, Guo L, Cheung W et al (2009) In vivo imaging of retinal cell apoptosis following acute light exposure. Ophthalmologe [epub ahead of print]
18. Eter N, Engel D, Meyer L et al (2008) In vivo visualization of dendritic cells, macrophages and microglial cells responding to laser-induced damage in the fundus of the eye. Invest Ophthalmol Vis Sci 49:3649–3658
19. Schmitz-Valckenberg S, Holz FG, Bird AC, Spaide RF (2008) Fundus autofluorescence imaging: review and perspectives. Retina 28:385–409
20. Bindewald-Wittich A, Han M, Schmitz-Valckenberg S et al (2006) Two-photon-excited fluorescence imaging of human RPE cells with a femtosecond Ti:Sapphire laser. Invest Ophthalmol Vis Sci 47:4553–4557
21. Han M, Giese G, Schmitz-Valckenberg S et al (2007) Age-related structural abnormalities in the human retina-choroid complex revealed by two-photon excited autofluorescence imaging. J Biomed Opt 12:024012

Index

SPRINGER NATURE

GPSR Compliance

The European Union's (EU) General Product Safety Regulation (GPSR) is a set of rules that requires consumer products to be safe and our obligations to ensure this.

If you have any concerns about our products, you can contact us on ProductSafety@springernature.com

In case Publisher is established outside the EU, the EU authorized representative is:

Springer Nature Customer Service Center GmbH
Europaplatz 3
69115 Heidelberg, Germany

Kolibri 360 GmbH
Ferdinand-Jühlke-Straße 7
99095 Erfurt, Deutschland
produktsicherheit@kolibri360.de